THE FOOT
AND ANKLE

**A Selection of Papers
from the American Orthopaedic
Foot Society Meetings**

THE FOOT
AND ANKLE

**A Selection of Papers
from the American Orthopaedic
Foot Society Meetings**

Editors

JAMES E. BATEMAN, M.D.

Surgeon-in-Chief
Orthopaedic and Arthritic
Hospital
Toronto, Ontario

ARTHUR W. TROTT, M.D.

Senior Orthopaedic Surgeon
Children's Hospital Medical
Center
Boston, Massachusetts

1980

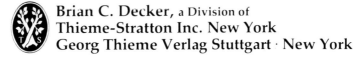
Brian C. Decker, a Division of
Thieme-Stratton Inc. New York
Georg Thieme Verlag Stuttgart · New York

Publisher: Brian C. Decker, a Division of
Thieme-Stratton Inc.
381 Park Avenue South
New York, New York 10016

The Foot and Ankle

ISBN 0-913258-71-7

Last digit is print number 9 8 7 6 5 4 3 2 1

CONTRIBUTORS

JAMES E. BATEMAN, M.D., F.R.C.S. (C).

Surgeon-in-Chief, Orthopaedic and Arthritic Hospital, Toronto, Ontario, Canada.

TERRENCE BECKER, M.D.

Assistant Professor of Radiology; Los Angeles County, University of Southern California Medical Center, Los Angeles, California.
Foot Injuries in Karate Experts

WALTER M. BRAUNOHLER, M.D.

Associate Clinical Professor, Department of Orthopaedics, Michigan State University School of Medicine, Lansing, Michigan.
Arthroplasty of the Great Toe with a Silicone Implant

THOMAS D. BROWN, PH.D.

Orthopaedic Research Laboratory, University of Pittsburgh School of Medicine, Pittsburgh, Pennsylvania.
Support Phase Kinematics of the Foot

HILTON BUGGS, M.A., Director

Peripheral Vascular Laboratory, Rancho Los Amigos Hospital, Downey, California.
Syme's Amputation of the Diabetic Foot

MARK B. COVENTRY, M.D.

Professor of Orthopedic Surgery, Mayo Medical School; Consultant Orthopedic Surgery, Mayo Clinic, Rochester, Minnesota.
Post-Traumatic Peroneal Tendinitis

GENEVIEVE DEGROOT SWANSON, M.D.

Associate in Research and Staff Plastic Surgeon
Blodgett Memorial Hospital
Grand Rapids, Michigan

G. PAUL DE ROSA, M.D.

Associate Professor of Orthopaedics Surgery, Pediatric Orthopaedics, Dept. of Orthopaedic Surgery, Indiana University School of Medicine; Chief of Neuro-muscular Disease (Orthopaedics), James Whitcomb Riley Hospital for Children, Indianapolis, Indiana.

EDWARD A. DYKSTRA, M.D.

Orthopaedic Surgeon, Steindler Orthopaedic Clinic, Iowa City, Iowa
Surgical Correction of the Resistant Club Foot

PHILLIP M. EVANSKI, M.D.

Associate Professor, Department of Orthopaedic Surgery, New York University Medical Center, New York, New York.
Tibiopedal Motion after Ankle Fusion and Arthroplasty

ROBERT H. FITZGERALD, JR., M.D.

Consultant, Orthopedic Surgery, Mayo Clinic; Assistant Professor of Orthopedic Surgery, Mayo Medical School, Rochester, Minnesota.
Post-traumatic Peroneal Tendinitis

DEBRA FORRESTER, M.D.

Associate Professor of Radiology; Los Angeles County, University of Southern California Medical Center, Los Angeles, California.
Foot Injuries in Karate Experts

NICHOLAS J. GIANNESTRAS, M.D. (Deceased)

Formerly Professor of Orthopaedic Surgery, University of Cincinnati School of Medicine, Cincinnati, Ohio.
Grice Arthrodesis in Nonparalytic Flexible Flat Feet

PETER A. GODSICK, M.D.

Associate Orthopaedic Surgeon, Hospital for Joint Diseases; Associate Orthopaedic Surgeon, St. Clare's Hospital, New York, New York
Quadruple Arthrodesis with Iliac Bone Graft

DONALD R. GORE, M.D.

Associate Clinical Professor of Orthopaedic Surgery, Medical College of Wisconsin, Milwaukee, Wisconsin; Consultant, Department of Surgery, Wood Veterans Administration Hospital, Wood, Wisconsin; Attending Staff and Chairman, Department of Surgery, Sheyboygan Memorial Hospital and St. Nicholas Hospital, Sheyboygan, Wisconsin.
Keller Bunionectomy with Opening Wedge Osteotomy of the First Metatarsal

JOHN S. GOULD, M.D.

Associate Professor of Orthopaedic Surgery; Chief, Section of Hand Surgery, Division of Orthopaedic Surgery, The University of Alabama in Birmingham; Director, Congenital Hand and Foot Clinic, State Crippled Children's Service, Birmingham, Alabama.
Surgical Reconstruction of the Talipes Equino Varus Deformity

JOHN L. HAGY, O.R.E.

Gait Analysis Laboratory, Shriners Hospital, San Francisco, California
Running, Jogging and Walking: A Comparative Electromyographic and Biomechanical Study

HAMILTON HALL, M.D., F.R.C.S. (C).

Assistant Professor, Department of Surgery, University of Toronto Faculty of Medicine; Staff Orthopaedic Surgeon, Toronto General Hospital; Consulting Orthopaedic Surgeon, Hillcrest Hospital and The Ontario Workmen's Compensation Board Rehabilitation Centre; Toronto, Canada.
A Simplified Workable Classification of Ankle Fractures

J. PAUL HARVEY JR., M.D.

Chief Physician, Department of Orthopaedic Surgery, Los Angeles County University of Southern California Medical Center, Los Angeles, California.
Fractures and Dislocations of the Tarsometatarsal Joint

RODRIGO HIDALGO, M.D.

Orthopaedic Staff, Venice Hospital, Venice, Florida.
Partial Excision of the Os Calcis in the Treatment of Lesions of the Calcaneous

JAMES G. HOEHN, M.D.

Assistant Professor, Division of Plastic Surgery, The Albany Medical College of Union University, Albany, New York.
Replantation of a Severed Foot

M. MARK HOFFER, M.D.

Chief, Children's Orthopaedics, Rancho Los Amigos Hospital, Downey, California.
Surgical Correction of Hallux Valgus in Cerebral Palsy

BARRY D. HOOTMAN, M.D.

Research Fellow, Department of Orthopaedics, University of Pittsburgh School of Medicine, Pittsburgh, Pennsylvania.
Forces Under the Foot: A Study of Walking, Jogging and Sprinting Force Distribution Under Normal and Abnormal Feet

L. HUNKA, M.D., F.R.C.S. (C).

Orthopaedic Fellow, Shriners Hospital of Montreal, Canada.
Ankle Fusions: A Current Study

RICHARD L. JACOBS, M.D.

Professor and Head, Division of Orthopaedic Surgery, The Albany Medical College of Union University, Albany, New York.
Replantation of a Severed Foot

MELVIN H. JAHSS, M.D.

Clinical Professor of Orthopaedic Surgery, Mount Sinai School of Medicine; Attending and Chief Orthopaedic Foot Services, Hospital for Joint Diseases and Mount Sinai Hospital, New York, New York.
Quadruple Arthrodesis with Iliac Bone Graft

ALLASTAIR KARMODY, M.D.

Associate Professor, Department of Surgery, The Albany Medical College of Union University, Albany, New York.
Replantation of a Severed Foot

JAMES KNAVEL, M.D.

Senior Resident in Orthopaedic Surgery, Medical College of Wisconsin, Milwaukee, Wisconsin.
Keller Bunionectomy with Opening Wedge Osteotomy of the First Metatarsal

GARY LaTOURETTE, M.D.

Private Practice, San Bernadino, California
Fractures and Dislocations of the Tarsometatarsal Joint

HOWARD LEVIN, M.D.

Senior Resident, Hospital for Joint Diseases, New York, New York.
Quadruple Arthrodesis with Iliac Bone Graft

ROBERT M. LUMSDEN II, M.D.

Affiliated Bone and Joint Surgeons, Phoenix, Arizona.

LOWELL D. LUTTER, M.D.

Clinical Associate Professor, Department of Orthopaedics, University of Minnesota, Minneapolis, Minnesota; St. Anthony Orthopaedic Clinic, Sports Medicine Division, St. Paul, Minnesota.
Orthopaedic Management of Runners

ROGER A. MANN, M.D.

Director, Gait Analysis Laboratory, Shriners Hospital; Associate Clinical Professor, Orthopaedic Surgery, University of California Medical School, San Francisco, California.
Running, Jogging and Walking: A Comprehensive Electromyographic and Biomechanical Study.

JOHN MAZUR, M.D.

Associate Director, Gait Analysis Laboratory, The Children's Hospital Medical Center, Boston, Massachusetts.
Ankle Arthrodesis: Long-Term Follow-Up with Gait Analysis

JAMES H. McMASTER, M.D.

Chief, Department of Orthopaedics, Allegheny General Hospital, Pittsburgh, Pennsylvania.
Forces Under the Foot: A Study of Walking, Jogging and Sprinting Force Distribution Under Normal and Abnormal Feet

WALLACE E. MILLER, M.D.

Professor, Department of Orthopaedics and Rehabilitation, University of Miami School of Medicine, Jackson Memorial Hospital Medical Center, Miami, Florida.
Operative Intervention for Fracture of the Talus

TILLMAN M. MOORE, M.D.

Assistant Professor, Orthopaedic Surgery, Indiana University School of Medicine, Indianapolis, Indiana.
Fractures and Dislocations of the Tarsometatarsal Joint

STANLEY H. NAHIGIAN, M.D.

Division of Orthopaedic Surgery, St. Luke's Hospital, Cleveland, Ohio.
Wire Loop Fixation of the Lateral Malleolus in Ankle Fractures

INDONG OH, M.D.

Department of Orthopaedic Surgery, Massachusetts General Hospital, Harvard Medical School, Boston, Massachusetts.
Wire Loop Fixation of the Lateral Malleolus in Ankle Fractures

MICHAEL J. PATZAKIS, M.D.

Associate Professor, Department of Orthopaedic Surgery, University of Southern California School of Medicine, Los Angeles, California.
Fractures and Dislocations of the Tarsometatarsal Joint

JACQUELIN PERRY, M.D.

Professor Orthopaedic Surgery, University of Southern California, Los Angeles; Chief of Orthopaedic Surgery, Rancho Los Amigos Hospital, Downey, California.
Tarsometatarsal Joint

MARIO E. PORRAS, M.D.

Private Practice, Bone and Joint Surgery, Reno, Nevada.
Partial Excision of the Os Calcis in the Treatment of Lesions of the Calcaneous

JOSEPH QUINTANA, M.S.

University of New Mexico, Albuquerque, New Mexico
Partial Excision of the Os Calcis in the Treatment of Lesions of the Calcaneous

MICHAEL D. ROBACK, M.D.

U.S.A.F. Hospital, Manchester Air Force Base, California.
Foot Injuries of Karate Experts

JAMES RUSSO, M.D.

Senior Resident, Los Angeles County University of Southern California Medical Center, Los Angeles, California.
Syme's Amputation of the Diabetic Foot

ROBERT RUTKOWSKI, M.D.

Research Fellow, Department of Orthopaedics, University of Pittsburgh, School of Medicine, Pittsburgh, Pennsylvania.
Support Phase Kinematics of the Foot

EDWARD SAID, M.D., F.R.C.S. (C), C.S.P.Q.

Orthopaedic Surgeon, Lakeshore General Hospital, Pte. Claire, Quebec; Staff Orthopaedic Surgeon, Shriners Hospital of Montreal, Montreal, Canada
Ankle Fusions: A Current Study

A. A. SAVASTANO, M.D.

Clinical Professor, Orthopaedic Surgery, Brown University Medical School; Surgeon-in-Chief (Emeritus), Department of Orthopaedic Surgery, Rhode Island Hospital, Providence, Rhode Island.
Recurrent Dislocation of the Peroneal Tendons

WENDELIN W. SCHAEFER, M.D.

Attending Staff, Sheboygan Memorial Hospital and St. Nicholas Hospital, Sheboygan, Wisconsin.

PIERCE E. SCRANTON, JR., M.D.

Clinical Instructor, University of Washington School of Medicine, Seattle, Washington.
Forces Under the Foot: A Study of Walking, Jogging and Sprinting Force Distribution Under Normal and Abnormal Feet. Support Phase Kinematics of the Foot

JACK L. SEAQUIST, M.D.

Former Resident, Children's Orthopaedic Service, Rancho Los Amigos Hospital, Downey, California.
Surgical Correction of Hallux Valgus in Cerebral Palsy

DAVID SEGAL, M.D.

Director, Orthopaedic Surgical Service, Department of Orthopaedic Surgery, Boston City Hospital, Boston, Massachusetts.
Ankle Function: Measurement and Functional Bracing of the Fractured Ankle

T. N. SILLER, M.D., F.R.C.S. (C).

Orthopaedic Surgeon, Reddy Memorial Hospital; Orthopaedic Surgeon, Shriners Hospital of Montreal, Montreal, Canada; Lecturer of Surgery, McGill University, Canada.
Ankle Fusions: A Current Study

SHELDON R. SIMON, M.D.

Director, Gait Analysis Laboratory, The Children's Hospital Medical Center, Assistant Professor, Harvard Medical School; Associate, Orthopaedic Surgery, Peter Bent Brigham Hospital and The Children's Hospital Medical Center, Boston, Massachusetts.
Ankle Arthrodesis: Long-Term Follow-Up with Gait Analysis

RONALD W. SMITH, M.D.

Assistant Clinical Professor, Department of Surgery/Orthopaedics, University of California School of Medicine, Los Angeles, California
Grice Arthrodesis in Nonparalytic Flexible Flat Feet

ALFRED B. SWANSON, M.D.

Chief, Orthopaedic Surgery and Orthopaedic Research, Blodgett Hospital, Grand Rapids, Michigan.
Arthroplasy of the Great Toe with a Silicone Implant

ILAN TAMIR, M.D.

Private Practice, Beverly Hills, California.
Foot Injuries of Karate Experts

ARTHUR W. TROTT, M.D.

Senior Orthopaedic Surgeon; The Children's Hospital Medical Center, Boston, Massachusetts.
The Normal Human Foot: What is It?

F. WILLIAM WAGNER, JR., M.D.

Clinical Professor, Orthopaedic Surgery, University of Southern California School of Medicine, Los Angeles; Co-Chief, Orthopaedic-Diabetes Service, Rancho Los Amigos Hospital, Downey, California.
Syme's Amputation of the Diabetic Foot

STEPHEN WASILEWSKI, M.D.

Attending Orthopaedic Surgeon, Lahey Clinic Foundation, Boston, Massachusetts.
Management of Unstable Ankle Fractures

THEODORE R. WAUGH, M.D.

Professor and Chairman, Department of Orthopaedic Surgery, New York University Medical Center, New York, New York.
Tibiopedal Motion after Ankle Fusion and Arthroplasty

JOHN WEBB, M.D., F.R.C.S.

Fellow, Orthopaedic-Diabetes Service, Rancho Los Amigos Hospital, Downey, California.
Syme's Amputation of the Diabetic Foot

ISADORE G. YABLON, M.D.

Professor of Orthopaedic Surgery, Director of Research, Boston University School of Medicine; Visiting Surgeon, University Hospital, Boston, Massachusetts.
Management of Unstable Ankle Fractures

F. B. ZAHRAWI, M.D.

Division of Orthopaedic Surgery, St. Luke's Hospital, Cleveland, Ohio.
Wire Loop Fixation of the Lateral Malleolus in Ankle Fractures

PREFACE

One goal of the American Orthopaedic Foot Society is to provide the means by which physicians, especially orthopaedic surgeons, can keep current with respect to the management of the foot disorders. Publication of *The Foot and Ankle* is one of the Society's contributions to its educational objective.

The first volume represents a selection of some of the best original papers presented at Society's annual meetings in Las Vegas (1977) and San Francisco (1978).

Data reported in the chapters of this work are based on reports presented at the meetings; however, many of the authors revised their manuscripts to make them up-to-date as of July 1979. Current references were added, data on series of patients were extended, and illustrations were supplied to amplify the text. We have arrayed the chapters according to subject matter, resulting in six sections on trauma, forefoot, hindfoot and ankle, biomechanics, sports medicine, and congenital anomalies. In selecting articles for the book, we tried to choose those with current ideas and methodologies of practical use to the clinician. Our hope is that residents and fellows will find insights into mechanisms of injury as well as treatment protocols of seasoned clinicians.

The coeditors are grateful to the authors for their response in the preparation of the manuscripts, and to the publisher for his diligence in producing the volume.

James E. Bateman, M.D.
Arthur W. Trott, M.D.

CONTENTS

Chapter One

THE NORMAL HUMAN FOOT——WHAT IS IT?   1
ARTHUR W. TROTT, M.D.

Part One: Trauma

Chapter Two

A SIMPLIFIED WORKABLE CLASSIFICATION OF ANKLE FRACTURES   5
HAMILTON HALL, M.D., F.R.C.S. (C)

Chapter Three

MANAGEMENT OF UNSTABLE ANKLE FRACTURES 11
ISADORE G. YABLON AND STEPHEN WASILEWSKI, M.D.

Chapter Four

ANKLE FUNCTION: MEASUREMENT AND FUNCTIONAL BRACING OF THE FRACTURED ANKLE 20
DAVID SEGAL, M.D.

Chapter Five

WIRE LOOP FIXATION OF THE LATERAL MALLEOLUS IN ANKLE FRACTURES 24
STANLEY H. NAHIGIAN, INDONG OH, M.D. AND
F. B. ZAHRAWI, M.D.

Chapter Six

TIBIOPEDAL MOTION AFTER ANKLE FUSION AND ARTHROPLASTY 36
PHILLIP M. EVANSKI, M.D. AND THEODORE R. WAUGH, M.D.

Chapter Seven

**FRACTURES AND DISLOCATIONS OF THE
TARSOMETATARSAL JOINT** 40
GARY LATOURETTE, M.D., JACQUELIN PERRY, M.D., MICHAEL
J. PATZAKIS, M.D., TILLMAN M. MOORE, M.D., AND J. PAUL
HARVEY, JR., M.D.

Chapter Eight

**OPERATIVE INTERVENTION FOR FRACTURE OF THE
TALUS**.. 52
WALLACE E. MILLER, M.D.

Chapter Nine

REPLANTATION OF A SEVERED FOOT.................... 64
RICHARD L. JACOBS, M.D., JAMES G. HOEHN, M.D., AND
ALLASTAIR KARMODY, M.D.

Part Two: Hindfoot and Ankle

Chapter Ten

**ANKLE ARTHRODESIS: LONG-TERM FOLLOW-UP WITH
GAIT ANALYSIS** 73
SHELDON R. SIMON, M.D. AND J.OHN MAZUR, M.D.

Chapter Eleven

QUADRUPLE ARTHRODESIS WITH ILIAC BONE GRAFT... 93
MELVIN H. JAHSS, M.D., PETER A. GODSICK, M.D., AND
HOWARD LEVIN, M.D.

Chapter Twelve

POST-TRAUMATIC PERONEAL TENDINITIS............... 103
ROBERT H. FITZPATRICK, JR., M.D., AND
MARK B. COVENTRY, M.D.

Chapter Thirteen

**RECURRENT DISLOCATION OF THE PERONEAL
TENDONS**... 110
A. A. SAVASTANO, M.D.

Chapter Fourteen

**GRICE ARTHRODESIS IN NONPARALYTIC FLEXIBLE FLAT
FEET** 116
NICHOLAS J. GIANNESTRAS, M.D., AND
RONALD W. SMITH, M.D.

Chapter Fifteen

SYME'S AMPUTATION OF THE DIABETIC FOOT 127
F. WILLIAM WAGNER, JR., M.D., JAMES RUSSO, M.D.,
JOHN WEBB, M.D., F.R.C.S., AND HILTON BUGGS, M.A.

Chapter Sixteen

ANKLE FUSIONS: A CURRENT STUDY 131
E. SAID, M.D., F.R.C.S.(C), L. HUNKA, M.D., F.R.C.S.(C), AND
T.N. SILLER, M.D., F.R.C.S.(C)

Part Three: Forefoot

Chapter Seventeen

**ARTHROPLASTY OF THE GREAT TOE WITH A SILICONE
IMPLANT**... 137
ALFRED B. SWANSON, M.D., ROBERT M. LUMSDEN II, M.D.,
ALFRED A. BRAUNOHLER, M.D., AND GENEVIEVE DEGROOT
SWANSON, M.D.

Chapter Eighteen

**SURGICAL CORRECTION OF HALLUX VALGUS IN
CEREBRAL PALSY**...................................... 143
M. MARK HOFFER, M.D., AND JACK L. SEAQUIST, M.D.

Chapter Nineteen

**KELLER BUNIONECTOMY WITH OPENING WEDGE
OSTEOTOMY OF THE FIRST METATARSAL** 147
DONALD R. GORE, M.D., JAMES KNAVEL, M.D., AND
WENDELIN W. SCHAEFER, M.D.

Part Four: Sports Medicine

Chapter Twenty

ORTHOPAEDIC MANAGEMENT OF RUNNERS............. 155
LOWELL D. LUTTER, M.D.

Chapter Twenty-One

FOOT INJURIES OF KARATE EXPERTS.................... 159
MICHAEL D. ROBACK, M.D., ILAN TAMIR, M.D., DEBRA
FORRESTER, M.D., AND TERRENCE BECKER, M.D.

Part Five: Biomechanics

Chapter Twenty-Two

**RUNNING, JOGGING AND WALKING: A COMPARATIVE
ELECTROMYOGRAPHIC AND BIOMECHANICAL STUDY** .. 167
ROGER A. MANN, M.D., AND JOHN L. HAGY, O.R.E.

Chapter Twenty-Three

PARTIAL EXCISION OF THE OS CALCIS IN THE TREATMENT OF LESIONS OF THE CALCANEOUS 176
MARIO E. PORRAS, M.D., RODRIGO HIDALGO, M.D., AND JOSEPH QUINTANA, M.S.

Chapter Twenty-Four

FORCES UNDER THE FOOT: A STUDY OF WALKING, JOGGING AND SPRINTING FORCE DISTRIBUTION UNDER NORMAL AND ABNORMAL FEET 186
PIERCE E. SCRANTON, JR., M.D., BARRY D. HOOTMAN, M.D., AND JAMES H. MCMASTER, M.D.

Chapter Twenty-Five

SUPPORT PHASE KINEMATICS OF THE FOOT 195
PIERCE E. SCRANTON, JR., M.D., ROBERT RUTKOWSKI, M.D., AND THOMAS D. BROWN, PH.D.

Part Six: Congenital Anomalies

Chapter Twenty-Six

SURGICAL RECONSTRUCTION OF THE TALIPES EQUINO VARUS DEFORMITY 207
JOHN S. GOULD, M.D.

Chapter Twenty-Seven

SURGICAL CORRECTION OF THE RESISTANT CLUB FOOT 215
G. PAUL DE ROSA, M.D., AND EDWARD A. DYKSTRA, M.D.

Index ....

Chapter One

THE NORMAL HUMAN FOOT—WHAT IS IT?

Arthur W. Trott, M.D.

It is obvious that the present-day human, regardless of race, arose from a common ancestor, whether you believe in the Bible or in evolution. It is not sufficient to say that the foot is an adaptation of a prehensile organ which resulted from arboreal predecessors resorting to a terrestrial and biped habitat. According to Wood-Jones,[1] The English anatomist, the foot has undergone tremendous evolutionary change, and further, is still undergoing changes in response to stress.

The human population on this earth consists of vast multitudes; yet if one were to examine their feet, a remarkable similarity would be found. This is true whether they wear shoes or not, and climatic variations do not appear to have any effect. Minor variations do exist according to functional adaptation or genetic influences, but they are not of such magnitude as to cause wide deviations from the norm.

ANTHROPOLOGICAL CLASSIFICATION

However, it is difficult to determine what constitutes a normal human foot. Some authorities, especially anthropologists, try to classify normal on anatomic grounds. Slight variations in bony size and shape do not appear to have significant effects on function, at least clinically. Wood-Jones[1] and others have used a digital formula to classify types of feet to which classical terms have been applied. The Grecian foot has a great toe that is shorter than the second toe; it occurs in 18 per cent of the population. The Egyptian foot is characterized by a great toe longer than the second; this occurs in 74 percent of people. A third type has the great toe equal to the second in length and is known as a "squared foot;" it is seen in 8 per cent of people. From this simple classification, three variables have been introduced already, yet there is no evidence to date to indicate that one type is more subject to disease or mechanical disorders than another.

Adding another dimension to the problem, the relation in length of the great toe to the second toe does not necessarily have that same relation with respect to the lengths of the appropriate metatarsals. Thus a Grecian foot can have a first metatarsal that is shorter or longer than, or equal to the length of the second metatarsal. The same relative relationship applies to the Egyptian and the squared foot, so now we have nine variables to consider in normal feet, with only a small part of the anatomy involved so far. In fact, Wood-Jones states, "It is normal in man for the head of the second (Metatarsal) to be the most advanced member of the series." Viladot[2] of Spain has tried to establish some relationship of these latter variables to clinical conditions, the main aspect being the relative lengths of the first and second metatarsals, and he has had some success. Since not all feet that he considers as deviates from the norm develop clinical problems, this classification does not meet the criteria to define normality or abnormality.

It probably means that the human foot is remarkably adaptable to many types of stress. Again from Wood-Jones: "We must conclude that the bulk of humanity is condemned by the normal disposition of the bones of the foot to show some departure from the normal functioning of the foot."

FUNCTIONAL CLASSIFICATION

When we try to define a normal foot it does not make much sense to become involved in anatomic minutiae. The foot is involved primarily in stance and gait, yet the parameters of these functions have not been clearly defined or quantitated. At particular times during the gait cycle, the foot must be flexible and yet stable to be adaptive to irregularities in the terrain; it becomes a rigid lever system at other points in the gait cycle. However, it is not sufficient to consider the foot only with respect to its function, because tibial rotation in particular, and rotation of the knee, hip, pelvis, and femur play a role in how the foot functions in gait and stance. As shown by Roger Mann[3] and others, internal rotation of the tibia with the foot in ground contact causes pronation of the foot, while conversely, external rotation of the tibia produces supination or inversion of the foot. The significance of these parameters in a particular individual and with regard to clinical problems or complaints has not been evaluated as yet. Additional problems in this analysis consist of the relation of minor or major anatomic variations to serious alterations of basic functions of the foot.

"IDEAL FOOT"

Thus it would appear, at least at the present time, that a definition of a normal human foot is elusive and cannot be delineated accurately. The greatest obstacle is the immense variation in minor features which is present in the human race without detriment to normal function of the foot. It is a blessing that the foot is normally a flexible structure that can adapt to innumerable adverse situations with minimal or no structural or functional complications. What concerns us as orthopaedic surgeons are those feet that react adversely to stress and develop clinical problems.

Since it seems impossible at this time to define a normal foot, perhaps we should consider an "ideal foot." This is a poor concept, but probably the best we can do with present knowledge. The "ideal normal" foot should possess neutral anatomic contours, such as a heel that is perpendicular to the surface, neither in valgus nor varus. However, experience shows that a mild degree of heel valgus may occur in so-called normal feet without any observable effect. To proceed, the inner border of the foot should be straight from heel to great toe. The medial longitudinal arch should be a gentle, smooth curve from beneath the heel to an apex at the midfoot, and then should curve downward to reach the ground at the level of the metatarsal heads. Floor contact should be present on the plantar surface at the heel, lateral aspect of the foot, and at the ball of the foot. In addition, the foot should be asymptomatic under all conditions of adequate function and have no disease in the osseous or soft tissues. The squared type possesses a heel in apparent neutral, a moderate height to the medial arch, good weight distribution through the ball of the foot, and striaght toes. The posterior view reveals slight valgus of the heel which is of no functional or clinical significance and is probably a normal relation with respect to weight bearing. This type of foot should have no problems, be able to function in sports and daily activities consisting of considerable standing and walking without any complaints. If proper fit is provided, the type of footwear should present no problems to this individual, and this is about the closest we can come to a "normal" foot.

Why should we be so concerned with normal feet? If we can properly define the normal, the significant deviations will become more meaningful relative to anatomic and functional disorders. Medicine as practiced today is geared to crisis situations. The patient seeks medical attention only when he or she has symptoms of a problem. Solution of the problem leads eventually to an accumulation of cases which, when collected form the basis of a scientific paper. To make the approach to and the solution of the problem scientifically plausible, measurements are made, usually of angles between bones and joints, and deviations from an arbitrary norm are considered suitable for the particular surgical procedure under discussion. The problem with this approach is that an abnormal population of symptomatic or overstressed feet are being judged by an arbitrary norm. What about patients whose feet are abnormal as judged by such norms, who do not seek nor do they need medical attention because they have adequate function for their needs and are asymptomatic? Are they abnormal because they do not fit the criteria, or are they normal because they function well and have no symptoms? The scientific validity of measurements such as these is of doubtful significance.

A case in point is that of the abnormally short or atavistic first metatarsal as postulated by Dudley J. Morton.[4] This has been incriminated as the major defect in a number of foot disorders. The study by Harris and Beath[5] of Canadian soldiers revealed that over one third (35.5 per cent) had a short first metatarsal, but the vast majority of those with significant measureable shortening of the first metatarsal had no symptoms related to it, and furthermore, presented no evidence of disturbance in the weight distribution in their feet. Another finding in this study demonstrated that there was a wide variation and error in measurement by x-ray, since a valgus position of the foot increased the length of the first metatarsal, and a varus position decreased it. Finally, this same study revealed that "no strict parallelism exists between lowering of the longitudinal arch and impairment of function." Here we have a study of a supposedly normal population that exhibited obvious and measureable deviations from the norm, yet had no associated clinical problems. This leads to the question, should we treat all deviations from the norm, and if not, how do we determine those that require treatment?

Obviously, those individuals who are symptomatic require relief, but what about those who have similar foot deviations without complaints? Preventive medicine in regard to this problem would appear to be of questionable value on the basis of present data.

Another aspect of the problem of the normal foot relates to the footwear industry and standards-setting organizations, both voluntary and governmental. Recently, a problem arose in that segment of the footwear industry concerned with manufacture of steel-toe box safety shoes. Owing to the large influx of female workers in heavy industry, safety shoes for them became mandatory to meet safety standards. The steel-toe box for men did not lend itself cosmetically to acceptance by the women. To meet the objections and still provide adequate safety, it was necessary to measure the height of the great toe in both men and women and to develop normal values to help resolve the problem. The result was that the steel-toe box could be reduced in height by 1/16 of an inch for women and yet provide adequate margins of safety. The effect of the appearance of the resultant shoe was far greater than the slight difference in measurement would at first indicate.

The effect of the type of footwear on the stability and safety for the foot is the subject of another standards-setting organization. The greater aspect of this study probably relates to the interaction of the shoe with the weight-bearing surface, but to investigate it thoroughly, considerable aid is needed from the orthopaedic profession, especially in the field of biomechanics. What is needed is the reaction of the normal foot under the test circumstances, but if we do not or cannot define a normal foot, how do we relate the test results to the great majority of the population? In addition, is a type of footwear, or particular heel material, more suitable for normal feet, as compared with pronated or cavus feet?

The wide variablity and adaptability of the normal human foot is readily apparent to the footwear industry. The foreign imports, which include over 60 per cent of female shoes now sold, do not provide half-sizes and have generally only three widths: narrow, average, and wide. At present, data relative to any deleterious effects of such inadequate fitting are sparse. The American footwear industry is attempting to change the sizing of the shoe lasts, which has been based on the arithmetic mode in use since the twelfth century, to a geometric or proportional grading. This change is in part economic, designed to meet foreign competition, but again we have no objective data from the medical standpoint to determine if this is a beneficial change or not. These are some of the investigative channels that need to be pursued in order to derive some useful data relative to performance of normal feet under various external conditions.

The whole problem of children's footwear needs considerable investigation. We do not know what happens to children with pronated feet that are not treated. How many develop stable "normal" feet wearing regular shoes and canvas shoes is not known because generally they are not allowed to remain untreated. I suspect that a large number of children with asymptomatic flat feet would end up with essentially normal feet if not orthopaedically treated, but I cannot prove this except with a small number of cases which are not significant. Obviously, those with symptomatic flat feet require attention. What is needed is a prospective study to evaluate the effect of treatment on the course of *asymptomatic* flat feet in children. In addition, the value of the various modalities of treatment requires investigation, especially the need for and efficiency of reinforced extended heel counter shoes in these children.

Turning to the adult foot, there have been many methods of measurement based on the x-ray which have been utilized in the past. Many relate to disorders of the foot, so what is needed is a standardized set of measurements performed on a sufficiently large group of individuals with "normal" asymptomatic feet to provide a statistical base. In particular, the position of the foot during the radiologic examination is of great importance since inversion and eversion of the heel change the parameters in the remainder of the foot leading to errors of measurement. A standardized technique needs to be developed before meaningful values can be obtained. Such values can be applied to abnormal and symptomatic situations and correlated with significance, relevance, and magnitude. In this way, it is hoped that in spite of probable wide variations, some useful values will be obtained to understand the genesis of disorders of the foot and possibly aid in better management of these problems.

In addition, our colleagues in biomechanical investigation should be able to add valuable data to assist in more complete evaluation of the normal foot as well as to further delineate the disorders in function of the abnormal foot.

At one time, I thought it would be easy to define the normal foot. After many observations and consultations with various authorities it has become apparent that the normal foot is a nebulous entity at the moment, incapable of concrete definition. However, the necessary ingredients for a proper evaluation of the problem along the lines suggested do exist.

REFERENCES

1. Wood-Jones, F.: *Structure and Function as Seen in the Foot, 2nd ED.* , London: Bailliere, Tindall and Cox, 1949.
2. Viladot, A.: Metatarsalgia Due to Biomechanical Alterations of the Forefoot, *Orth. Clin. North Amer. 4:* 165–78, 1973.
3. Mann, R.: Personal Communication.
4. Morton, D.J.: *The Human Foot.* New York: Columbia University Press, 1936.
5. Harris, R.I. and Beath, T.: Army Foot Survey, Vol. I, Nat. Res. Council, Ottawa, Canada, 1947.

Chapter Two

A SIMPLIFIED WORKABLE CLASSIFICATION OF ANKLE FRACTURES

HAMILTON HALL, M.D., F.R.C.S. (C)

The first definitive description of fractures about the ankle was published by Sir Percival Pott in 1758.[1] His paper described a variety of fracture patterns in the lower tibia and fibula. Prior to this time all fractures in the area had been regarded as a single uniform injury. Pott's classification required refinement, but it was not until 1922 that Ashhurst and Bromer provided the first detailed classification of ankle fractures based upon the mechanism of injury.[2] They designated fractures by adduction, abduction, and lateral rotation. To each they added degrees of injury reflecting progressively more severe trauma. The authors completed their classification with fractures from vertical compression, direct violence, and the high fibular fracture first described by Maisonneuve in 1840.[3]

Extending the work of Ashhurst and Bromer, Lauge-Hansen provided a highly detailed classification of ankle injuries based upon cadaver studies. Fractures were classified as supination-adduction, supination-eversion, pronation-abduction, and pronation-eversion.[4] With varying degrees of modification the work of Ashhurst and Bromer and Lauge-Hansen has been the basis for every classification of ankle injuries published since.

Sir Astley Cooper first described a fracture of the posterior tibial margin in 1822.[5] This fracture has been described subsequently by several authors, and the impairment of ankle stability from fractures involving between one fourth and one third of the articular surface has been emphasized. Wilson[6] clearly differentiates between two types of posterior lip fractures: those with and those without an element of vertical compression.

Weber,[7] working with the Swiss Association for the Study of Internal Fixation, proposed a simplification of the Danis classification in an attempt to return to a more practical approach. Weber recognized three types of ankle injury based upon the fracture pattern. He also described a third type of posterior malleolar fracture, a posterior medial lip broken in conjunction with a shear fracture of the medial malleolus.

THE CLASSIFICATION

The simplified classification I propose is an attempt to further clarify the situation and to provide a practical and useful method of assessing fractures of the ankle. A good working classification must either

5

aid memory or direct treatment. In my opinion, a classification such as the one proposed by Lauge-Hansen does neither. Its considerable value lies in promoting a deeper understanding of the complexities of ankle injuries, but it offers little solace or support to the orthopaedic resident faced with an unclassified ankle fracture in the emergency room at 2:00 A.M.

The overwhelming majority of ankle fractures are caused by abduction, adduction, external rotation, or a combination of these three forces. Although direct violence and vertical compression occur, they are far less common. Therefore, their presence having been acknowledged, they can be excluded from this classification. The movements of adduction and internal rotation share common components. For this reason and because their separation serves no clinical purpose, I have used the term *inversion* to imply both. Similarly, though to a lesser degree, abduction and external rotation are related movements. The term

eversion is used here to include both of these. It is basically the amount of external rotation in the combined movement which determines the height of the fibular fracture above the ankle mortise.

TYPE A—INVERSION INJURY

Inversion injuries of the ankle produce an avulsion fracture of the fibula below the level of the joint line and a shear fracture of the medial malleolus extending obliquely upward from its junction with the horizontal tibial plafond. Figure 2-1 illustrates a Type A fracture. Because the transverse avulsion fracture of the fibula occurs below the level of the tibiofibular ligaments, there is no disruption in the articulation between the tibia and fibula. Both malleoli retain their ligamentus attachment to the talus and hindfoot. These intact ligaments create a potentially stable situation. In spite of its appearance (Fig. 2-2), Type A injuries

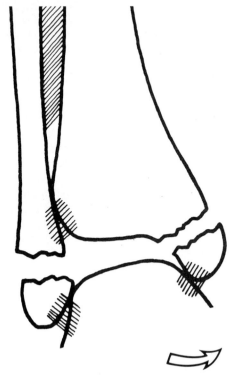

FIGURE 2-1 Type A fractures are produced by adduction and internal rotation. Fibula is avulsed below tibiofibular ligaments.

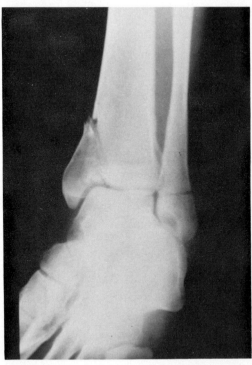

FIGURE 2-2 Long oblique fracture above medial malleolus is typical of Type A fracture. In this case closed reduction and below-knee cast immobilization produced a good result.

usually behave as two-part fractures, allowing reduction by closed methods and simple cast immobilization.

A posterior lip occurs infrequently with Type A fractures. Figure 2-3 indicates that the position of the posterior tibial fracture is medial, adjacent to the fracture of the medial malleolus. Here the posterior lip is broken by the same direct blow that caused the medial malleolar damage. This fracture bears no relationship to the posterior tibial fracture invariably seen with the Type B_2 injury.

TYPE B—EVERSION INJURY

Eversion injuries are considerably more common than the Type A inversion fractures. Two kinds of Type B fracture are identified. In each variety, however, there is an avulsion fracture of the medial malleolus at or below the level of the tibial pla-

fond and a shear fracture of the fibula laterally. Occasionally the medial malleolus may remain intact, as the eversion strain produces only a rupture of the deltoid ligament.

TYPE B₁—FIBULAR FRACTURE AT OR BELOW THE JOINT LINE

Fractures of Type B_1 have little external rotation component. The fibular fracture is generally a short oblique fracture that begins below the level of the tibiofibular ligaments. Figure 2-4 demonstrates the typical pattern. Although disruption of the lower portion of the anterior tibiofibular ligament usually occurs, the posterior syndesmotic ligament remains intact and there is no avulsion fracture of the posterior lip. B_1 fractures are bimalleolar only. As in the case of the Type A fractures, in spite of the x-ray appearance

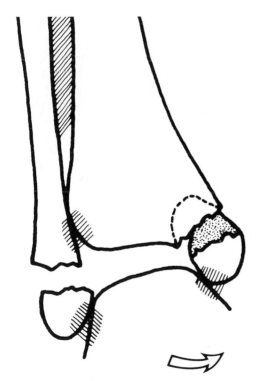

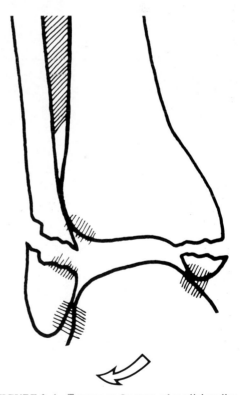

FIGURE 2-3 When the mechanism of Type A fracture includes excessive internal rotation, a medial portion of the posterior tibial lip may be fractured. This fragment is the result of direct blow and is unrelated to the avulsion fracture seen with eversion injuries.

FIGURE 2-4 Transverse fracture of medial malleolus at right angles to line of ligament pull marks it as avulsion injury. The common mechanism of both Type B fractures is eversion.

(Fig. 2-5) B₁ fractures can generally be treated successfully by closed means. The success of closed treatment lies in adequately restoring the fibular length and correcting lateral talar subluxation.

TYPE B₂—FIBULAR FRACTURE ABOVE THE JOINT LINE

Eversion injuries combined with a significant external rotation force produce fractures of the fibula above the level of the inferior tibiofibular syndesmosis. As shown in Figure 2-6, a fracture of the fibula above the joint line must be accompanied by the disruption of the tibiofibular ligaments and the creation of a diastasis. Care must be taken to differentiate high fibular fractures caused by trauma to the ankle from fractures through the midshaft of the fibula resulting from a direct blow.

Disruption of the posterior syndesmotic ligament virtually always takes the form of an avulsion fracture through the posterior tibial lip. This fracture occurs through the posterior lateral corner of the bone immediately adjacent to the fibula. As the diastasis increases, the avulsed fragment separates from the tibia but retains its proper relationship to the fibula (Fig. 2-7). This avulsion is by far the commonest form of posterior lip fracture. It can occur only with a diastasis of the inferior tibiofibular joint and specifically only with the disruption of the posterior syndesmotic ligament—that is, only with a B₂ fracture. The presence of the diastasis renders this type of ankle injury potentially unstable. For this reason internal fixation is more commonly indicated than with the other types. Successful reduction requires realignment of the lateral malleolus with restoration of fibular length and reapproxi-

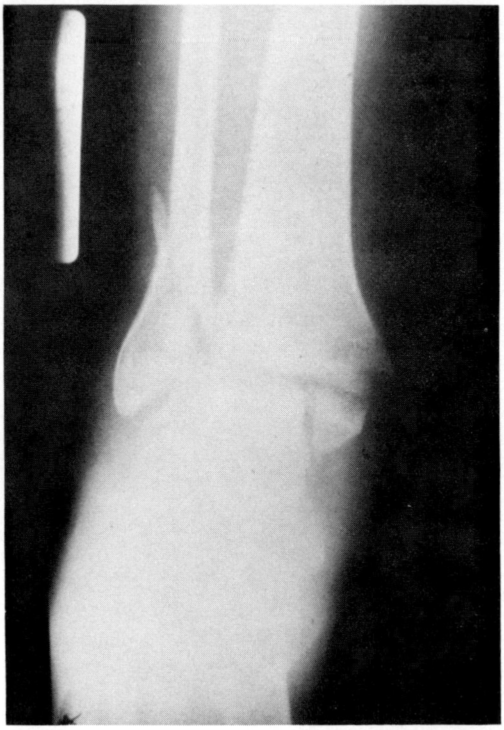

FIGURE 2-5 Notice that fibular fracture begins at joint line and extends upward. Posterior syndesmotic ligament remains intact, and there is no separation of posterior tibial lip. In this case fibular length could not be restored by closed manipulation and open reduction was required.

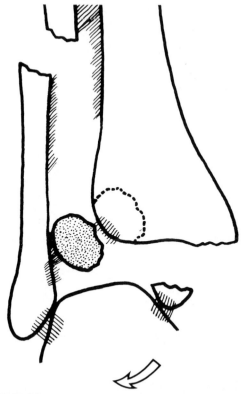

FIGURE 2-6 Interosseous membrane will be disrupted to height of fibular fracture. With loss of both tibiofibular ligaments this fracture pattern is particularly unstable.

mation of the tibiofibular joint. The success of the surgical approach depends upon correct handling of the lateral malleolus.

THE SIGNIFICANCE OF THE POSTERIOR TIBIAL LIP

The size of the posterior lip increases with the amount of vertical loading. It has been clearly shown by McLaughlin[8] and others that an unreduced posterior tibial lip fracture involving 25 per cent or more of the articular surface will lead to posterior talar subluxation. Fractures of this size are commonly recognized as a significant feature of the injury. However, the simple avulsion fracture of the B_2 type without vertical loading usually constitutes less than 10 per cent of the joint surface and its significance is frequently overlooked.

The presence of a posterior lip avulsion associated with a fibular fracture above the level of the joint line, including the Maisonneuve fracture through the fibular neck, indicates the presence of a diastasis. Displacement may not be apparent on x-ray. If the fractures of both the fibula and the "third malleolus" are undisplaced, actual separation of the tibia and fibula may not have occurred. Nevertheless, the potential for instability is present and must be taken into account during the fracture management. Isolated posterior tibial lip fractures rarely occur.[9] The appearance of a lip fracture on lateral x-ray (Fig. 2–8) should always initiate a search for the high fibular fracture confirming the presence of a Type B_2 ankle injury.

Because the posterior lip fragment retains its anatomic relationship to the fibula, the displacement of the fracture is an excellent guide to the displacement of the lateral malleolus. Shortening of the fibula places the broader distal end of the bone against the mortise on the lateral side of the tibia. Without restoration of length

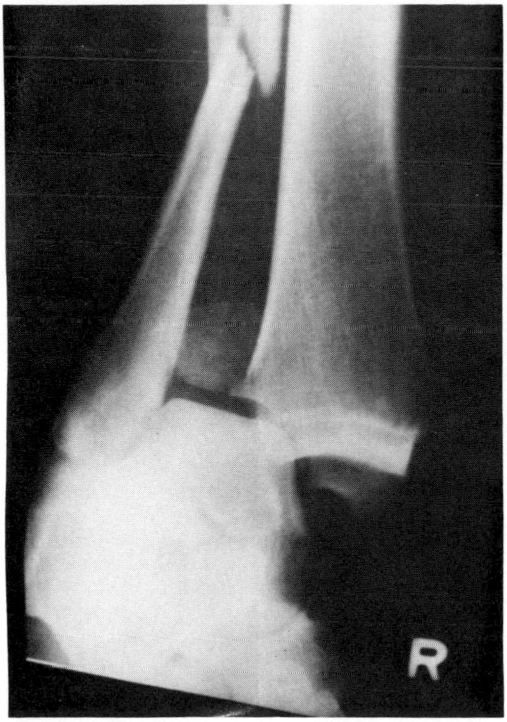

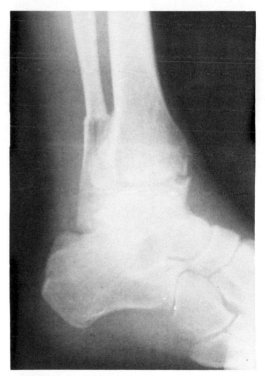

FIGURE 2–7　Fragment of bone lying above talus is posterior lip of tibia in correct alignment with fibula. Notice that degree of external rotation has produced a lateral view of tibia with anteroposterior view of talus.

FIGURE 2–8　Large posterior tibial lip is easily recognized. In this case there is no difficulty locating fibular fracture. The same avulsion of tibial lip will occur when height of fibular fracture places it above the limit of routine ankle x-ray.

proper reduction of the tibiofibular joint is impossible, and widening of the ankle mortise with lateral subluxation of the talus is inevitable. X-ray views of the fibula (Fig. 2-9) may not clearly demonstrate the degree of shortening, but the amount of posterior lip elevation seen on the lateral x-ray is usually easy to assess. The amount of elevation corresponds to the amount of fibular shortening. As the fibula is reduced, generally by open means, the posterior tibial fracture will be drawn back into position. Because of its intact ligamentus attachment to the fibula, internal fixation of even a small posterior tibial fragment can add additional stability to the fixation of the lateral malleolus and help to prevent late lateral talar subluxation.

interpret the injury. To achieve a precise description they forfeit much practical application.

This short article describes a simple workable classification of ankle injuries which offers a practical method of directing treatment. Ankle fractures are simply classified as Type A (inversion fractures) or Type B (eversion fractures). The more common Type B injuries are subclassified into fractures of the fibula at or below the syndesmosis—Type B_1—or fractures of the fibula above the syndesmosis—Type B_2. Type B_2 fractures are associated with a disruption of the distal tibiofibular syndesmosis and are potentially unstable. Fractures of the posterior tibial lip are generally associated only with the Type B_2 injuries and are of diagnostic significance.

SUMMARY

Most ankle fracture classifications use detailed anatomy and pathophysiology to

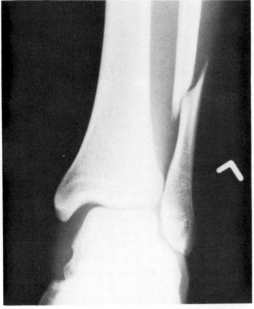

FIGURE 2-9   Fibular shortening may be underestimated owing to spiral nature of fracture. In addition to posterior lip fracture visible on lateral projection, marked subluxation of talus indicates excessive fibular shortening.

REFERENCES

1. Pott, P.: *Some Few General Remarks on Fractures and Dislocations.* London: Hawes, Clarke and Collins, 1758. Reprinted in Bick, E.M.: *Classics of Orthopaedics.* Philadelphia: J.B. Lippincott Co., 1976.
2. Ashhurst, A.P.C. and Bromer, R.S.: Classification and Mechanism of fractures of the leg bone involving the ankle. *Arch. Surg.* For: 51-129, 1922.
3. Maisonneuve, J.G.: Recherches sur la fracture du péroné. *Arch. Gen. de Med.* 7:165-87, 1840.
4. Lauge-Hansen, N.: Fractures of the ankle, II. Combined experimental—surgical and experimental—roentgenologic investigations. *Arch. Surg.* 60:957-85, 1950.
5. Cooper, A.P.: *On Dislocation of the Ankle-Joint.* London: Hurst, Rees, Orme and Broure, 1822. Reprinted in Bick, E.M.: *Classics of Orthopaedics.* Philadelphia: J.B. Lippincott Co., 1976.
6. Wilson, F.C.: Fractures and Dislocations of the Ankle. In Rockwood, C.A. and Green D.P. (Ed.): *Fractures.* Philadelphia: J.B. Lippincott Co., 1975, p. 1380.
7. Müller, M.E., Allgöwer, M. and Willenegger, H.: *Manual of Internal Fixation.* New York: Springer-Verlag, 1970, p. 196.
8. McLaughlin, H.L. and Ryder, C.T.: Open reduction and internal fixation for fractures of the tibia and ankle. *Surg. Clin. North Amer.* 1523-34, 1949.
9. Bonnin, J.G.: *Injuries to the Ankle.* Darien, Connecticut: Hafner Publishing Co., 1970.

Chapter Three

MANAGEMENT OF UNSTABLE ANKLE FRACTURES

Isadore G. Yablon, M.D.
Stephen Wasilewski, M.D.

THE ROLE OF THE LATERAL MALLEOLUS

In following patients who had sustained displaced bimalleolar fractures of the ankle, it was noted that a number of these developed late degenerative changes occurring from three to eight years after their injury. In an attempt to find a common denominator that would shed some light on the etiologic factors of this unfortunate complication, it was noted that there was incomplete reduction of the lateral malleolus in all of the patients who developed degenerative changes. To assess the role of the lateral malleolus the experiments described below were performed.

Materials and Methods

Laboratory Studies

Fresh human cadaveric ankles were stripped of skin, muscles, and tendons. Two K-wires were inserted transversely through the talus to stabilize the subtalar joint. These K-wires were perpendicular to the long axis of the fibula and parallel to the tibial plafond in order that rotatory and valgus-varus instability could be measured. Four separate studies were done to assess the effects on ankle stability after (1) isolated division of the deltoid ligament; (2)

isolated division of the fibular collateral ligaments; (3) transverse osteotomy of the medial malleolus of the level of the joint with all ligaments intact; and (4) short oblique osteotomy of the lateral malleolus distal to the anterior tibiofibular ligament.

Another series of experiments was undertaken to determine the mechanisms responsible for incomplete talar reduction. Using additional specimens, the lateral and medial malleoli were osteotomized and the foot was externally rotated to simulate the presenting appearance of these injuries. The ankle was then placed in valgus and 30° of external rotation. Manual reduction was then attempted by applying a varus stress and internally rotating the ankle as would be done clinically.

Clinical Studies

In order to determine whether primary reduction of the medial malleolus would be sufficient to afford an anatomic reduction of the ankle, seventeen patients with bimalleolar fractures had the medial malleolus reduced and fixed with a screw in the conventional manner. Intraoperative roentgenograms were then obtained, and these revealed that in fourteen patients there was an incomplete reduction of the talus and lateral malleolus. The screw in the medial malleolus was removed and the lateral mal-

11

leolus was reduced with a four-hole plate without replacing the screw in the medial malleolus, following which intraoperative stress roentgenograms were obtained.

Results

Laboratory Studies

When the deltoid ligament alone was divided no instability resulted. Osteotomizing the medial malleolus at the level of the joint line allowed for 10° to 15° of rotatory displacement, but very little valgus instability resulted. When the lateral collateral ligament complex was divided there were 30° of external rotation and 10° of inversion (Fig. 3-1). After division of the lateral malleolus distal to the anterior tibiofibular ligament there were 40° of external rotation and 20° of inversion (Fig. 3-2).

When the medial malleolus was reduced with the screw after creating bimalleolar fractures in cadaveric ankles the position of the talus was generally improved, but anatomic reduction was not achieved because the lateral malleolus impinged upon the proximal fibular fragment (Fig. 3-3). The talus could be accurately repositioned only by applying an internal rotatory force. However, this resulted in marked stretching of the fibular collateral ligaments because the lateral malleolus remained unreduced (Fig. 3-4). The talus followed the displacement plane of the lateral malleeous, and only by accurately reducing the lateral malleolus could the talus resume its anatomic position.

Clinical Studies

In those fractures where there was incomplete reduction of the talus after the medial malleolus was reduced, the talus could be anatomically repositioned only when the lateral malleolus was reduced by the application of a four-hole plate (Figs. 3-5 through 3-8). Intraoperative stress films indicated that the talus remained stable despite the fact that no fixation was used for the medial malleolus (Fig. 3-9).

The results in fifty-three patients who

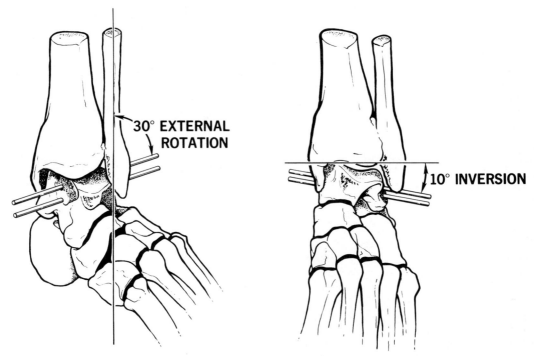

FIGURE 3-1   Demonstrates amount of instability after division of fibular collateral ligaments.

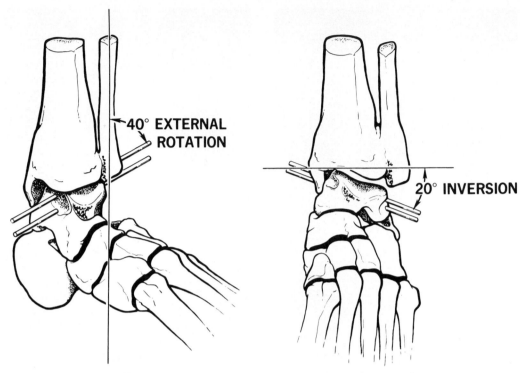

FIGURE 3–2 Demonstrates instability after osteotomy of lateral malleolus.

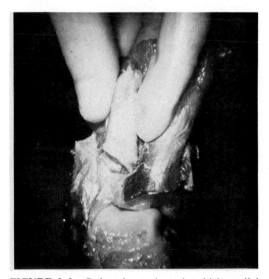

FIGURE 3–3 Cadaveric specimen in which medial and lateral malleoli have been osteotomized and ankle abducted and externally rotated. Medial malleolus was securely fixed with a compression screw. Talus has been incompletely reduced because of impingement of lateral malleolus on fibular shaft, preventing complete reduction.

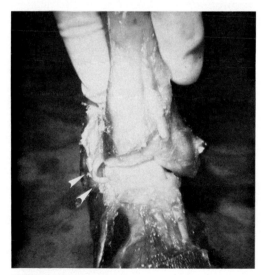

FIGURE 3–4 Cadaveric specimen demonstrating that anatomic reduction of talus can be achieved by forced internal rotation. Note that because lateral malleolus is still unreduced, fibular collateral ligaments (arrows) are stretched to permit position of the talus.

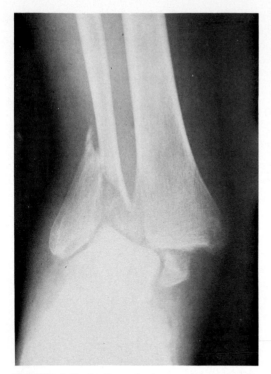

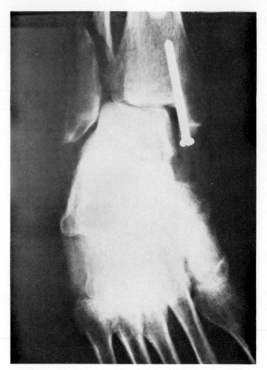

FIGURE 3–5 Radiograph demonstrating unstable bimalleolar fracture of the ankle.

FIGURE. 3–6 Intraoperative radiograph in which medial malleolus has been reduced and held in place with a screw. Complete reduction of talus has not been achieved and there is residual displacement of lateral malleolus.

were treated by open reduction and internal fixation of the lateral malleolus showed that the talus was anatomically reduced in each case. Follow-up was from six months to nine years, and there were no late degenerative changes. There were two postoperative infections that responded to débridement, antibiotic therapy, and closed suction irrigation. There was one case of superficial skin necrosis because the leg was not elevated postoperatively.

DISCUSSION

It was surprising to observe that the ankle was stable after division of the deltoid ligament. However, in reviewing the literature no references could be found describing talar instability as a result of rupture of this ligament only, without other associated injuries. In addition, very few surgical procedures are available for the repair of a torn deltoid ligament.

DuVries[2] has described a surgical procedure in which a cruciate incision is made in the deltoid ligament, with the edges being subsequently resutured. The indications for this procedure, however, were more for relief of pain rather than for instability. Wiltberger and Mallory[8] described an operation for reconstruction of the deltoid ligament utilizing a portion of the posterior tibial tendon. These authors did not provide evidence that their operation was used for instability resulting only from a ruptured deltoid ligament. Some of the cases they presented showed residual talar displacement following a fracture of the lateral malleolus and a tear of the deltoid ligament in which the lateral malleolus remained incompletely reduced.

It was noted that the ankle was relatively stable after division of the medial malleolus. Clinical proof of this observation is noted in Figure 3–10. The patient had sustained a fracture of the medial mal-

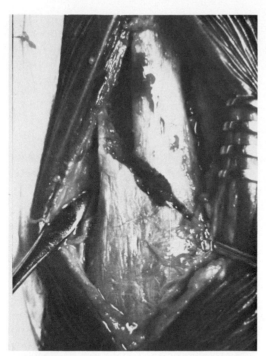

FIGURE 3-7 Intraoperative photograph showing displacement of lateral malleolus.

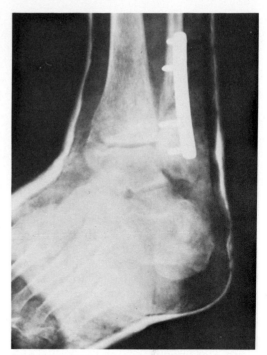

FIGURE 3-8 Postoperative radiograph in which lateral malleolus has been accurately reduced with a four-hole plate. Talus is also reduced.

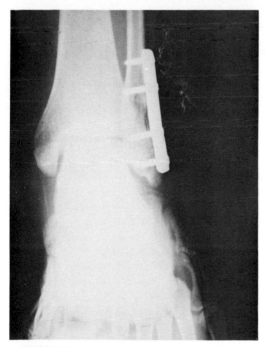

FIGURE 3-9 Intraoperative stress radiograph demonstrating that ankle is stable once lateral malleolus is securely fixed. No displacement of talus is present despite the fact that medial side of ankle has not been internally fixed.

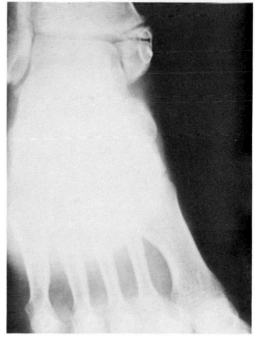

FIGURE 3-10 Radiograph of patient who sustained fracture of medial malleolus twenty-five years earlier. Fibrous union has occurred, but despite this ankle is stable.

leolus twenty-five years earlier. Fibrous union had occurred, but despite this the talus was perfectly stable. If the medial malleolus was vital in maintaining stability of the ankle then fibrous union would be inadequate to provide this support, just as fibrous union is inadequate to support the tibia or femur. Figure 3–11 demonstrates an intraoperative stress photograph. The patient had an osteochondral fracture of the dome of the talus on the medial side. In order to expose the fragment, the medial malleolus had to be osteotomized at the level of the joint. There was slight rotatory displacement between the talus and the tibia but no valgus or varus instability was present.

The results of these studies indicate that in displaced bimalleolar fractures the talus follows the displacement plane of the lateral malleolus.[3] Reducing only the medial malleous may still leave the talus unstable because of incomplete reduction of the lateral malleolus.[5] Forced reduction of the talus can occur by stretching the fibular collateral ligaments, but when immobilization is discontinued the talus is potentially unstable because the fibular collateral ligaments remain in a stretched posi-

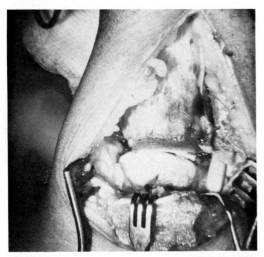

FIGURE 3–11 Intraoperative stress photograph of patient who had an osteochondral fracture of superior and medial bone of talus. An osteotomy of medial malleolus was done to provide exposure. A valgus and external rotation stress has been applied. There are about 5° of rotatory instability but no valgus instability.

tion. This results in a predisposition to late degenerative changes, since the talus bears more weight per unit area than any other bone in the body and anatomic restoration is therefore mandatory.

THE ISOLATED FRACTURE OF THE LATERAL MALLEOLUS

Since the previous studies emphasized the importance of the lateral malleolus in injuries of the ankle, and since incomplete reduction of the lateral malleolus indicated residual talar instability, a question arises regarding the management of the isolated fracture of the lateral malleolus in which the talus remains in its anatomic position. Figure 3–12A is an example of just such a case. There is a minimally displaced fracture of the lateral malleolus without any talar displacement (Fig. 3–12B). This injury was treated by the application of a below-knee cast. Ten days later an abnormal talar tilt was present (Fig. 3–13). The talus is not displaced laterally but appears tilted owing to rotatory displacement. During surgery the deltoid ligament was explored and was found to be intact. When the lateral side of the ankle was opened, in addition to the fracture of the lateral malleolus there was a complete tear of the anterior tibiofibular ligament. The lateral malleolus was fixed with a four-hole plate, which restored stability of the ankle. Because the significance of the anterior tibiofibular ligament appears not to have been fully appreciated the following study was undertaken.

Materials and Methods

Eight cadaveric ankles were utilized. The specimens were stripped of skin and soft tissues and the anterior tibiofibular ligament was exposed. An oblique osteotomy was created in the lateral malleolus and talar instability was tested. The anterior tibiofibular ligament was then divided with the lateral malleolus intact and with the lateral malleolus osteotomized. Stability of the ankle was determined by applying valgus and varus rotatory stresses after sutur-

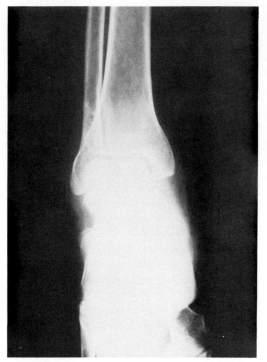
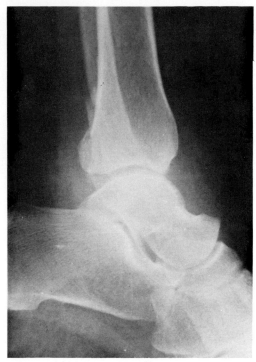

FIGURE 3-12 (A) Radiograph of patient who sustained fracture of lateral malleolus. The talus remains in its anatomic position. (B) Lateral radiograph of same patient demonstrating the fracture of lateral malleolus.

ing the anterior tibiofibular ligament and after fixing the lateral malleolus with a plate.

Results

Osteotomy of the lateral malleolus with the anterior tibiofibular ligament in-

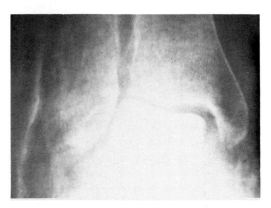

FIGURE 3-13 Radiograph of same patient demonstrating a talar tilt ten days after application of plaster cast.

tact did not result in any talar instability (Fig. 3-14). However, when the anterior tibiofibular ligament was divided after osteotomizing the lateral malleolus, a talar tilt was present (Fig. 3-15). When either the ligament was repaired or the lateral malleolus was reduced with a plate, stability of the ankle was restored (Figs. 3-16 and 3-17).

DISCUSSION

When radiographs indicate a fracture of the lateral malleolus alone it may create an enigma with regard to subsequent management. It has been adequately stressed that fractures of the lateral malleolus may be accompanied by a rupture of the deltoid ligament that could result in subsequent talar displacement, despite the fact that the initial radiographs indicate a normal position of the talus.[7] However, talar displacement may occur in those instances where the deltoid ligament is intact but in which a

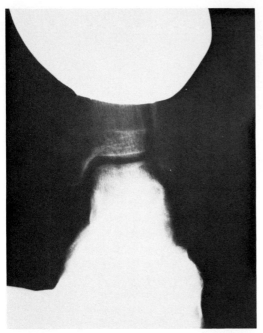

FIGURE 3–14 Stress radiograph of a cadaveric specimen in which lateral malleolus was osteotomized proximal to anterior tibiofibular ligament. Tibiofibular ligament was not divided. Note that ankle is stable.

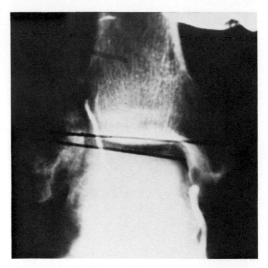

FIGURE 3–15 Stress radiograph of cadaveric specimen in which lateral malleolus was osteotomized and anterior tibiofibular ligament divided. Talar tilt is present.

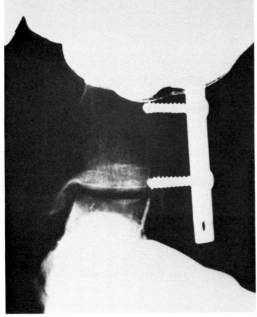

FIGURE 3–16 Stress radiograph of cadaveric specimen. Lateral malleolus was fixed with a plate. Although anterior tibiofibular ligament was not repaired, restoring stability to lateral malleolus restores stability to ankle.

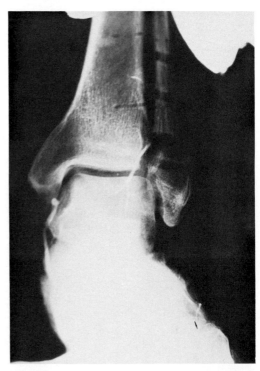

FIGURE 3–17 Stress radiograph of same specimen as in Figure 3 = 16. Plate was removed from lateral malleolus, and anterior tibiofibular ligament was repaired with nonabsorbable sutures. Ankle is stable.

tear of the anterior tibiofibular ligament exists. Cedell,[1] Iselin,[3] Magnusson,[4] and Solonen and Lauttamus,[6] have stressed the importance of this ligament in maintaining ankle stability. Based on the studies described in this paper, it would appear that ankle instability can occur in the presence of an intact deltoid ligament if a fracture of the lateral malleolus is accompanied by a tear of the anterior tibiofibular ligament.

We can conclude, therefore, that fractures of the lateral malleolus alone are stable only if no other ligaments are torn. Fractures of the lateral malleolus alone are unstable if either the deltoid or anterior tibiofibular ligaments are torn. In isolated fractures of the lateral malleolus the integrity of the deltoid and anterior tibiofibular ligaments should be verified. Injury to the deltoid ligament can be ascertained by pain on palpation and by the presence of ecchymosis. Injuries of the anterior tibiofibular ligament may be more difficult to detect but can be determined by the presence of pain in the interval between the tibia and fibula. In some instances it may be necessary to infiltrate the ankle with a local anesthetic and perform stress tests. Arthrography may also be helpful to demonstrate the rupture of the anterior tibiofibular ligament. If these ligaments are intact the injury may be treated conservatively by the application of a below-knee walking cast for about six weeks. If, however, these ligaments are not intact, an attempt should be made to accurately reduce the lateral malleolus by manipulation and the extremity should be immobilized in a long-leg cast. Frequent radiologic assessment is necessary to determine whether talar displacement has occurred. If displacement occurs, open reduction and internal fixation of the lateral malleolus are recommended.

REFERENCES

1. Cedell, C.A.: Supination-outward rotation injuries of the ankle. A clinical and roentgenological study with special reference to the operative treatment. *Acta Orthop. Scand.,* Supplementum 110, 1967.
2. DuVries, M.L.: *Surgery of the Foot* (2nd Ed.,). St. Louis: C.V. Mosby Co., 1965.
3. Iselin, M. and DeVellis, H.: La primaute du péroné dans les fractures du cou-de-pied. *Mem. Acad. Chir.* 87:399–408, 1961.
4. Magnusson, R.: On the late results in non-operated cases of malleolar fractures. A clinical-roentgenological-statistical study. 1. Fractures by external rotation. *Acta Chir. Scand.,* Supplementum 84, 1944.
5. Mueller, M.E., Allgower, M. and Willenegger, H.: *Manual of Internal Fixation.* Berlin: Springer, 1970.
6. Solonen, K.A. and Lauttamus, L.: Operative treatment of ankle fractures. *Acta Orthop. Scand.* 39:223–37, 1968.
7. Staples, O.S.: Injuries to the medial ligaments of the ankle. Result study. *J. Bone Joint Surg.* 42A:1287–1307, 1960.
8. Wiltberger, B.R. and Mallory, T.M.: A new method for the reconstruction of the deltoid ligament of the ankle. *Ortho. Rev.,* 1:37 41, 1972.

Chapter Four

ANKLE FUNCTION: MEASUREMENT AND FUNCTIONAL BRACING OF THE FRACTURED ANKLE

DAVID SEGAL, M.D.

The ankle is the most congruous joint of the lower extremity[6]; it enables us to dorsi- and plantar flex the foot through an oblique axis that inclines laterally and posteriorly. The axis can be defined quite accurately at the tips of the medial and lateral malleoli. In evaluating this function, one needs a standard method of examination, which as yet has not been defined. The methods presently recommended are outlined in the *Manual of Orthopedic Surgery* and in text books in which the motion of the ankle is examined by actively dorsi- and plantar flexing the foot with the knee either straight or bent.[1,2,5] The figures obtained for the ankle can vary from 20° to 35° of dorsiflexion and from 30° to 50° of plantar flexion. This method of examination and measurement is grossly inaccurate. Physiologically, most of the dorsiflexion takes place after midstance phase and is a pure passive movement. The dorsiflexors of the foot and toes are inactive as seen on the electromyograms.[3,4] Active dorsiflexion to a much lesser degree takes place during swing phase to clear the toes off the ground. Therefore, it is my opinion that dorsiflexion should be measured in the weight-bearing position.

In the proposed method of examination, the patient stands on the foot to be examined, holding on to the examining table or cabinet for balancing purposes only. By bringing the weight of the body over the leg to be examined and bending the knee, the angle measured between the tibia and sole of the foot is subtracted from 90° and represents the amount of dorsiflexion of the ankle (Fig. 4-1). During the examination the heel and sole should not be lifted off the floor. Squatting is not an adequate position for measurement, as the gastrocsoleus is contracted, preventing dorsiflexion of the ankle beyond neutral.

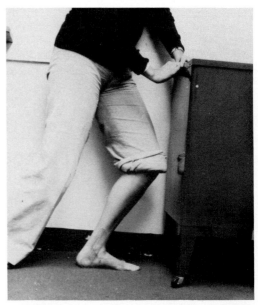

FIGURE 4-1 Measuring dorsiflexion in weight-bearing position. Goniometer is parallel to tibia and sole of foot

Plantar flexion is done with the patient sitting or lying, actively or passively plantar flexing the foot. The measurement is conducted on the medial side of the foot, the axis being distal to the tip of the medial malleolus (Fig. 4-2). The angle is measured between the hindfoot and the tibia and subtracted from 90°. Previous methods of measurement[1,2] of plantar flexion were inaccurate, as they included motion present at the mid- and forefoot. In cadaveric experiments, after transfixing the os calcis and talus to the tibia, one can demonstrate 15° to 20° of motion present at the mid- and forefoot. Similarly, by superimposing x-rays taken in maximum dorsi- and plantar flexion, one can demonstrate 20° of motion present at the mid- and forefoot (Fig. 4-3). This unique approach to the measurement of ankle motion will eliminate inaccuracies, standardize the method of examination, and provide a uniform method of documentation.

With the availability of this new method of examination of ankle motion, stiffness was found in most of the ankle fractures that were immobilized in a cast. During the last two years the orthopaedic Department at Boston City Hospital treated unstable ankle fractures with open reduction. In patients with unstable fractures requiring open reduction and internal fixation, stability is achieved by using screw and plate fixation because circlage wires or Rush pins do not provide enough internal stability and require additional fixations with a cast. In unstable fractures where the lateral malleolus is displaced, associated with tear of the deltoid ligament, the lateral

malleolus is reduced and the deltoid ligament repaired as well. If syndesmotic ligament tears are present, a syndesmotic screw is used to maintain proper alignment of the distal tibiofibular joint. In all patients, following surgery the leg is immobilized in a short leg cast and elevated. The cast is bivalved forty eight hours postoperatively and active assisted range of motion of the ankle is initiated. The patient uses Kerlix or an Ace bandage to assist in active dorsiflex-

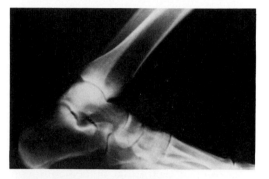

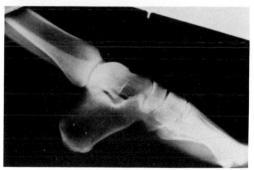

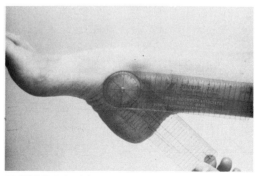

FIGURE 4-2 Plantar flexion of ankle is measured with goniometer parallel to hindfoot and tibia.

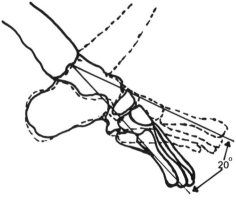

FIGURE 4-3 (A and B) Lateral projection of normal ankle in maximum dorsi-and plantar flexion: (C) Superimposition of x-rays of A and B; 20° of plantar flexion in mid- and forefoot.

ion of the ankle. Between exercises, the bi-valved cast is used to immobilize the ankle in a neutral position. A short leg brace is applied on the fifth to eighth postoperative day (Fig. 4-4). The surgical treatment provides anatomic reduction and stability, and the brace is designed to enable dorsi- and plantar flexion and to minimize rotation (Figs. 4-5 and 4-6). While in the brace, the patient is encouraged to ambulate, bearing weight as tolerated, and to regularly perform dorsiflexion exercises.

At Boston City Hospital in the past two years, 278 ankle fractures were seen, of which 112 required open reduction and internal fixation. At the time of this report there were over fifty patients who underwent open reduction, among them some who required syndesmotic screw fixation. All were treated with the short leg brace and immediate weight bearing; not one developed hardware failure or nonunion of the lateral malleolus; and only three had a nonunion of the medial malleolus in conjunction with a figure-of-8 fixation. Eleva-

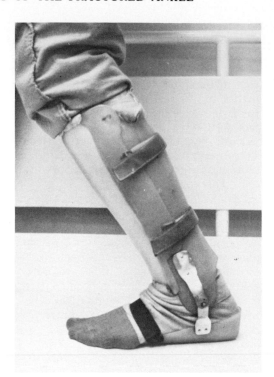

FIGURE 4-5 Rigid hinges and tight fit of brace allow for dorsiflexion.

tion of the leg is constantly stressed as the single most important factor in rehabilitation of the ankle, and the syndesmotic screw is routinely removed after six weeks. The brace is maintained for a total of twelve weeks; for the first six weeks it is worn day and night and for the last six weeks only during the day. It has been our experience that immediate weight bearing

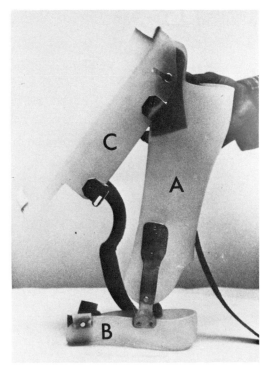

FIGURE 4-4 The three components of brace are shown: (A) posterior shell; (B) plastic shoe insert, (C) anterior section.

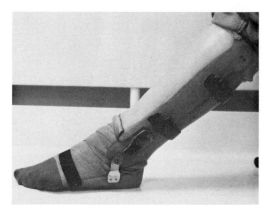

FIGURE 4-6 Same patient as in Figure 4-5, demonstrating plantar flexion.

and bracing of fractured ankles reduces bone and muscle atrophy as well as joint stiffness and pain, and the patient's comfort is significantly enhanced. I have noted that patients with 10° of dorsiflexion have unrestricted ambulation, excluding athletic activities. Early weight bearing and dorsiflexion exercises are the key factors for obtaining it; plantar flexion will always accompany the dorsiflexion, usually with 3 to 5 additonal degrees.

APPENDEX

Custom-Made Short Leg Brace

The custom-made short leg brace has been used in over fifty patients following surgical treatment of ankle fractures. A cast mold of the lower leg and foot is taken on the fourth or fifth postoperative day once the swelling subsides and with the medial and lateral malleolus outlined. A thin strip of cotton webbing is placed over the anterior surface of the tibia for easy removal of the cast mold. The orthosis is fabricated from a positive cast mold and is constructed of three parts, the first of which is a posterior shell (Fig. 4-4A) that extends over the gastrocsoleus muscle and medial and lateral malleolus with a cutout over the achilles tendon. The posterior shell surrounds the lower leg over the medial, lateral, and posterior surfaces. A plastic shoe insert (Fig. 4-4B) for foot support is attached with metal hinges to the posterior shell at the level of the malleoli. The third part of the brace consists of an anterior section (Fig. 4-4C) applied to the anterior surface of the tibia and attached to the posterior shell with Velcro straps. The proximal part of the anterior section (C) is attached to the posterior shell (A) by a keyhole slot that fits over a stud. Adjusting the straps, the patient can tighten the brace around the lower leg with the rigid hinges, enabling unrestricted dorsi- and plantar flexion and minimizing rotation. The brace can easily fit into a sneaker, shoe, or walking boot. The patient is encouraged to ambulate with crutches bearing weight as tolerated, and routinely perform dorsiflexion exercises. Ace bandages or anti-inflammatory drugs are given as indicated. The brace is removed for bathing and skin care and is worn for the first six weeks day and night and for the second six weeks only during the day.

REFERENCES

1. D'Ambrosia, R.D.: *Musculosketal Disorders: Regional Examination and Differential Diagnosis.* Philadelphia: J.B. Lippincott, 1977.
2. Manual of Orthopedic Surgery. The American Orthopaedic Association.
3. New York University Postgraduate Medical School: *Prosthetics and Orthotics: Lower Limb Prosthetics.* New York, 1975 rev., p. 101.
4. Perry, J.: Kinesiology of lower extremity bracing. *Clin. Ortho.* 102:18, July-Aug., 1974.
5. Schatzker, J. et al.: Irreducible fracture disolocation of the ankle due to posterior dislocation of the fibula. *J. Trauma* 17:397, 1977.
6. Simon, W.H., et al.: Joint congruence: a correlation of joint congruence and thickness of articular cartilage in dogs, *J. Bone Joint Surg.* 55A:1614, 1973.

Chapter Five

WIRE-LOOP FIXATION OF THE LATERAL MALLEOLUS IN ANKLE FRACTURES

Stanley H. Nahigian, M.D.
Indong Oh, M.D.
F.B. Zahrawi, M.D.

In displaced bimalleolar or trimalleolar fractures of the ankle, a slight malreduction or nonanatomic position of the lateral malleolus is frequently thought to be acceptable as long as the medial or large posterior malleolar fragment has been well reduced and stabilized. The belief that ankle function is not materially affected whatever the roentgenographic appearance of the lateral malleolus reduction has commonly prevailed even to the present. Recently, the importance of an anatomic reduction of the lateral malleolar fracture by open methods, restoring normal ankle joint mechanics, has been receiving greater emphasis.[1,3,5,7,23] The biomechanical importance of the fibula in the dynamic function of the ankle has been studied anatomically in normal athletes by telephoto motion studies and cineroentgenograms by Weinert and associates,[20] who showed an active fibula to be vital to normal ankle function and not merely a rudimentary strut.

EXPERIMENTAL AND CLINICAL STUDIES

Experimental studies have shown that even a minute displacement, rotation, or shortening of the lateral malleolar fragment resulted in displacement of the vertical axis of the talus.[21,23] Because of the closed, compact anatomic configuration of the tibiotalofibular articulation, minor displacement of the talus in either the anteroposterior or mediolateral plane considerably reduces the contact surface between the tibia and the talus.[15] Lambert[11] showed that the fibula was not merely a lateral buttress but a weight-bearing bone and an integral part of the static supportive architecture of the leg. Maintenance of the original length of the distal fibula is a key factor in restoring the normal congruity of the ankle joint. Thus the precise fit between the articular ridge of the tibia plafonde and the corresponding articular groove on the talar dome cannot be disturbed without leading to incongruity dysfunction and the late development of post-traumatic arthritis.[1,5,9,22] For purely mechanical reasons, closed reduction with cast immobilization for displaced fractures seldom can produce an anatomic reconstitution of the ankle joint. Often partial interposition of fascial, ligamentous, and periosteal soft tissue or even small bone fragments hinder an anatomic reduction. Of course, even with a nonanatomic reduction, the fractures will usually reunite but with the surrounding lateral ligaments in a displaced position, which may cause an incongruity of the oblique talofibular articulation. Several studies[10,14,19] demonstrated that incomplete reduction of the lateral malleoulus was a major cause of failure in ankle fracture management. The very few comparative studies of conservative and operative treatment of ankle fractures report varying results. Wilson's[22] series showed slightly better results in operative treatment, and the frequency of post-traumatic arthritis in closed management as reported in Magnusdn's[13] series was twice that in the operative management as reportedby Cedell.[4] The recent report of Yablon and colleagues[23] showed no instance of degenerative arthritis when the lateral malleolus fracture was reduced anatomically and fixed by an open method.

RATIONALE OF WIRE-LOOP FIXATION

In principle, an anatomic closed reduction and casting of the fracture is the desirable method of treatment. When open reduction is indicated the tissue damage should be minimal. Most ankle fractures are further immobilized by a plaster cast following closed reduction alone or even after internal fixation. When external immobilization is employed, the internal fixation need be sufficient only to resist the stresses to which the fracture fragments will be exposed before the consolidation has taken place. Therefore, a simple, effective internal fixation device that can stabilize the fracture fragments with minimal further damage to the already disrupted blood supply in the area is desirable. Wire-loop fixation for suitable fractures of the lateral malleolus can accomplish this goal.

The cerclage fixation in long bone fractures has been condemned in the belief that it devitalizes bone fragments by strangling the blood vessels and inhibiting extension of periosteal callus over the fracture site.[6] During fracture healing the blood vessels of the periosteal callus are arranged perpendicular to the surface of the cortex;

therefore, the cerclage wire would not block the periosteal vessels[18,17] which are derived from the main vessels of the limb.[12] Encircling wires over the cortical surface would not disturb medullary circulation, which supplies the inner two thirds or three quarters of the cortex. A wire, being round in cross-section, has minimal contact with the cortical surface so that osseous callus grows over the wire without erosion or fibrous formation when the wire remains secure.[18]

The reasons for poor surgical results with cerclage wire fixation are much more likely to be from careless periosteal stripping, excessive damage to the surrounding soft tissue, and insufficient or incorrect application of the wire loops. Successful cerclage fixation for human tibia fractures has been reported.[2]

The A-0 group advocates total stable anatomic reconstitution of the joint with rigid fixation and no plaster immobilization.[14] This method entails considerable dissection, a time-consuming procedure, and a rather large metallic device on a small area of bone. This increases the chance of disturbing the blood supply, damaging surrounding soft tissue, and the possibility of technical error.

An intramedullary device is used for certain fractures, but it is difficult to control the rotatory forces and overriding malposition common in oblique fractures. Moreover, these methods usually require a second operation for removal of the fixation device. The wire loop can be left in without any ill effects. The single or multiple small screws can be used as well but generally require more extensive surgical exposure, and the holding power of the threads of the screw is less than the wire loop(s) which circumscribe the entire external cortical surface.

Indications

The wire-loop fixation is suitable for displaced, oblique, or spiral fractures (Fig. 5-1) of the lateral malleolus which cannot be reduced anatomically and maintained with plaster immobilization alone. Ideally,

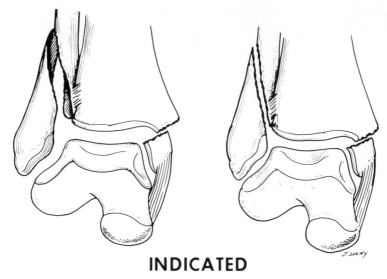

INDICATED

FIGURE 5-1 These are suitable malleolus fracture sites for wire-loop fixation because of the obliquity, location, and intact anterior tibiofibular ligament.

the length of the oblique fracture should be at least twice as long as the diameter of the bone at the fracture site. In certain comminuted fractures of the distal fibula with large butterfly fragments we have used the wire loop alone or in combination with an intramedullary device (Fig. 5-2). Wire-loop fixation is not suitable for a very short oblique or transverse fracture (Fig. 5-3). If internal fixation is needed for this type

of fracture an intramedullary rod or a long screw can be used.

Operative Technique and Postoperative Management

A longitudinal incision is made over the posterolateral border of the fibula over the ankle. The length of the incision need

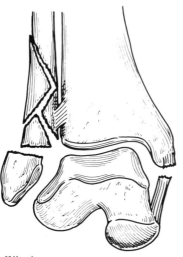
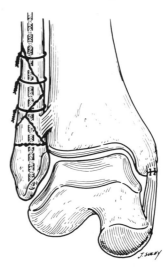

FIGURE 5-2 Wire loops are a necessary component to the intramedullary device to restore reduction and maintain length in this type of comminuted fracture.

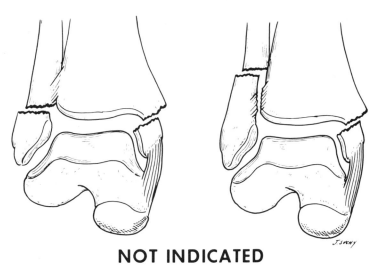

NOT INDICATED

FIGURE 5-3   These fractures are not suitable for wire-loop fixation.

be sufficient only to allow for examination of the anterior tibiofibular ligament integrity and to view the fracture completely so that any interposed soft tissue or bony fragments can be cleared away. The fracture is reduced and a curved wire passer or aneurysm needle is used to place one to three wires around the fibula close to the bone but extraperiosteally. Ideally, the wires are placed at a distance apart that is greater than the diameter of the fibula at the fracture site. Only one wire can be used in certain relatively short oblique fractures. Two or three wires are applied when required to achieve stability. Eighteen-guage (1.0236 mm) or occasionally 20-gauge (0.8128 mm) wire is suitable for the fibula. The anatomic reduction is secured under direct vision and the wire loops are completed in proper tension with a mechanical twister-type wire tightener of the Rhinelander type.[16,18]

The method of fixation of the medial and/or posterior malleolar fragments depends on the judgment and preference of the surgeon. We have used bone nails (Palmar nails), screws, tension band wires, and threaded pins in the medial malleolus. In bimalleolar fractures the fibula is fixed first before the medial malleolus is stabilized. The medial ankle ligaments and capsular tears are repaired after fibula fixation is completed. When a large posterior malleo-

lar fragment is present it is reduced and fixed first, then the fibula, and lastly the medial aspect is stabilized. Intraoperative x-rays are taken.

After wound closure, an above-the-knee, three-plane posteromediolateral plaster splint with a compression dressing is applied with the ankle in the neutral position. Antibiotics are not routinely used in closed fractures. Elevation of the limb and an active exercise program for limb control is begun as soon as possible postoperatively. Five to ten days later, when the edema has subsided, a well-fitted, below-the-knee cast is applied. No weight bearing is allowed for six weeks after surgery. X-rays are then taken in plaster, and progressive weight bearing in the cast is permitted for the next two to three weeks. The cast is removed, the ankle x-rayed, and no further immobilization is needed eight weeks after injury. If there is insufficient healing, possibly for further weeks of crutch protection is needed. Ankle and foot exercises for limb rehabilitation and methods to control the swelling are necessary.

Clinical Experience

From 1964 through 1976 there were fifty cases of ankle fractures in which the wire loop was used by the authors for treatment of displaced fractures of the lateral malleolus. In six of the fifty cases the wire loop was used in conjunction with an intramedullary device to secure and anatomically reduce the fibular malleolus. In the remaining forty-four cases the wire loop(s) alone was used on the lateral malleolus as the internal fixation.

In the forty four cases, twenty nine were female, fifteen were male, and the age range was from thirteen to seventy seven years with an average age of forty years. The type of injury included twenty one trimalleolar, twelve bimalleolar (one open fracture on the medial aspect), ten lateral malleolar fractures with rupture of the deltoid ligaments and capsule, and one lateral and posterior malleolar fracture.

In twenty one trimalleolar fractures, six had all three malleolar fractures operated and fixed internally: fourteen cases had the medial and lateral malleolus fixation and one had the lateral malleolus only stabilized by three wire loops (Fig. 5-4A-C). All of the twelve bimalleolar

fractures had internal fixation for the medial malleolus and one or more wire loops on the lateral malleolus. The wire-loop fixation was used in ten lateral malleolar fractures with ruptured deltoid ligaments (Figs. 5-5A, 5-6B,C). All these cases had the soft tissue repair after the lateral malleolus had been stabilized. In the one lateral and posterior malleolar fracture, the lateral malleolus was fixed by wire-loop fixation and two screws were used to fix the large posterior malleolar fragment.

The lateral malleolar fractures were reduced in anatomic position and maintained by one wire in eleven cases; two wires were used in twenty nine cases; and in four cases three or four wire loops were used for the long oblique or spiral fractures.

All fractures healed in anatomic position without loosening or breakage of the wires except in two cases. One patient bore full weight on the leg during and after the hospital stay, against advice, destroying the

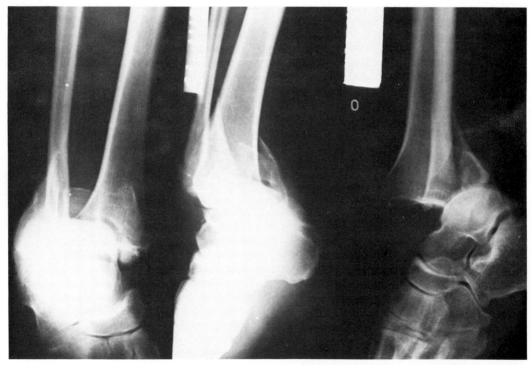

FIGURE 5-4 (A) 33-year-old male with torsional injury caused by fall while wearing high platform shoes; he sustain trimalleolar fracture dislocation of right ankle.

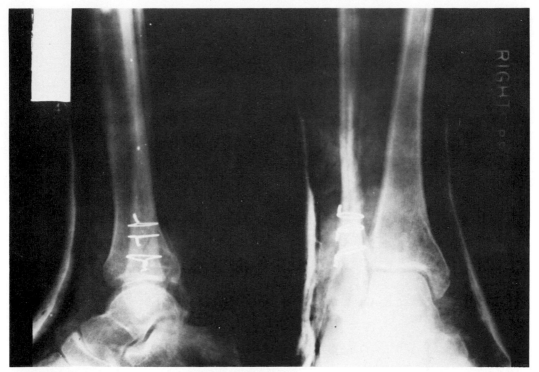

FIGURE 5-4 (B) X-rays following open reduction with three wire loops placed on lateral malleolus. No internal fixation of medial malleolus was possible because of extensive comminution.

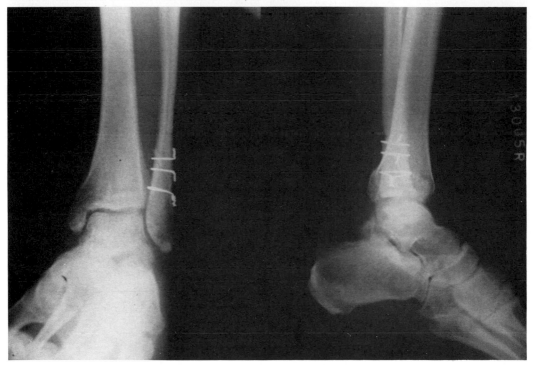

FIGURE 5-4 (C) Followpyp xprays after plaster removal before returning to work.

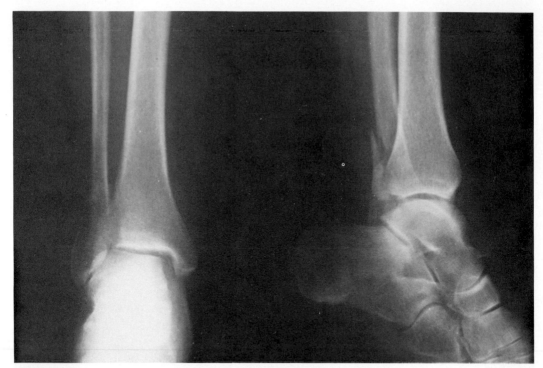

FIGURE 5-5 (A) 64-year-old female injured when she slipped on ice. Fracture dislocation of her right ankle involved lip of posterior malleolus with rupture of all medial supporting ligaments.

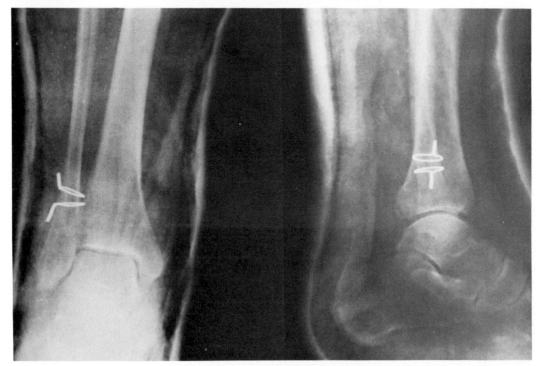

FIGURE 5-5(B) X-rays following open reduction with two wire loops laterally to stabilize fibula. Deltoid ligament and anterior capsule were surgically repaired.

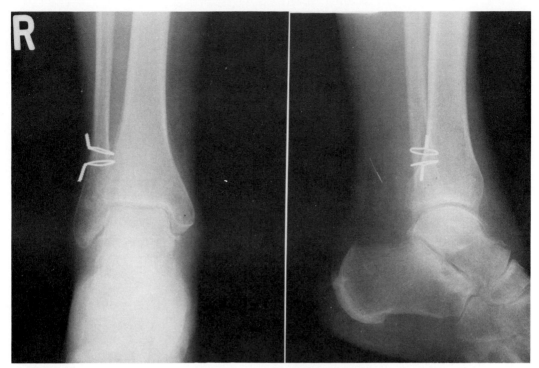

FIGURE 5-5   (C) Follow-up x-rays after plaster was removed She is asymptomatic on follow-up examination twenty months after injury.

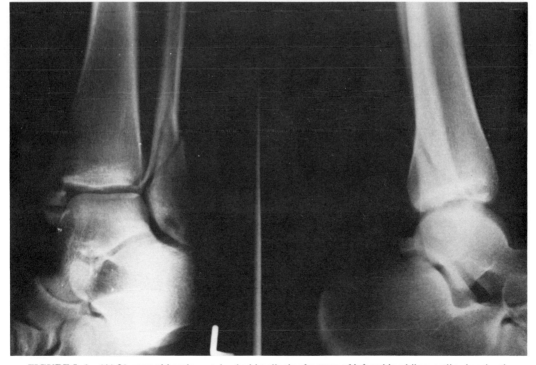

FIGURE 5-6   (A) 21-year-old male sustained a bimalleolar fracture of left ankle while wrestling in school.

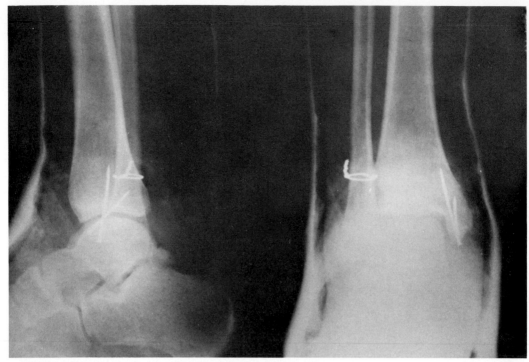

FIGURE 5–6   (B) X-rays immediately after open reduction; only a single wire loop was needed laterally. Palmar bone nails were used in medial malleolus.

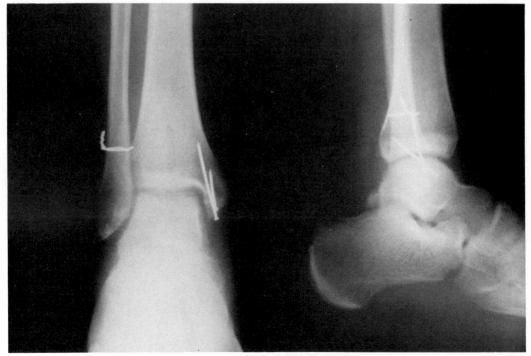

FIGURE 5–6   (C) X-rays after cast had been removed. On follow-up two years later he is asymptomatic and actively participates in athletics.

plaster cast on several occasions with complete loss of position. Seven months later a successful tibiotalar arthrodesis was performed for the painful malunion. The second case was a brittle juvenile diabetic who initially healed without difficulty but who, four months after the injury, gradually developed painless swelling in the ankle and had a rapid deterioration with Charcot-type joint destruction without significant discomfort. This unstable ankle had to be braced and he eventually underwent a total ankle replacement at another institution eighteen months after injury.

The complications were all of a minor nature and had nothing to do directly with the wire-loop fixation (Table 5-1). Some patients had tenderness on deep palpation over the knotted areas of the wire loop, but, it was not severe enough to warrant removal. To date no wires have been removed. There were no delayed unions or nonunions of the fibula.

The follow-up was for two months to 12.5 years with an average of forty three months. Eleven patients were lost to follow-up less than six months after injury— all were lost track of shortly after the plaster was removed. Thirty-three cases were followed for one year or longer and eighteen of these thirty three cases were followed for three years or longer.

The results of treatment were based on the subjective and objective assessment. The concepts of "excellent," "good," or "poor" were tabulated in the table (Table 5-2). There were thirty one cases of "excellent" or "good" and two "poor" re-

TABLE 5-1   Complications

2 Superficial medial aspect wound infections
1 Postoperative pneumonitis
1 Skin ulceration at the proximal cast margin—Treated with small skin graft one month after fracture
1 Causalgia pain of four months duration, successfully treated with physical therapy

sults. In the eighteen cases followed three years or longer all were considered "good" or "excellent." The two "poor" cases deteriorated within one year following injury.

DISCUSSION

Comparison studies of results of treatment of ankle fractures are virtually impossible because of the myriad patterns and severity of injuries and the variation of treatment patterns owing to concurrent injuries. The most important factor is the inability to evaluate the exact nature and magnitude of the injury at the moment of the trauma. Most of the evaluation for study purposes is based on the first x-ray films taken shortly after arrival in the hospital. This view is often misleading because the gross malalignment or dislocation has been improved, if not reduced, by the patient, emergency ambulance personnel, nurses, x-ray technicians, or emergency room physicians. This makes any prospective study comparing modes of treatment vis-a-vis the lesion involved inaccurate, for there is no prior knowledge of the *exact*

TABLE 5-2   Results of Treatment

25 CASES—"EXCELLENT"	6 CASES—"GOOD"

No:
Pain
Limp
Swelling
Discernible loss of motion
    (Clinically or by measurement)
Further surgery* or appliance
Medications
	Occasional:
	"Barometer" pain
	Swelling—No treatment required
	Discernible loss of motion
	    (None of practical importance)
	
	No:
	Further surgery* or appliance
	Medication
	Limp

*Surgery for removal of asymptomatic screw not included.

mechanism and the extent of the injuries at the time of the impact. The soft-tissue damage or defect is too infrequently documented by accurate photographs for study purposes.

The damage to the articular cartilage of the talus, fibula, and/or tibia with severe cuts, avulsions, and fragments of the hyaline cartilage loose in the joint is not seen on x-ray and may contribute to a post-traumatic change regardless of the type of fixation used to achieve stability.

Recent experimental studies have verified the importance of anatomically reducing the fibula, and clinically we have noticed its importance in achieving and holding the anatomic reconstitution of the ankle joint congruity when the fibular malleolus is fixed. We feel that this comparatively simple, atraumatic, effective technique should be adopted by those subscribing to the concept of an anatomic stabilization of the lateral malleolus fracture. More is being learned about the role of the lateral malleolus in the dynamic ankle function. Exactly how strong the fibular fixation must be in maintaining the reduction needs further biomechanical study. Clinically, wire-loop fixation gives a trouble-free method of adequate stabilization of the lateral aspect of suitable ankle lesions with no symptoms referrable to the lateral column support. This form of treatment, to our knowledge, had not been previously reported in any significant number of cases. With the increasing emphasis on open reduction an internal fixation of the lateral malleolus, different types of fixation should be reported and encouraged so that they can be added to other techniques already known to surgeons dealing with these problems.

CONCLUSION

Displaced bimalleolar, trimalleolar and oblique or spiral fractures of the lateral malleolus associated with medial ligament damage seldom can be anatomically reduced and/or maintained by closed reduction and plaster immmobilization alone. When open reduction is indicated, the lateral malleolar fracture should be anatomically reduced and fixed internally to restore a normal ankle joint.

Wire-loop fixation for indicated displaced oblique or spiral fractures of the lateral malleolus is a simple and effective way of internal fixation with a minimal amount of metal implanted. The anatomically reduced fracture is further protected for eight weeks in a below-the-knee cast. There were no inherent complications, no delayed or nonunions in treating a suitable lateral malleolar fracture by this wire-loop technique. No second operation has been necessary for removal of the wires. Minimal instrumentation is needed.

This method does not completely preclude the development of post-traumatic arthritis, especially if there is damage to the articular surface at the time of injury. We feel that there is increasing evidence in the surgical and biomechanical literature which shows the importance of the fibula in weight bearing and as an *active* stabilizing force of the ankle joint. This series supports the concept that an accurate anatomic reduction of the lateral malleolus will lessen the change of post-traumatic changes after this type of injury.

REFERENCES

1. Brodie, I.A.O.D. and Denham, R.A.: The treatment of unstable ankle fractures. *J. Bone Joint Surg.* 56B: 256–62, 1974.
2. Buhler, J.: Percutaneous cerclage of tibial fractures. *Clin. Ortho.* 105:276–82, 1974.
3. Burwell, N.H. and Charnely, A.D.: The treatment of displaced fractures at the ankle by rigid internal fixation and early joint movement. *J. Bone and Joint Surg.* 47B: 634–60, 1965.
4. Cedell, C-A.: Supination outward injuries of the ankle. *Acta Ortho. Scanl. Suppl.:* 110, 1967.
5. Cedell, C-A.: Ankle lesions. *Acta. Ortho. Scand.* 46: 425–45, 1975.
6. Charnley, J.: *The Closed Treatment of Common Fractures* (3rd Ed.). Baltimore: The Williams and Wilkins Co., 1961, pp. 24–26.
7. Danis, R.: *Les Fractures Malleolaires.* In *Theorie et Pratique de l'osteosynthese.* Paris: Masson, 1949.
8. Gothman, L.: Local arterial changes associated with experimental fractures of the rabbit's tibia treated with encercling wires (cerclage)—a microangiographic study. *Acta Chir. Scand.* 123:1–11, 1962.

9. Gregory, J., Patzakis, M.J. and Harvey, J.P., Jr.: Precise evaluation of the reduction of severe ankle fractures. *J. Bone Joint Surg.* 56A: 979–93, 1974.

10. Kleiger, B.: The treatment of the oblique fractures of the fibula. *J. Bone and Joint Surg.* 43A: 969–79, 1961.

11. Lambert, K.L.: The weight-bearing function of the fibula. *J. Bone Joint Surg.* 53A: 507–13, 1974.

12. MacNab, I. and De Hass, W.G.: The role of periosteal blood supply in the healing of fractures of the tibia. *Clin. Ortho.* 105: 27–33, 1974.

13. Magnusson, R.: On the late results in nonoperated cases of malleolar fractures. I. Fractures by external rotation. *Act Chir. Scand. Suppl.:* 84, 1944.

14. Mueller, M.E. and Allgower, M.: *Technique of Internal Fixation of Fractures.* New York: Springer-Verlag, 1965.

15. Ramsey, P.L. and Hamilton, W.: Changes in tibio-talar area of contact caused by lateral talar shift. *J. Bone and Joint Surg.* 58A: 356–57, 1976.

16. Rhinelander, F.W.: Instruments for use with flexible steel wire in bone surgery. *J. Bone Joint Surg.* 40A: 365–74, 1958.

17. Rhinelander, F.W.: The normal microcirculation of diaphyseal cortex and its response to fracture. *J. Bone Joint Surg.* 50A: 784–880, 1968.

18. Rhinelander, F.W.: Minimal internal fixaton of tibial fractures. *Clin. Ortho.* 107: 188–220, 1975.

19. Solonen, K.A. and Lauttamus, L.: Operative treatment of ankle fractures. *Acta Ortho. Scand.* 39: 223–37, 1968.

20. Weinart, C.R., McMaster, J.H., Scranton, P.R., Jr. and Ferguson, R.J.: *Foot Science* Bateman, J.E. Philadelphia: W.B. Saunders Co., 1976, pp. 1–6.

21. Willenegger, H.: Die Behandlung der Luxationsfrakturen des oberen Sprunggelenkes nach Biomechanischen Gesichtspunkten. *Helvet. Chir. Acta* 28:225–39, 1961.

22. Wilson, F.C., Jr. and Skilbred, L.A.: Long-term results in the treatment of displaced bimalleolar fractures. *J. Bone and Joint Surg.* 48A: 1065–78, 1966.

23. Yablon, I.G., Heller, F.G. and Shouse, L.: The key role of the lateral malleolus in displaced fractures of the ankle. *J. Bone Joint Surg.* 59A: 169–73, 1977.

Chapter Six

TIBIOPEDAL MOTION AFTER ANKLE FUSION AND ARTHROPLASTY

PHILLIP M. EVANSKI, M.D.
THEODORE R. WAUGH, M.D.

Ankle arthrodesis is traditionally recognized as the accepted operative procedure for treatment of severe arthritis of the ankle. The results of arthrodesis of the ankle have varied considerably. Koch reported on 132 ankle fusions for traumatic arthritis.[4] Eighty-five per cent of the patients had pain relief, and complications were few. Morris and Herrick reviewed sixty three cases of ankle arthrodesis using nine major surgical methods.[7] Satisfactory results were attained in 82.5 per cent of patients; 17.5 per cent had poor results. Rimoldi reviewed forty nine Charnley ankle joint arthrodesis procedures with an average postoperative observation time of twelve years.[9] Thirty-six patients (73 per cent) expressed satisfaction with the result of the operation.

The results of other series have not been as satisfactory. Johnson and Boseker reviewed 140 ankle fusions and obtained follow-up data on 114.[3] Twenty-one procedures failed: fifteen ended in a pseudoarthrosis and six in amputation. An additional nineteen patients (17 percent) were considered to have only a fair result because of a constant limp and inability to perform their old job. Lance and colleagues, in reviewing 190 ankle fusions, reported a 22 percent nonunion rate and 31 percent unsatisfactory results.[6] Finally, Huckell and Fuller reported on twenty eight patients with ankle arthrodesis and noted that twenty

three patients complained of a limp, nineteen had pain, and only fourteen were pleased with the result.[2] They concluded that the results of their series were poor enough to consider the development of an alternative procedure.

This study is concerned with two aspects of ankle fusion versus ankle arthroplasty: First, the residual tibiopedal motion after fusion or arthroplasty. Secondly, patient assessment of satisfaction following fusion or arthroplasty.

CLINICAL MATERIAL AND METHODS.

Thirty-four ankle arthrodeseses performed at the University of California, Irvine, between January 1969 and December 1974 were reviewed. Twenty patients with unilateral arthrodesis were available for follow-up raidographic and physical examination. All fusions were by an anterior sliding bone graft, modified Charnley compression, or a combination of both methods.

Radiographic measurement of normal and residual tibiopedal motion after ankle fusion was performed on both the normal and fused sides. Dorsiflexion was measured in weight bearing, while plantar flexion was determined without weight bearing. The angle of motion was determined by a line drawn through the axis of the tibia, and a line drawn between the most inferior projection of the os calcis and the first metatarsal head as shown in Figure 6-1.

All patients were clinically examined and evaluated. Patient assessment of ankle arthrodesis was done by having the patient pick from one of five categories—much better, better, unchanged, worse, and much worse—when comparing their present status to their preoperative status.

Between May 1974 and December 1977, sixty-two ankle arthroplasties were performed at the University of California, Irvine. Twenty patients were randomly chosen and reviewed; the same techniques were used as for the previous group of ankle fusions. Tibiopedal motion was again determined by weight bearing in dorsiflexion and non-weight bearing in plantar flexion. Patient assessment of the result of arthroplasty was also evaluated on the same five-point scale comparing pre-and postoperative status as was used for ankle fusion.

RESULTS

The results of tibiopedal motion in normal ankles and in those treated with arthrodesis and arthroplasty are listed in Table 6-1. In the normal ankle, total motion was 60°, while with arthrodesis it was reduced to 18°, and arthroplasty allowed 45°. Dorsiflexion and plantar flexion were very nearly equal in the normal ankle, while dorsiflexion was comparatively reduced in ankles treated with arthrodesis or arthroplasty.

Patient assessment of the success of surgery in arthrodesis and arthroplasty is shown in Table 6-2. It is seen that seventeen patients (85 percent) considered themselves improved by arthroplasty, while eight (40 percent) noted improvement after arthrodesis.

DISCUSSION

In this study, tibiopedal motion in the normal foot averaged 60°; this is higher

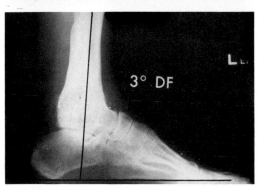
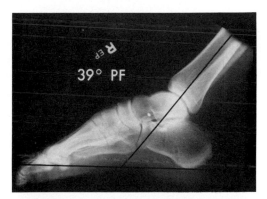
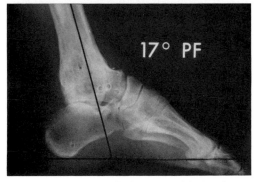

FIGURE 6-1 (A) Maximum dorsiflexion weight bearing; (B) maximum plantarflexion non-weight bearing on the normal side; (C) fusion side in maximum dorsiflexion;(D) fusion side in plantar flexion.

TABLE 6-1   Tibiopedal Motion in Normal, Arthrodesis, and Arthroplasty and Ankle*

ANKLE	DORSIFLEXION (AVG.)	PLANTAR FLEXION (AVG.)	TOTAL	RANGE
Normal	28°	32°	60°	40°–82°
Arthrodesis	7°	11°	18°	5°–38°
Arthroplasty	18°	27°	45°	23°–65°

*N = 20

than that previously reported by Wesley or Sammarco.[10,14] Presumably the differences are due to sample size and techniques. In this study patients were encouraged to dorsiflex until the heel cleared the ground. Large differences were noted in the patient population in the studies of Wesley and Sammarco. This was confirmed in this study, where the range was noted to be between 40° and 82° for normal individuals. Finally, our results agree with Sammarco's in that equal amounts of dorsiflexion and plantar flexion are present in the normal foot and ankle. The measurement of dorsiflexion without weight bearing leads to the clinical observation that dorsiflexion is much less than plantar flexion.

Table 6-1 shows the marked loss of motion when the normal side is compared with the arthrodesis side, from 60° to 18°, a loss of 70 percent. The importance of this significant loss of motion is made clear when investigations of normal walking are reviewed. Many authors have investigated tibiopedal motion during normal gait[5,8,11,12,15] The results listed in Table 6-3 do not cover all the literature but can be considered representative. Note that approximately 29° of tibiopedal motion occurs in normal walking. We feel that one

function of the foot in walking is energy absorption, and motion is required for this function.

The above partially explains why the results of ankle arthroplasty, as assessed by the patient, are superior to results of ankle fusion as shown in Table 6-2. At follow-up, when patients with ankle fusion were questioned they admitted to relief of ankle pain, but this was offset by complaints of pain in other areas of the foot and loss of overall function.

The surgical technique and early results of ankle replacement at the University of California, Irvine, have been reported.[1,13] The design of the ankle prosthesis used permits motion to physiologic limits and is restrained only by soft tissue. Figure 6-2 shows the amount of motion possible after arthroplasty. Forty-four of the sixty-two ankle arthroplasties done prior to December 1977 have recently been reviewed. The average follow-up is one and one-half years. Twenty-two patients (50 per cent) consider themselves much better, fifteen (34 per cent) are better, while four (9 percent) are unchanged, and three (7 per cent) are worse.

CONCLUSION

A comparison of ankle arthrodesis and ankle arthroplasty shows that arthro-

TABLE 6-2   Patient Assessment of Result Comparing Preoperative Status to Postoperative Status*

CONDITION	AFTER ARTHRO-DESIS	AFTER ARTHRO-PLASTY
Much better	4	9
Better	4	8
Unchanged	8	2
Worse	4	1
Much worse	0	0

*N = 20.

TABLE 6-3   Tibiopedal Motion in Normal Walking

AUTHOR	NUMBER CASES	TOTAL MOTION
Murray (1964)	60	28°
Sutherland (1972)	9	28°
Winter (1974)	12	35°
Stauffer (1977)	5	24°

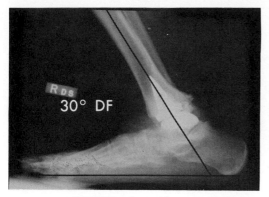 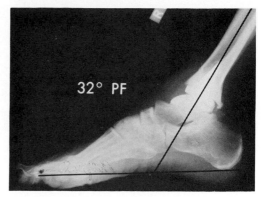

FIGURE 6-2 Ankle motion after arthroplasty—(A) dorsiflexion; (B) plantar flexion.

plasty preserves 75 per cent of normal tibiopedal motion, while arthrodesis preserves only 30 per cent. Patient assessment of the end result shows improvement in 85 per cent after arthroplasty and in 40 per cent after arthrodesis. Ankle arthroplasty is thus a useful procedure in the treatment of ankle arthritis.

References

1. Evanski, P.M. and Waugh, T.R.: Management of arthritis of the ankle: An alternative to arthrodesis. *Clin. Ortho.* 122:110, 1977.
2. Huckell, J.R. and Fuller, J.: In *Foot Science* Bateman, J.E., Ed. W.B. Saunders Co., Philadelphia: 1976, pp. 156-61.
3. Johnson, E.W. and Boseker, E.H.: Arthrodesis of the ankle. *Arch. Surg.* 97:766, 1968.
4. Koch, F.: The *Arthrodesis in the Restoration of Working Ability* Chapchal, G., Ed. Acton, Massachusetts: Thieme, Publishing Sciences Group, Inc., 1975.
5. Lamoreaux, L.W.: Kinematic measurements in the study of human walking. *Bull. Prosthet. Res.* 10:3, 1971.
6. Lance, E.M., Pavel, A., Patterson, R. L. Jr., Frico, L. and Larsen, I.J.: Arthrodesis of the ankle: A follow-up study. *J. Bone Joint Surg.* 53A: 1030, 1971.
7. Morris, H.D. and Herrick, R.T.: *In In Foot Science* Bateman, J.E., Ed. W.B. Saunders Co., Philadelphia: 1976; pp. 136-149.
8. Murray, M.P., Drought, A.B. and Kory, R.C.: Walking patterns in normal men. *J. Bone Joint Surg.* 46A: 335, 1964.
9. Rimoldi, M.: *The Arthrodesis in the Restoration of Working Ability* Chapchal, G. Ed. Acton, Massachusetts: Thieme, Publishing Sciences Group, Inc., 1975.
10. Sammarco, G.J., Burstein, A.J. and Frankle, V.H.: Biomechanics of the ankles: A kinematic study. Ortho. Clin. *North Amer.* 1973.
11. Stauffer, R.N., Chao, E.Y.S. and Brewster, R.C.: Force and motion analyses of the normal, diseased, and prosthetic ankle joint. *Clin. Ortho.* 127:189, 1977.
12. Sutherland, D.H. and Hagy, J.L.: Measurement of gait movement from motion picture film. *J. Bone Joint Surg.* 54A: 787, 1972.
13. Waugh, T.R., Evanski, P.M. and McMaster, W.C.: Irvine ankle arthroplasty, prosthetic design and surgical technique. *Clin. Ortho.* 114:180, 1976.
14. Weseley, M.S., Koval, R. and Kleiger, B.: Roentgen measurement of ankle flexion-extension motion. *Clin. Ortho.* 65:167, 1969.
15. Winter D.A., Quanbury, A.O., Hobson, D.A., Sidwall, H.G., Reimer, G., Trenholm, B.G., Steinke, T. and Shlosser, H.: Kinematics of normal locomotion—a statistical study based on T.V. data. *J. Biomech.* 7:479, 1974.

Chapter Seven

FRACTURES AND DISLOCATIONS OF THE TARSOMETATARSAL JOINT

GARY LATOURETTE, M.D.
JACQUELIN PERRY, M.D.
MICHAEL J. PATZAKIS, M.D.
TILLMAN M. MOORE, M.D.
J. PAUL HARVEY, JR., M.D.

Dislocation at the tarsometatarsal joint with or without fracture seems to be a problem for all concerned. The injury occurs so rarely that most practitioners are not familiar with the anatomy or methods of handling the problems. Also, if one examines the patients carefully for end results, one finds more trouble than might be expected.

The tarsometatarsal joint has been known as Lisfranc's joint ever since that French surgeon described an amputation done swiftly through this site *Sur l'amputation du pre dans l'articulation tarsometatarsienne.*

This area includes the five metatarsal bones, three cuneiform bones, and the cuboid bone. The cuboid articulates with the fourth and fifth metatarsals. The medial three metatarsals each articulate with one of the cuneiforms. The second metatarsal is the longest and the second cuneiform is the smallest and shortest of the cuneiforms; an indentation is formed in the line of the cuneiforms, and the long metatarsal fits into this. Thus one has a mortise with the base of the second metatarsal recessed between the first and the third cuneiform, with the second being the base of the mortise. This mortise stabilizes the area.

Further stability is provided because the second, third, and fourth metatarsals are wider on the dorsal surface than on the plantar surface. The first and fifth metatarsals have broad bases which to some degree overlap the adjoining metatarsal on the plantar surface.

In viewing this joint end on, one sees that the fifth metatarsal is lowest, literally resting on the supporting surface. The remainder of the bones rise to the highest joint at the dorsum of the first and second metatarsals. Thus as one looks superiorly, one sees an arch effect. If one looks anteriorly, again one sees the arch, Roman in type, with the bones like keystones, narrow inferiorly and wide superiorly, fitting closely when weight is applied superiorly (Fig. 7–1).[5]

Also necessary for stability are the ligaments and capsules of the joints. There are transverse ligaments joining the second, third, fourth, and fifth metatarsals to each

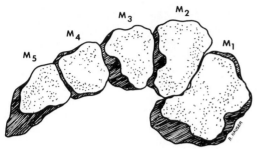

FIGURE 7-1 Note narrowing of width from superior to inferior of M2 and M3. Modeled after Lenczner et. al. *J. Trauma* 14: 12, 1974.

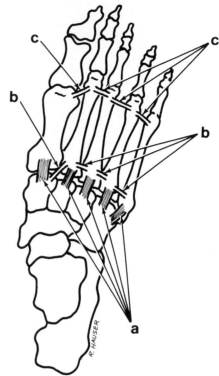

FIGURE 7-3 Note capsular structure around each metatarsal and the appropriate cuneiform(A); transverse ligament between metatarsal five and metatarsal four, metatarsal four and metatarsal three, metatarsal three and metatarsal two, and between metatarsal two and the first cuneiform (Lisfranc's ligament)(B).

Metatarsal one has no transverse ligament except at the distal end where there are transverse ligaments connecting all the metatarsal heads(C).

other, but none between the first and second metatarsals. There is a ligament between the first cuneiform and the second metatarsal known as Lisfranc's ligament (Fig. 7-2).[10] This helps to hold the lateral four metatarsals to the medial side of the foot. But it is obvious that the first metatarsal is relatively unattached to the other metatarsals at its proximal end. The tendons, short foot muscles, and plantar fascia also help to hold the foot together, but the ligaments are quite important for maintenance of actual juxtaposition of the bones (Fig. 7-3).

TYPES OF INJURIES

The injuries that occur in this area are dislocations and fractures associated with dislocations. Various classifications have been suggested, but a simple one was proposed by Quenu and Kuss[8] which is quite useful. It divides these fractures into three groups as follows: (1) homolateral dislocation in which all five metatarsals are dislocated in a coronal plane; (2) an isolated dislocation in which one or two metatarsals are dislocated in a coronal plane; and (3) a divergent dislocation in which there is displacement in the sagittal as well as the coronal plane.

A second method of understanding the injuries is to consider the source of the

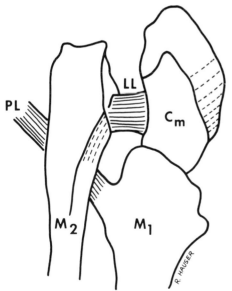

FIGURE 7-2 PL, peroneus longus; M2, second metatarsal; M1, first metatarsal; CM, first cuneiform; LL Lisfranc's ligament. Modeled after Figure 3 of Taussig and Hunter: *Ann. Chir.* 23: 1969.

trauma. The force can be classified as direct or indirect.[1,7] Dislocation due to direct force occurs in the plantar direction secondary to traumas such as a truck running over the foot or a heavy weight being dropped directly on the foot. Soft-tissue damage is extensive, and multiple open fractures are common.

Dislocation associated with indirect violence[1] follows several patterns that are largely dependent upon the position of the foot at the time of injury. The injury may seem trivial compared with that caused by direct trauma, but it usually has the force resulting from body weight times acceleration of the body at the time of injury. Such injuries occur when the foot is compressed by body weight when plantar flexed against the floorboard of a car that stops suddenly, as in an accident. It also occurs if the foot is caught in a hole and the patient falls, thus markedly distorting the foot by the weight of the falling body. With any of these injuries, the second metatarsal may fracture in the groove, thus permitting the dislocation to occur.[4,12,13]

METHODS

The purpose of our study was to review those injuries seen at Los Angeles County Hospital and to determine the end result of our treatment. From 1971 to 1976 we found about a thousand instances of foot injury involving bones and joints among admitting diagnoses for hospital patients in this period. Patients seen in the emergency room and treated only as outpatients are not counted. We have no available record of this type of patient. Of those admitted, forty-four were identified as having dislocation of the tarsometatarsal joints to some degree. Perhaps some minimal dislocations were not recognized. These forty-four patients form the basis of our study.

Twenty-eight patients were available for follow-up examination. One patient died of unstated cause; one was in military service overseas; and fourteen could not be found, making up the total of forty-four patients. Twenty-seven were interviewed personally by one of the authors. One pa-

tient was in a state prison; he was evaluated by the prison physician using our criteria. Twenty-two of these patients appeared for physical and x-ray examinations. Sixteen of these underwent gait analysis at Rancho Los Amigos Hospital Gait Laboratory, under the direction of Dr. Jacquelin Perry.

The length of follow-up ranged from ten months to five years, with a mean of three and one-half years. The ages ranged from eight to sixty-five years; twenty-five years was the median age. There were no deaths. Two partial and one Syme's amputation resulted from severe crush injuries with extensive soft-tissue damage. The dorsalis pedis artery was not found to be compromised in any of these instances. None of the closed fractures treated by open reduction became infected. Of the six open fractures, five became infected with results as previously mentioned. Both extremities were involved with equal frequency; however, males outnumbered females 3.1 to 1.

The circumstances through which the accident occurred are listed in Table 7-1. It is obvious that 50 percent are caused by some form of motor vehicle accident.

The types of dislocations and fractures resulting from these accidents are listed in descending order of frequency in Table 7-2. Lateral displacement of metatarsals two, three, four, and five account for 48 percent of the injuries described (Fig. 7-4A). Fracture of the base of metatarsal two (the keystone) was present 90 percent of the time (seventeen patients). This could be a large or small fragment. Other metatarsals were involved to a much lesser degree. Lateral displacement of all five meta-

TABLE 7-1   Circumstances of Injury

Automobile accident	14
Motorcycle accident	8
Tripped	8
Fell from height	5
Caught foot in boxcar coupling	2
Slid into second base	1
Mugged and dragged	1
Dropped heavy object on foot	1
Fell from horse	1
Cause unknown	3
Total	44

TABLE 7-2
Types of Fracture Dislocation

Lateral displacement of metatarsal 2, 3, 4, 5 with or without fracture	20
Lateral displacement of metatarsal 1, 2, 3, 4, 5 with fracture	12
Medial displacement of metatarsal 1	4
Medial displacement of metatarsal 1 with fracture	2
Crush injuries	3
Unknown	3
Total	44

tarsals was accompanied by a fracture of one or more of the metatarsals in all cases (Fig. 7-4B). Medial dislocation is rather uncommon and accounted for only six of the patients (Fig. 7-4C) in this group (14 percent). Of this group of six, only two patients had associated fracture of metatarsals two, three, four, or five or any combination of them. Fractures of the bones of the foot associated with these injuries were second metatarsal base, other metatarsal shafts, other metatarsal bases, cuboid, cuneiform, calcaneus, and navicular (Fig. 7-4D).

The treatment given is listed in Table 7-3. Open reduction and internal fixation was done using Kirschner wires. These wires remained in place an average of 6.7 weeks, with the earliest removal being at 4 weeks and the latest being at 16 weeks.

Patients began weight bearing on an

TABLE 7-3   Treatment Rendered

Open reduction internal fixation	24
Closed reduction internal fixation	6
Closed reduction external fixation	5
No reduction—cast only	4
Irrigation débridement	2
Open reduction external fixation	1
Unable to comment	2
Total	44

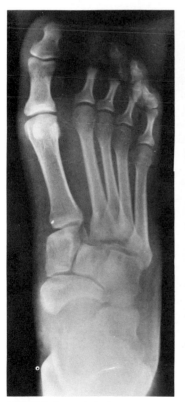
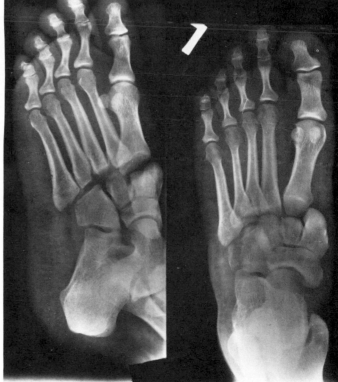

FIGURE 7-4 (A) & (B)   (A) Note small fracture at base of metatarsal 2 and Dislocation of metatarsals 2, 3, 4, and 5. (B) Note lateral dislocation of metatarsals 1, 2, 3, 4, and 5.

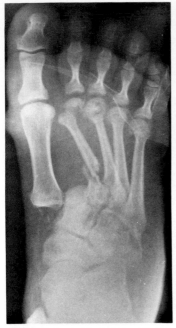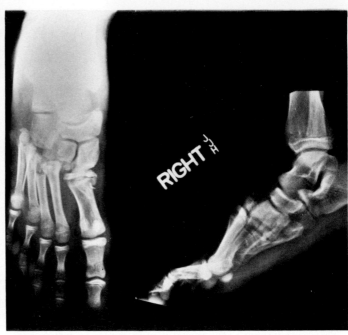

FIGURE 7=4 (C) & (D)   (C) Note medial dislocation of metatarsal 1 with fracture metatarsal 2 and 3 With medial displacement of fragment. (D) Crush-type injury with dorsal dislocation of metatarsal with fracture base of metatarsals 1, 2, and 5.

average of 7.6 weeks after injury, with the earliest attempt at 2 weeks and the latest at 20 weeks.

External fixation was removed an average of 9.2 weeks after application. The shortest period of immobilization was 4 weeks and the longest was 20 weeks. In reviewing the figures, there seemed to be a trend that showed that those patients spending less time in plaster and with early pin removal tended to have a greater number of points at last examination, and therefore a better result. However, this could not be proven statistically.

The twenty-two patients personally seen were evaluated at their last visit. An evaluation was devised based on employment history, physical examination, radiographic appearance, and kinesiology for some of the patients. Pain as reported by the patient was given ten points with arbitrary evaluation as noted in Table 7-4. Distance walked as reported by the patient was given ten points, again with arbitrary evaluation. Life-style comparing the pre-injury to the post-injury period was as-signed ten points. Physical examination as evaluated by limp when walking was given twenty points. Range of motion of ankle, subtalar and forefoot joint circumference of thigh and calf, and size of foot were all examined, but upon evaluation these were not found to show any significant statistical difference pre- or postoperatively. Therefore, only limp as noted by the examiner was evaluated. Of the twenty-two patients, sixteen had their gait recorded on videotape and can be reviewed at any time. X-ray examination was given twenty points, with points removed for increasing severity of findings of osteoarthritis (Table 7-4).

The overall findings based upon the evaluation of our patients as outlined above were ten patients with a good end result, two patients with a fair end result, and ten patients with a poor end result. Table 7-5 gives these results according to treatment. There was no statistically significant correlation (P = 0.1) between the results achieved and the method of fixation.

TABLE 7-4
Criterion for Standard Rating

PAIN—Ten points possible	POINTS
No pain	10
Occasional night pain	9
Consistent night pain	8
Pain after walking a long distance	7
Pain after walking a short distance	6
Constant Pain	4
Intolerable pain	0

DISTANCE ABLE TO WALK—Ten points possible

Walks one mile or more	10
Walks six to ten blocks	8
Walks only two or three blocks	6
Indoors only	4
Cannot walk	0

**RETURN TO PRE-INJURY LIFE-STYLE—
Ten points possible**

Return to full activity	10
Somewhat limited	8
Moderately limited	6
Severely limited	4
Disabled	0

LIMP—Twenty points possible

No limp	20
Limp barely visible	16
Limp readily seen	10
Needs device of some sort	6
Cannot walk	0

X-RAY—Twenty points possible

Normal as compared with uninvolved foot	20
A poor reduction of 2nd metatarsal cuneiform joint	−4
Two or more joints with severe involvement	−4
Joint space narrowing any joint	−3
Spurs or osteophytes	−3
Joint margin sclerosis	−3
Disuse atrophy	−3

TABLE 7-5 Treatment

	RESULT BY STANDARD RATING		
	Good	Fair	Poor
No reduction, cast only	1		3
Open reduction internal fixation anatomic after operation	3		1
Open reduction internal fixation not anatomic after operation	3	1	7
Closed reduction percutaneous pinning anatomic after operation	2		
Closed reduction percutaneous pinning not anatomic after operation			1
Closed reduction external fixation not anatomic	1		
Total	10	1	12

(Table 7-7). The patients with good results could walk an unlimited distance. The patients with fair and poor results walked less far. All patients could walk at least a block or two. Two of those in the poor category could walk appreciable distances but were downgraded because of complaints of pain and because the x-ray showed severe loss of anatomy and findings of osteoarthritis. All patients complained of swelling after walking.

The category noted as return to pre-injury life-style was a rather subjective evaluation on the part of the observer, with judgment made after talking to patients

FACTORS EVALUATED

Almost all twenty-two patients interviewed complained of pain (Table 7-6). This pain was usually described as dull and aching, and with few exceptions was located in the central and dorsal area of the foot at the region of the second and third metatarsal cuneiform joint. Another pain radiating posterolaterally toward the cuboid bone often accompanied this pain. Only one patient complained of plantar pain, and he had an unreduced plantar dislocation of his cuboid bone.

Distance walked is our next factor

TABLE 7-6 Pain

	PATIENTS	SCORE	AVERAGE
Good Results	4	10	
	2	9	9
	4	8	
Total	10		
Fair Results	1	5	
	1	8	6.5
Total	2		
Poor Results	3	6	
	2	5	
	4	4	4.6
	1	2	
Total	10		

TABLE 7-7   Distance Walked

SCORE BREAKDOWN BY NUMBER OF PATIENTS			
	Patients	*Score*	*Average*
Good Results	*10*	*10*	
Total	*10*	*10*	*10*
Fair Results	*1*	*6*	
	1	10	*8*
Total	*2*		
Poor Results	*1*	*8*	
	2	6	
	3	5	*4.9*
	3	4	
	1	2	
Total	*10*		

about their life-styles (Table 7-8). One patient stated she could not wear shoes. Two patients wore only tennis shoes, since others were too uncomfortable. One patient wears only wedge-heeled shoes, although this could be considered at the present time as acceptable style. Most of the patients could no longer run and four females stated that they could no longer dance, since the involved foot was too uncomfortable. Five patients were still on disability pensions; however, two of these patients had been injured a short time ago—one ten months and the other one year. In general, those with poor results had to modify their pre-injury life-styles.

TABLE 7-8   Lifestyle

SCORE BREAKDOWN BY NUMBER OF PATIENTS			
	Patients	*Score*	*Average*
Good Results	*8*	*10*	
	1	9	*9.7*
	1	8	
Total	*10*		
Fair Results	*1*	*10*	*9*
	1	8	
Total	*2*		
Poor Results	*2*	*6*	
	1	5	
	2	4	*3.7*
	4	2	
	1	0	
Total	*10*		

Limp as an end result seemed important to these observers; therefore, a larger value was assigned to it (Table 7-9). Also, this category seemed to separate the patients most clearly, although there was some overlap of the fair category, with the point rating of sixteen being present in all three categories at adjacent levels.

The patients were concerned about limp and noticed this most readily; it also caused changes in shoe wear. Approximately one half of the patients noted that their shoe wear was uneven, with shoes wearing out laterally on the involved extremity first. As noted in the category of life-style, some had to change their type of shoe, a concern in this style-conscious era.

X-ray evaluation, like limp, was thought to be of importance. Therefore, twenty points were assigned for the evaluation (Table 7-10). Points were subtracted for malunion of fractures and incomplete reduction of dislocation, particularly of the second metatarsal tarsal joint as measured by the relatively straight line along the medial (tibial) border of the first metatarsal and the medial (tibial) border of the second cuneiform bone as described by Foster and Foster.[3] Also, points were subtracted for various signs of osteoarthritis, sclerosis of subchondral bone of joint, loss of joint space, spur formation, and fusion of joints. Again, the patients with better results had x-rays most similar to the preoperative picture.

An important new approach was the

TABLE 7-9   Distance Walked

SCORE BREAKDOWN BY NUMBER OF PATIENTS			
	Patients	*Score*	*Average*
Good Results	*7*	*20*	*18.8*
	3	*16*	
Total	*10*		
Fair Results	*2*	*16*	*16*
Total	*2*		
Poor Results	*2*	*15*	
	4	14	*11.0*
	4	8	
Total	*10*		

TABLE 7-10   X-ray Evaluation

SCORE BREAKDOWN BY NUMBER OF PATIENTS

	Patients	Score	Average
Good Results	2	17	
	4	16	
	1	14	14.9
	1	13	
	2	12	
Total	10		
Fair Results	1	16	10.5
	1	5	
Total	2		
Poor Results	1	12	
	1	10	
	1	9	
	4	8	
	1	6	7.5
	1	6	
	1	4	
	1	2	
Total	10		

study of gait by means of foot switches attached to the sole of the shoe and contact being made when weight was placed on the foot. Switches were applied to particular sites, under the heel, under the head of the fifth metatarsal, under the head of the first metatarsal, and under the great toe. As the patient walks, weight is applied to the switch, closing it. Then current flows to a telemetry set that sends signals to a receiver attached to a computer. Times are therefore provided for weight bearing on the different areas of foot in the exact sequence. At the same time, the patient is photographed by a videotape machine and the material from the foot switch is also applied to the tape as a bar graph. Thus one can tell exactly in sequence of gait where weight is being born.[2,9,11]

The material is provided by a computer as a percentage of time of one gait cycle for one foot—the time from heel strike to heel strike. We have evaluated the results by comparing the percentage of time of weight bearing of one area to the same area of uninvolved foot. All segments of the gait cycle in the stance phase showed obvious differences between involved and uninvolved foot for the time of heel strike

and time of fifth metatarsal, first metatarsal, and great-toe weight bearing. But the most consistent differences were in time of weight bearing on the heel and distal fifth metatarsal area and during total foot flat (heel and distal fifth and first metatarsal areas). Therefore, these two phases were evaluated and compared at both standard gait (that is, the patient's comfortable gait) and fast gait (that is, asking the patient to actually walk faster than comfortable). Times for each area comparable for both feet during weight-bearing cycle were rated as good; when the times were very unequal, the results were considered to be poor. Using a scale of ten points (Table 7-11), values were assigned for increasing difference in time spent weight bearing between the involved and uninvolved foot.

The comparison of time spent on weight bearing on the heel and fifth metatarsal at free cadence is seen best in Figure 7-5A. Figure 7-5, 5A, B, C, and D graphically illustrate this difference for different gaits and different sites as noted. Most of the patients spent time on the heel and fifth metatarsal, hesitating to go forward onto their first metatarsal as well, since this would be painful because force would be exerted through the metatarsal tarsal cuneiform joints.[5] In fast cadence (Fig. 7-5B), the patients with a poor rating are still hesitating and spending more time on the hindfoot of the involved side, whereas patients with better results are

TABLE 7-11   Kinesiologic Evaluation

SCORE	% AGE DEVIATION*
10	0- 3
9	4
8	5
7	6
6	7-8
5	9-11
4	12-14
3	15-16
2	17-21
1	22-30
0	over 30

*Deviations is the difference in the percentage of the weight-bearing cycle born on a specified site between uninvolved foot and involved foot.

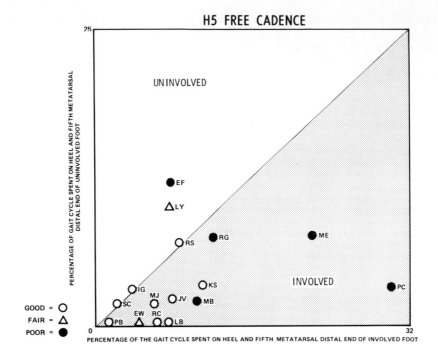

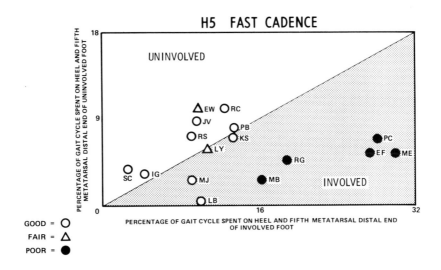

FIGURE 7–5   (A = D) Comparison of time spent on weight bearing on heel and fifth metatarsal at free cadence for varying gaits and sites.

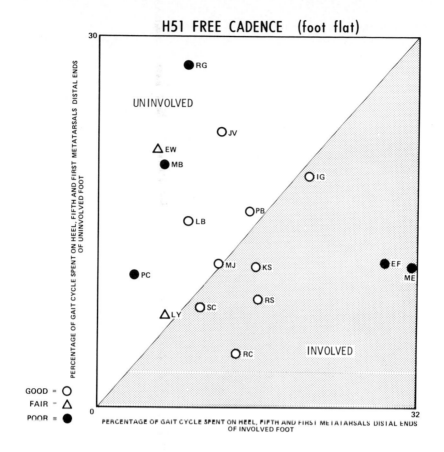

H51 FREE CADENCE (foot flat)

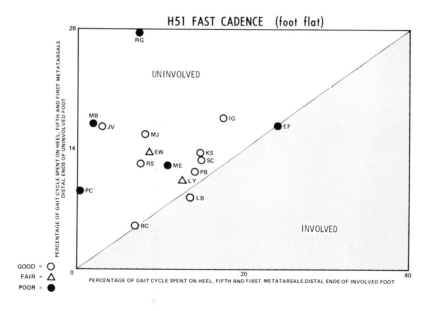

H51 FAST CADENCE (foot flat)

spending almost equal time on both feet or actually hurrying off the involved foot.

Figure 7–5C shows us that during foot-flat weight bearing (i.e., heel, fifth, and first metatarsal), the patients seem to spend a relatively equal time on each or move off the involved foot earlier. The reasons why two patients do not show this pattern cannot be readily understood. These two patients have the shortest follow-up—eight months and one year, respectively. When the patients walked at a fast cadence (Fig. 7–5D), they showed an even greater difference in total foot-flat weight bearing time. The result is that the patients hurried off the involved foot. Now the two problem patients also show a shift to the uninvolved side.

Comparing the end results (Table 7–12) based on conventional evaluation and kinesiology, the good categories had the same group of patients in it, except for one patient who moved from fair by stand-

ard method to good as measured by kinesiology. This patient had little limp, and other evaluations were all in the good category except for x-ray, which was graded low because of osteoarthritic findings. Perhaps these x-ray findings were overrated. The patient bore weight especially on both sides at slow gait; in fast gait, there was a slight difference with more time on the heel. Perhaps there was a slight pain noted in metatarsal tarsal joints.

The fair category changed most; it increased in number with kinesiologic studies. Three patients moved from good by standard classification to fair by kinesiologic classification. One of them had high values in all standard categories but could wear only platform shoes. Looking at gait study, patients walked at slow cadence with more time on the hindfoot of the involved side and less in total foot flat with weight on the first metatarsal. At fast cadence, the patient moved off the involved foot rapidly because of pain at the metatarsal cuneiform area of injury. Two other patients had similar patterns.

Using kinesiologic methods, two patients rated poor by standard methods were moved up to fair. One of these was a patient who had spent time in jail, who stated there was much pain, and who could walk only a short distance; yet kinesiology showed relatively equal time weight bearing. We felt this patient had something to gain from complaints. Finally, one patient was moved from poor by standard classification to fair by kinesiologic classification. He was an alcoholic who could walk only a relatively short distance and complained of pain. He had some claudication and also was relatively hard to evaluate. gait studies showed relatively equal weight-bearing times, but perhaps the short distance in the test situation allowed normal feeling, while longer distances tended to give more trouble.

TABLE 7–12   Standard Method of Evaluation Versus Kinesiologic Methods

STANDARD		KINESIOLOGIC	
Patients	*Good Score,* 55–70	*Patients*	*Good Score* 8–10
I.G.	57	I.G.	10
R.C.	61	R.C.	9.5
M.J.	62	R.S.	8.5
J.V.	62	S.C.	10
L.B.	61	K.S.	8
R.S.	64	P.B.	8
S.C.	67	L.Y.	9.5
K.S.	60		
P.B.	67		
Patients	*Fair Score,* 40–54	*Patients*	*Fair Score,* 6–7.9
L.Y.	42	M.J.	7.5
E.W.	48	E.W	7.0
		J.V.	6.5
		R.G.	6.5
		L.B.	6.0
		E.F	6.9
Patients	*Poor Score,* 0–39	*Patients*	*Poor Score,* 0–5.9
M.B.	38	M.B.	3.5
M.E.	36	M.E.	4.5
R.G.	32	P.C.	2.5
E.F.	31		
P.C.	29		

SUMMARY

We have provided an end result study on a series of patients with dislocations of the tarsometatarsal joint. We have used a standard classification and compared it with gait study. The use of gait study is a more scientific evaluation of the patients and, in our opinion, provides a better method of truly evaluating the end result in the patient.

We would suggest that care be taken to obtain anatomic reductions by whatever means possible in injuries at the tarsometatarsal joint. We would also suggest that early removal of fixation devices (without jeopardizing fixation) and early ambulation may provide better end results.

REFERENCES

1. Aitken, A.P. and Poulson, D.: Dislocations of the tarsometatarsal joint. *J. Bone Joint Surg.* 45A: 246-60, 1963.
2. Curry, C.L.: Stride characteristics of normal adults. Masters Thesis, USC School of Physical Therapy, March 1976.
3. Foster, C. and Foster, R.: Lisfranc's tarsometa- tarsal fracture-dislocation. *Radiology* 120:79-83, 1976.
4. Jeffreys, T.E.: Lisfranc's fracture-dislocation. A clinical and experimental study of tarsometa- tarsal dislocations and fracture dislocation. *J. Bone Joint Surg.* 45B: 546-51, 1963.
5. Lenczner, E.M., Waddell, J.P. and Grahams, D.: Tarsal metatarsal (Lisfranc's) dislocation. *J. Trauma* 14 (12): 1012-20, 1974.
6. Manter, J.T.: Distribution of compression forces in joints of the human foot. *Anat. Rec.* 96: 313-21, 1946.
7. O'Regan, D.S.: Lisfranc's dislocations. *J. Med. Soc. N.J.* 66: 575-77, 1969.
8. Quenu, E. and Kuss, G.: Etude sur les luxations du metatarse. *Rev. Chir.* 1909: 39/40, 281-336; 720-91.
9. Rousek, R.: Stride characteristics of normal adults. Masters Thesis, USC School of Physical Therapy, November 1976.
10. Taussig, G. and Hautier, S.: Les fractures- luxations de l'articulation de Lisfranc. *Ann. Chir.* 23: 1131-41, 1969.
11. Waters, R.: Personal communication.
12. Wiley, J.J.: The mechanism of tarsometatarsal joint injuries. *J. Bone Joint Surg.* 53B: 474-82, 1971.
13. Wilson, W.D.: Injuries of the tarsometatarsal joints. *J. Bone Joint Surg.* 54B: 677-86, 1971.

Chapter Eight

OPERATIVE INTERVENTION FOR FRACTURE OF THE TALUS

Wallace E. Miller, M.D.

In the majority of instances, the concern regarding operative intervention in injuries of the talus involves a decision as to whether the injury has caused a complete fracture across the neck or the body of the talus. Giannestras and Sammarco[2] have recommended a manipulation for closed fractures immediately after injury. If manipulation is unsuccessful, open reduction is immediately done with smooth Kirschner-wire fixation. If the fracture is an open injury, the same K-wire fixation is done, but the skin is not closed. The guidelines are clear and the plans for care are without fault. However, utilizing the same techniques and judgment, differing results are reported. Mindell[8] claims 20 percent avascular necrosis and 75 percent subtalar arthritis in his series. Pennal[10] reported 30 percent avascular necrosis and 60 percent subtalar arthritis. The discrepancy probably exists in variations of case material included in statistical series reports from McKeever[7] up to the present time.

Hawkins[5] classification clarified some of the confusion in results by delineating three types of fractures of the neck of the talus. For example, his Group I fracture is a complete but undisplaced vertical fracture through the neck of the talus. He reports union in all of these fractures and no incidence of avascular necrosis. In his Group II type, the vertical fracture of the neck of the talus must be displaced and the subtalar joint subluxed or dislocated.

Again union occurred in all of the Group II fractures, but there was 42 percent avascular necrosis. The Group III type was a fracture with all the features of Type II but with the additional dislocation of the body of the talus from the ankle (the fracture line frequently entered the body of the talus). Avascular necrosis jumped to 91 percent and nonunion was further identified in three of these patients. Pennal[10] noted 100 percent incidence of avascular necrosis and Mindell found that 70 percent of this type had unsatisfactory results. Hawkins' overall incidence of 58 percent avascular necrosis of all three types is a statistical percentage that may be compared with series not using his classification. The value of his classification is the predictability of what to expect from each type.

Another helpful contribution of Hawkins'[5] was his finding (now identified as Hawkins' sign) of subchondral atrophy in the dome of the talus. It is a black line on the anteroposterior roentgenogram (Fig. 8-1). This view is made with the foot out of plaster and is best demonstrated between the sixth and eighth week following the trauma. The finding is on the lateral view as well but is sometimes not seen as clearly on the six-week films. Hawkins feels that the presence of this black line is a good sign and that it eliminates the diagnosis of avascular necrosis. The same findings have been observed in our series. This sign does seem to reflect his observations. It is im-

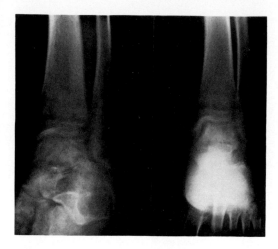

FIGURE 8-1 This anteroposterior view of talus shows Hawkins sign of revascularization as a black line immediately under dome of talus present at six weeks after injury. No avascular necrosis ensued.

portant to determine if it is there so as to plan future care. Those patients who do not show this line are going to have avascular necrosis.

STUDY SERIES

To delineate decisions of care, a study series (Table 8-1) was undertaken. It was not intended that the study should either prove or disprove other well-documented series. The intent was to emphasize and bring to the forefront some inherent principles of care.

A review of severe fractures of the neck and body of the talus at the University of Miami Medical Center, including private patient fractures of the clinical faculty and greater Miami area, over ten years (1966-1976) revealed twenty-eight fractures in twenty-six patients; there were bilateral talus fractures in two instances. Dislocations of the talus without fracture were excluded. Small fractures that did not involve the integrity of the talus were also excluded. One patient was lost to follow-up shortly after hospitalization and five others had a follow-up of up to only eight months before they too were lost. This left a total of nineteen patients for a study series with an average follow-up of three and one-half

years. There were four patients followed up to two years; five patients were followed up to three years; and ten patients were followed up to five years. The youngest patient was seventeen, the oldest patient was sixty-eight. The average age was 32.8 years, and the mean age was 27. This is a fracture of the young adult in most instances and is most commonly seen after a severe contact accident, as occurs in an automobile or airplane accident.

Fourteen of the fractures were treated closed and fourteen had operative intervention. Of the fractures treated closed, all had a simple manipulation and cast application. One of the more difficult closed fractures required three manipulations and still ended up with a good result. One of the closed fracture cases had a delayed union, which finally did heal with a good result after two years. The only other one of the closed fractures that was delayed in union was treated at two years after trauma with two screws and a bone graft, with union occurring finally in the third year and resulting in a slightly limited range of motion. There were some roentgenographic residual alterations of shape of the talus with hypertrophic spurring and early degenerative joint changes in 85 percent of those treated closed; however, these patients were usually active and had returned to some form of activity or occupation without the use of external support. The implication was that most of the closed fractures seemed to do well, but patients were left with evidences of their injury both clinically and on follow-up roentgenograms. The good results were identified in individuals who had no pain, no limp, no swelling, no limitation of activity, and ability to return to their former level of activity or occupation. However, there were definite roentgenographic findings of degenerative joint change in all but two instances. Therefore, *excellent* was not selected to identify these results; instead, *good* was used to identify our best results.

Using Hawkins' classification criteria, there were sixteen of Type I, five of Type II, and five of Type III. All of the poor results were in Type II and Type III. The pattern of good results seemed to be pre-

TABLE 8-1 Study Series: Talus Fractures

	NAME	AGE	SEX	FRACTURE CLASSIFICATION (HAWKINS')	INJURY DATE	MECHANISM OF INJURY	TALUS FRACTURE DIAGNOSIS	TREATMENT	COMPLICATIONS AND COMMENTS	FOLLOW-UP TIME	RESULTS	OCCUPATION RESUMED
1	C.W.	23	F	I	1/ 4/66	Auto accident	Closed Fracture, neck of talus, right	Closed reduction, cast 14 weeks	10% loss of joint motion, midtarsal	20 months	Good	Teacher: Yes
2	B.D.	39	F	I	6/29/68	Fell at home	Open contaminated fracture mid talus, right	Reduction; cast 24 weeks	Union delayed until 25 months	8 years 4 months	Good	Housewife: Yes
3	R.S.	28	M	II and III (bilateral)	3/ 3/69	Auto accident	Bilateral closed fractures; right more comminuted involving head and neck	Closed reduction; Cast 4 months	Partial ant talectomy of right talus 3 weeks after injury	15 months	Good Lt. Poor Rt.	Salesman: Yes
4	A.H.	68	M	I	6/19/71	Fell down stairs	Fracture, mid body talus, right	Closed reduction; cast 4 months	Fractured ankle 1 month out of cast additional cast immobilization)	5 years 4 mosths	Good	Retired
5	K.T.	39	M	II	7/17/69	Fell down elevator shaft	Fracture, mid neck talus, right	Open reduction 8 weeks; 2 K-wire fixation; weight bearing 12 weeks	Painful ankle; stiffness	7 years 4 months	Fair	Formerly construction now maintenance
6	P.G.	17	F	II	4/ 9/71	Auto accident	Open fracture, mid talus, right	Debride, reduction; cast 5 months	Slow recovery; part. weight bearing 1 year; pain, limp, some loss foot mobility	5 years 7 months	Fair	Student: on feet 6-8 hours no ext. sup.
7	S.P.	24	F	I	6/18/71	Auto accident	Fracture, mid neck talus Lacerated right ankle (talus fracture side)	Closed reduction; cast (IM rod fem. same side)	Weight bearing 7 weeks tenderness	5 years 4 months	Good	Housewife: On feet 8-9 hours
8	G.B.	45	F	III	9/17/72	Auto accident	Open, gross contaminated fracture, waist talus and ankles, right	Debride, reduction; K-wire fixation	Cmp'd site drain. 8 months; slight loss of ankle motion	3 years 5 months	Good	Housewife: On feet all day
9	A.S.	58	F	III	9/14/72	Fell from ladder	Closed fracture, midtalus, left; assoc. medial malleolus fracture	Open reduction; 2 K-wires: screw in malleolus	Avascular necrosis	4 years 2 months	Poor	Housewife: On feet but refuses fusion
10	A.R.	37	M	I	10/19/72	Motorcycle accident	Closed fracture, talus, right	Closed reduction; cast 10 months	Delayed union 24 months; iliac bone graft and 2 screws at 25 months gave union in 3 months	8 years 4 months	Fair	Salesman: Active
11	P.K.	28	M	II	2/24/73	Auto accident	Crush injury fracture, os calas/mid talus, and torn lig. ankle, right	Closed reduction; cast 4 months	Pain, stiffness, some loss flex.	3 years 7 months	Fair	Machinist: Full time
12	R.W.	18	M	III	4/24/73	Caught in conveyor belt	Open fracture, midtalus; assoc. skin loss, right	Open reduction; skin grafts; K-wire fixation	Pain, swelling, stiffness; needs cane; talus viable and fracture healed	3 years 6 months	Poor	Comp. inj.: Unemployed poor motivation
13	G.M.	24	M	I	9/ 1/ 73	Motorcycle accident	Closed fracture, mid talus and ankle, right	Open reduction; screw fixation	Pain, swelling, limp; x-ray shows revascularized talus	3 years 2 months	Fair	Service advisor: On feet 8-10 hours
14	R.D.	26	M	I	11/17/73	Auto accident	High neck fracture, margin of body of talus, right	Closed reduction; cast 6 months	Full weight bearing; no support 9 months	3 years	Good	Teacher: Fully active
15	O.B.	25	F	II	5/10/74	Auto accident	Cmp'd talus and dome fracture/skin graft lat. ankle, left	Debride; pin fix 6 weeks; non-weight bearing 8 weeks	Stiffness, loss of motion, fibrous ankylosis; no pain w/1" heel	30 months	Poor	Housewife: Unable to be active
16	S.W.	49	M	I	7/ 9/74	Fall from ladder: 20'	Closed fracture, talus, Left mid neck; assoc. fractures, right os cal., T9., L2 vert.	Closed reduction; walk. heel 6 weeks; cast off 14 weeks	Pain; heel lock and click; limited motion 5-10° dorsiflexion; inversion and eversion	2 years 4 months	Fair	Unemployed, Completely disabled
17	M.K.	24	M	I	3/ 5/75	Fell 14 stories	Midtalus neck fracture, Left; Left carpal navic. Right ankle dislocation; lumbar fracture L1, 2, 3	Open reduction; 2 K-wire fixation; cast 14 weeks	No limp or loss of motion	20 months	Good	Works 8 hours: Some swelling
18	R.B.	19	M	I	6/10/75	Motorcycle accident	Fracture, high neck of talus near ant. dome edge, right	Closed reduction; cast 20 weeks; Par weight bearing 6 months; full weight 9 months	Pain, swelling, limited motion; partial talectomy 8 months after injury	17 months	Poor	Gas station attend: Stays on job, limps
19	J.R.	28	M	I and II (bilateral)	10/22/75	Auto accident	Bilateral displacement (mark. right); fracture displacement left hip, avulsion left medial malleolus tib. and 4, 5 left metatarsals	Open reduction; 2 K-wires	Weight bearing in stand. table at 10 months; revascularization needed; pain On right	14 months	Fair left Poor right	Unemployed: Complications, poor motivation

dictable in those patients who had both a Type I fracture and a closed procedure of treatment.

Perhaps the most interesting observation was that there was only one instance of a painful avascular necrosis (Fig. 8-2). This occurred in a patient with a Type III fracture and following open reduction. There were five other instances of roentgenographic appearance of avascular necrosis noted for several months and up to three years after the initial injury, but this observation had to be reconciled with asymptomatic patients who were functioning satisfactorily. In addition, nonunion was really not a problem either. In one instance, a bone graft was used to stimulate union after two years of delayed union, and in another instance union finally occurred spontaneously at twenty-five months.

The finding of only one instance of avascular necrosis and only two instances of delayed union problems was balanced in a negative sense by the flood of residual complaints from the patients when they were contacted after they had discontinued medical care. Eight patients were willing to say they were doing well. Frequently the patient was unhappy with his limited range of motion, even though pain was not a feature. Stiffness definitely hampered activities. When pain was present, it was usually at the tips of the malleoli and at the ankle joint level. When stiffness of the foot was a complaint, pain was more often noted in the midtarsal joint region. Only one patient resorted to external support (cane).

In the majority of instances in the fourteen open reductions, Kirschner wires and Steinmann pins were used for fixation. Usually two pins were used; occasionally,

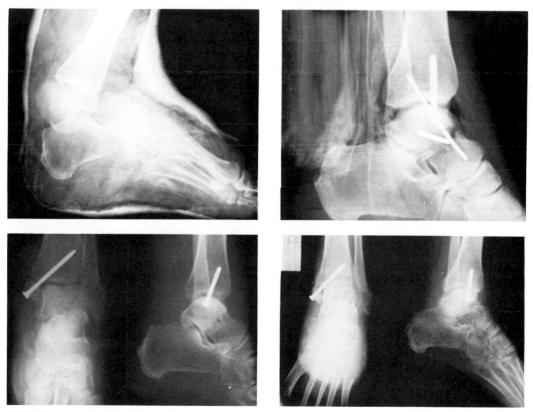

FIGURE 8-2 (A) Avascular necrosis developed after this severe injury to talus. Initial view shows amount of displacement although the fracture was closed. (B) Two months postoperative. No complication. (C) Three months after injury. Fixation pins removed. (D) Five months after injury. Avascular necrosis changes are present now.

one pin was used; and in one instance, three pins were used. They were all placed longitudinally through the entire length of the talus to maintain the reduction. In one additional instance, a vertical pin was used directly up through the os calcis and into the tibia. In one reduction a screw was used. In two instances no fixation at all was necessary. The solution for one other of these open reductions was a partial talectomy initially (a partial talectomy was also done as a salvage procedure later in one of the poor results).

In the follow-up study there were eight good results, seven fair results, and six poor results (in twenty-one fractures in nineteen patients). All of the poor results were in patients who had had open reduction. This partially reflects the severity of the injury requiring the open reduction rather than a direct bad effect of the surgery. A patient's result was classified as (excellent) good when he returned to his previous level of activity and occupation with no swelling, stiffness, or pain. A fair classification was used when a patient had stiffness, swelling, and aching discomfort but would be on the foot for a six- to eight-hour time period. Poor results had all of the noted features not present in the good results, plus presence of features on roentgenogram that were predictable abnormalities for future complaints.

DISCUSSION

The implication in this study is that the treatment plan needs to be directed toward accuracy of contact of bone of the talus, whether open or closed, and that bone healing will occur and is directly proportional to the restoration of bone contact. Circulation restoration is also directly proportional to the accuracy of the reduction, with the assumption that this restoration occurs reasonably close in time to the original injury.

The puzzling discrepancy in low avascular necrosis in this series compared with others might be a reflection of fewer severe fractures, but the typing classification obviated some of this if there is a variation in patients in this series. The possibility of the poor results being in the group of lost patients also needs to be considered; but many of these patients were seen for three, four, five, and even eight months after injury. Certainly there should have been some indication that there was going to be nonunion or avascular necrosis as a problem in that length of time, even though it was too short a time to allow the statistics to be clouded by including these cases in the report. A more likely possibility is that there has been less attention given and little concern on our part when the roentgenograms showed findings of "avascular necrosis." The lack of clinical correlation of pain and the tolerance of the patient to the allowed activity and weight bearing seemed to contraindicate the use of the term "avascular necrosis," at least in its usual context of being a bad omen.

VASCULAR SUPPLY

The initial surge of restoration of blood supply more usually occurs through the medial surface of the body, the anterior lateral vessels, and the tarsal canal arteries, according to Mulfinger and Trueta.[9] It is their observation that most fractures of the neck of the talus do not cause avascular necrosis of the body, but they further note that this condition seems to occur with dislocation or fracture-dislocation or arterial occlusion from surrounding soft-tissue damage. This most recent study of the vascular supply of the talus is a final statement of authority, in most respects supplementing and building on observations by Kelly and Sullivan[6] and Haliburton, Kelly, and Wildenauer.[3] The conclusion of all of these detailed studies adds to Wildenauer's[11] original finding, which was that the talus has a rich blood supply even though more than three fifths of its surface is articular cartilage. The implication in the work of Mulfinger and Trueta[9] is that Hawkins' sign might better be thought of as an indication that the blood supply to the talus was allowing for revitalization of the dome through an intact or restored artery of the tarsal canal. If the presence of subchondral atrophy is a good sign then it must be reflecting a near normal vascular supply of the small end arterioles demonstrated by these authors as originating from the artery of the tarsal canal in twenty out of thirty of their specimens. The other supply of blood for the body of the talus might be deltoid branches entering the body medially or the lateral branches from the artery of the tarsal sinus. The anatomic studies favor Hawkins' sign being a reflection of a functioning tarsal canal artery.

AVASCULAR NECROSIS

A common problem in any consideration of avascular necrosis is just what is meant by the term. Studies done by Harris[4] of radiographic interpretation of avascular bone as reported in 1960 seemed to correlate with our own clinical observations that there has been a misconception of what is going on in substance after a temporary separation of a major bone segment, such as a femoral head. Experimentally, these authors divided the ligamentum teres, dislocated the femoral head, and severed the head from the neck. This was done in rabbits. Avascular necrosis was evidenced by empty lacunae, absence of osteogenic cells, and atrophy of marrow. The significance of the study was that "avascular bone which was not re-ossified showed no change in density;" whereas, "areas of avascular bone being repaired by new appositional bone showed an increase in density." The implication in the situatio

located the femoral head, and severed the head from the neck. This was done in rabbits. Avascular necrosis was evidenced by empty lacunae, absence of osteogenic cells, and atrophy of marrow. The significance of the study was that "avascular bone which was not re-ossified showed no change in density;" whereas, "areas of avascular bone being repaired by new appositional bone showed an increase in density." The implication in the situation of the talus is that when one finds increasing density in radiographs, it is a sign of increasing reossification rather than of increasing necrosis (Fig. 8-3).

BONE IMPLANTS

There is considerable advantage in being able to approach the talus from the medial side and removing the medial malleolus to do so, as noted by Garcian and Parkes.[1] This technique was employed twenty-five years ago for a bone graft study done in three instances, with a follow-up in all three patients (two years, four years, and fifteen years) noting no avascular necrosis (Table 8-2).

In 1952 an interlocking bone graft was inserted medially in three patients *within* the talus itself (i.e., not as an exposed implant that could be visualized once the talus was reduced). The graft seemed to function both as an internal fixation device and as an implant that may have acted as a template for increasing bone production. All three of these cases did well, as can be

TABLE 8-2   Study Series: Primary Treatment and Talus Bone Implant

	NAME	AGE	SEX	FRACTURE CLASSIFICATION (HAWKINS')	INJURY DATE	MECHANISM OF INJURY	TALUS FRACTURE DIAGNOSIS	TREATMENT	COMPLICATIONS AND COMMENTS	FOLLOW-UP TIME	RESULTS	OCCUPATION RESUMED
1	L.P.	27	F	I	7/13/52	Automobile accident	Closed Fracture, left high neck fracture of talus at margin of dome	Open reduction 11 days after injury	Iliac graft site and foot wound healed per primum; cast removed 12 weeks; full weight bearing 20 weeks	15 years	Good	Housewife: 1½" heel on shoe; can wear canvas shoe
2	R.H.	44	M	II	11/ 9/54	Comp. inj.; fall from scaffold	Closed Fracture, right talus; gross deformity and swelling	Closed reduction; circulation improved; open reduction 4 days later	Iliac graft site and foot wound healed per primum; cast removed 12 weeks; full weight bearing 24 weeks	3 years 6 months	Good	9 months: Returned to job; no complaints 2 years later
3	R.C.	28	F	III	5/ 2/55	Automobile accident	Closed Fracture, Comminution and dislocated ankle joint, severe deformity	Open reduction immediately, as swelling not present at that time	Iliac graft site and foot wound healed per primum; cast removed 14 weeks; full weight bearing 22 weeks	2 years 2 months	Good	Housewife: 1" heel; slight swelling

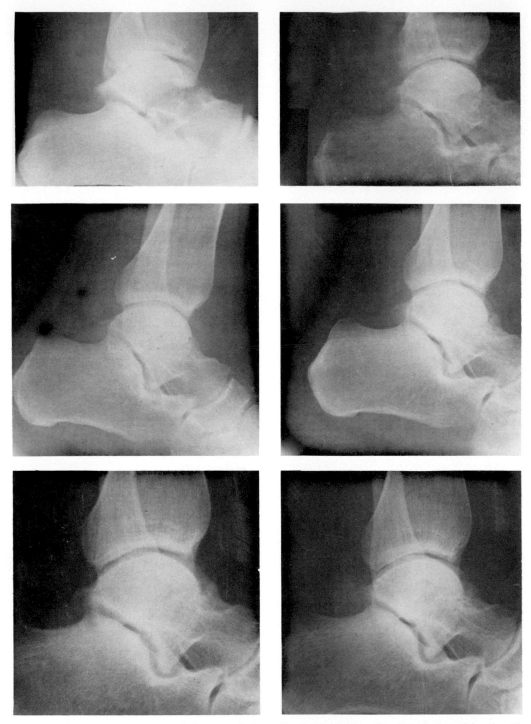

FIGURE 8-3 (A) Initial fracture. (B) Four months later. Fracture healed but talus shows increased den sity. (C) One year later. No avascular necrosis. (D) Two years later. No loss of talus but note that subtalar changes are present. (E) Five years later. (F) Seven years later. This was a fair result with return to his occupation as a construction worker. There are sub talar arthritic changes to correspond with stiffness and localized pain over subtalar joint; however, patient is not incapacitated, nor does he require a fusion, and no avascular necrosis is present.

noted in the later follow-up films (Figs. 8-4, 8-5, 8-6). No clear-cut evidence that the bone implants did any more than skillfully placed Kirschner wires would do led to reluctance in pursuing use of this graft.

Hawkins[5] noted that in over half of his cases the replacement of the dead bone began on the medial side of the talus and advanced laterally. The supposition is that the re-establishment of blood supply through the medial surface of the talus can be a major factor in the healing process no matter whether a graft is inserted or not (Fig. 8-7). However, if one can place the graft early and establish template action as a part of maintaining viability of the injured talus, it may be a better choice to do grafting early rather than to wait for the lack of a Hawkins sign to initiate intervention, since this would be two to three months after injury.

Two of Hawkins' patients had cortical bone grafts used primarily for internal fixation. The details of these cases are not known, but it was noted that segmental necrosis appeared above the grafts in the body of the talus and collapse of a portion of the dome of the talus followed. The implication is that two Steinmann pins for accurate reduction is a better choice. Bone grafting was done for avascular necrosis in four of Hawkins' patients to accelerate bone replacement; but it was his feeling that the grafts did not accomplish this purpose. The concern in this observation is that the grafts may well have been done at a time when the surrounding substance of the talus was not able to respond to the stimulus of the implant, and that they should have been done at an earlier time or initially. A similar conclusion might be drawn from the poor result in the one bone graft described by Mindell,[8] since it was done one year after injury for both nonunion and avascular necrosis.

CONCLUSION

This study series of twenty-eight displaced fractures of the neck and body of the talus without dislocation at the ankle joint in comparison with reported other series led to some general observations. All three types of fractures (utilizing Hawkins' classification) were represented, that is Type I (twenty), Type II (five), and Type III (three) in a follow-up of nineteen patients which was sufficient to draw conclusions. The following findings and impressions evolved:

1. Union of the fractures occurred in all patients in this series and in a high percentage in other series' reports.

2. Avascular necrosis of the talus occurred in only one patient in this series, a low incidence in relation to exact anatomic reductions.

3. Full weight bearing would be better avoided until the fracture line is completely obliterated, since resorption and deformity of the talus are more likely to occur with weight bearing before ten weeks—a reflection of inadequate fracture healing rather than the effect of avascular necrosis.

4. Weight bearing after four months, with fracture union but suspected avascular necrosis, will have little adverse effect on the eventual outcome.

5. The ability to obtain and maintain an anatomic reduction (closed or open) is the most important factor in predicting good results in fractures of the Hawkins' Group II type. Group III dislocation injuries are not predictable as to outcome; but rather than the displacement factor or severity of the original injury, it is the original reduction that counts most.

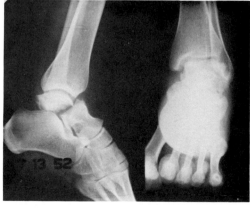

FIGURE 8-4 (A) This talus fracture has a poorer prognosis, since it is a high neck fracture at margin of head of talus.

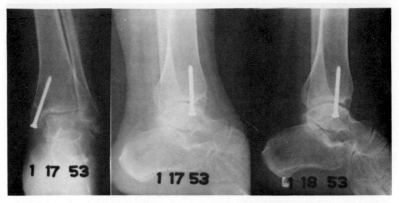

FIGURE 8-4 (B) Six months after open reduction and insertion of iliac bone implant for fixation, no fracture line is noted and there is no evidence of graft outline.

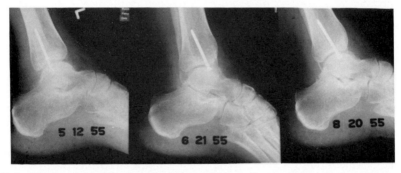

FIGURE 8-4 (C) Three-year follow-up films show a viable, well-restored talus. Patient has no complaints.

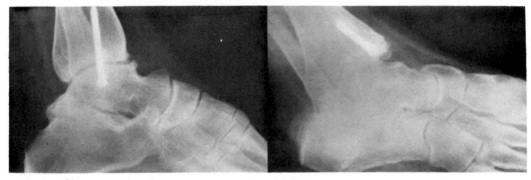

FIGURE 8-4 (D) Fifteen-year follow-up film shows no residual of bone implant, but there are joint changes that indicate degenerative narrowing is present now, although patient is still without complaints.

6. Pin fixation (Kirschner wire or Steinmann pin) is sufficient to hold a reduction.

7. A bone implant (iliac) through a medial approach (medial malleolar osteotomy) can be used to hold an anatomic reduction and as an agent of fixation. An advantage is that the graft does not have to be removed at a later date should any other type of procedure be indicated that would require "bone stock." There is no proof that the presence of the implant negates the

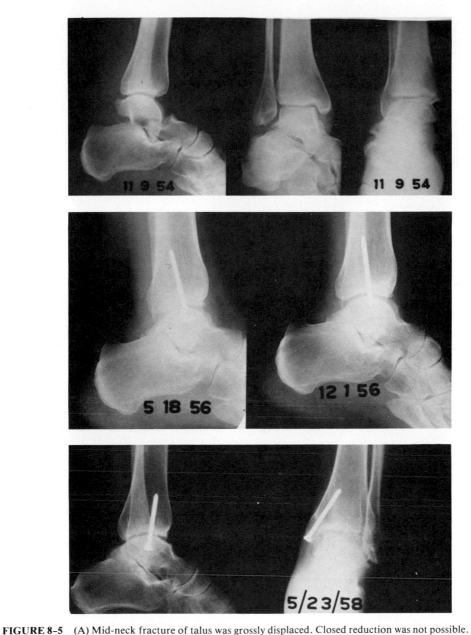

FIGURE 8-5 (A) Mid-neck fracture of talus was grossly displaced. Closed reduction was not possible.

(B) Lateral views at eighteen months and two years show good revascularization of talus after open reduction and insertion of iliac bone implant for fixation.

(C) Three and one-half years after injury there are no symptoms, no residual signs of injury, and no avascular necrosis. Patient was injured on the job and had no residual impairment and no disability.

possibility of avascular necrosis.

I wish to acknowledge the contributions of the following orthopaedic surgeons who offered their case material for study: Mark Brown, M.D., Alan Cohen, M.D., Claude Holmes, M.D., Richard Levitt, M.D., Elwin Neal, M.D., Arturo Ortiz, M.D., Neil Rohan, M.D., Hugh Unger, M.D. and Herbert Virgin, M.D.

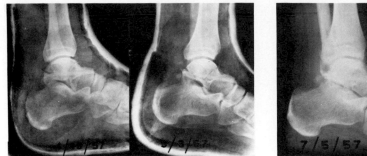
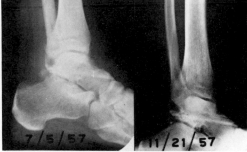

FIGURE 8-6 (A) The more cortical the implant, the more the shadow is visible over a prolonged time period. (B) Incorporation of bone implant as a tem plate remains distinct at three months and eight months after surgery. A cancellous graft will give a more normal talus appearance.

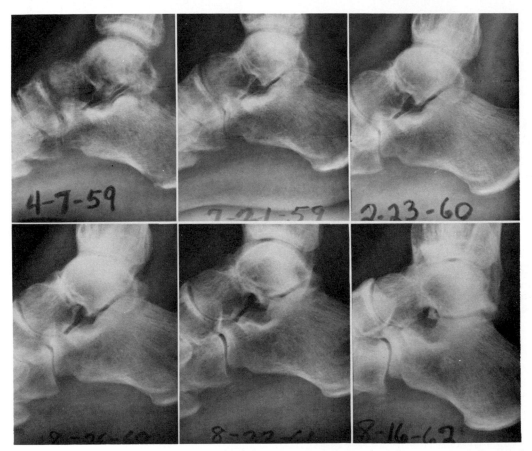

FIGURE 8-7 Revascularization of talus is identified here in a series of views extending over a three-year period. Fracture line in this situation of a closed reduction is still visible two years later, and only after three years does it finally disappear. Avascular necrosis was of concern at each successive visit but did not develop. Weight bearing was allowed at three months (second view—upper middle).

REFERENCES

1. Garcia, A. and Parkes, J.C.,II: *Fractures of the Foot*. In Giannestras, N.J. (Ed.): *Foot Disorders, Medical and Surgical Management* (2nd Ed.). Philadelphia: Lea and Febiger, 1973.
2. Giannestras, N.J. and Sammarco, G.J.: *Fractures and Dislocations in the Foot* (Chap. 19). In Rockwood and Green: *Fractures*, Vol. 2. Philadelphia: J.B. Lippincott, 1975, p. 1446.
3. Haliburton, R.A., Sullivan, C.R., Kelly, P.J. and Peterson, L.F.A.: The extraosseous and intraosseous blood supply of the talus. *J. Bone Joint Surg.* 40A: 1115-20, 1958.
4. Harris, W.R. and Bobechko, W.P.: Radiographic density of avascular bone. *J. Bone Joint Surg.* 42B: 626-36, 1960.
5. Hawkins, L.G.: Fractures of the neck of the talus. *J. Bone Joint Surg.* 52A: 991-1002, 1970.
6. Kelly, P.J. and Sullivan, C.R.: The blood supply of the talus. *Clin. Ortho.* 30: 37-44, 1963.
7. McKeever, F.M.: Treatment and complications of fractures and dislocations of the talus. *Clin. Ortho.* 30: 45-52, 1963.
8. Mindell, E.R., Cisek, E.E., Kartalian, G. and Dziob, J.M.: Late results of injuries to the talus. *J. Bone Joint Surg.* 45A: 221-45, 1963.
9. Mulfinger, G.L. and Trueta, J.: The blood supply of the talus. *J. Bone Joint Surg.* 52B: 160-67, 1970.
10. Pennal, G.F.: Fractures of the talus. *Clin. Ortho.* 30: 53-63, 1963.
11. Wildenauer, E.: Die Blutversorgung des Talus. *Zeitschr Anat.* 115: 32-36, 1950.

Chapter Nine

REPLANTATION OF A SEVERED FOOT

RICHARD L. JACOBS, M.D.
JAMES G. HOEHN, M.D.
ALLASTAIR KARMODY, M.D.

Replantation of severed extremities has been reported with increasing frequency since the original report by Malt and McKhann.[17] With few exceptions, these have documented replantation of various amputations of the upper extremity. The philosophy concerning replantation of the lower extremity and foot has been stated by Harris: "There are but few indications for replantation of a severed lower extremity."[10] However, there have been scattered reports of successful lower extremity replantations which appear to be functioning successfully,[3,19,21,23,26] along with apocryphal reports of miracles.[28] When faced with the amputated member, many surgeons turn to prostheses.

Since we successfully replanted a forefoot in a young boy following a power mower injury,[25] the advantages of replantation over acceptance of the deformity have become apparent. It is our purpose to relate our experiences in this case and to urge that more interest be given to replantation after lower extremity injuries.

CASE REPORT

A two-and-one-half-year-old boy slipped on wet grass and thrust his right foot into the blades of a rotary lawn mower (Fig. 9-1). His right foot was cleanly amputated at the level of Chopart joint(s).

A neighborhood physician obtained hemostasis by direct pressure and then retrieved the forefoot, placed it in a clean plastic bag, and packed it in ice. A rescue squad rapidly transported the patient to our emergency room.

Débridement

Within ninety minutes, general anesthesia started and the teams began the pro-

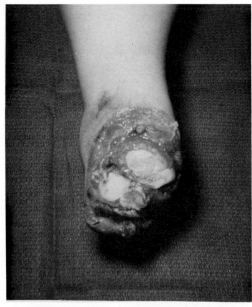

FIGURE 9-1 Hindfoot before débridement.

cess of determining the suitability for replantation. One surgical team examined, débrided, and identified structures in the amputated forefoot; the other performed the same exploration on the patient's amputation site. In both areas, the skin margins and the subcutaneous tissues were sharply débrided and the tendons identified. Identification of the dorsalis pedis artery and the posterior tibial artery was followed by inspection of their lumina with the operating microscope.

The proximal end of the artery was flushed by release of the microsurgical clamps. The distal arterial tree was gently flushed with dilute chilled heparin solution. The wound was irrigated with 1 percent neomycin solution.

Bone Shortening

Inspection of the bony surfaces of the severed forefoot revealed the absence of the tarsal navicular. To débride and to provide adequate bone shortening for tension-free vascular repairs, it was decided to excise the proximal articular surfaces of the cuneiforms (Fig. 9-2) and the cuboid. On the hindfoot, débridement and shortening

was by excision of the exposed articular surfaces of the talus and the calcaneus. Total foot shortening produced by these débridements was estimated at 2 m.

All members of the replantation team inspected the foot and decided to proceed with the attempt.

Bone Fixation

With the forefoot held in proper relationship to the hindfoot (Fig. 9-3), two Kirschner wires were introduced through the forefoot into the hindfoot, slightly angled toward each other to achieve firm fixation. The entire foot was then dorsiflexed and maintained in the position by the introduction of a third Kirschner wire through the heel into the distal tibia. This immobilized the ankle joint and prevented tension on the proposed vascular repair.

Arterial Repair

Inspection of the porta pedis and the

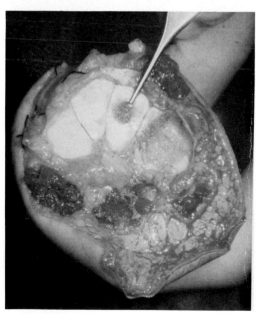

FIGURE 9-2   Cuneiforms were seen in forefoot.

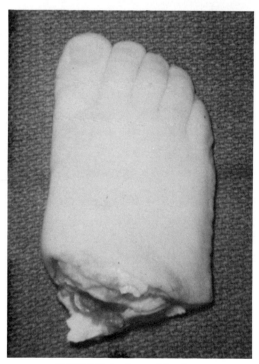

FIGURE 9-3   Severed forefoot.

posterior tibial vessels revealed two arteries with small lumina buried deep in the cleft between the reapproximated surfaces. It was decided not to repair the posterior tibial vessels, and they were ligated.

Attention was turned to the dorsalis pedis artery, which was estimated to have an internal lumen of 3 mm. A fine Fogarty catheter was used on the proximal arterial tree to insure absence of clots, and the artery was flushed satisfactorily. The distal artery had been perfused previously. Both ends were trimmed in preparation for anastomosis. The repair was done under magnification with running and interrupted sutures of 9-0 nylon. When the arterial clamps were released, circulation seemed to be re-established. Within ten minutes, however, flow was obviously decreasing and the arteriotomy was reopened. No evidence of clot was found, and the artery was flushed proximally and distally again. After the arteriotomy was repaired again, the extensor retinaculum was released at the ankle and on the dorsum of the forefoot. After this release, good flow returned and persisted three and one-half hours from the start of surgery.

Venous Repair

After arterial inflow was established, the only satisfactory vein was repaired with 9-0 nylon suture in a fashion similar to the arterial repair. Prolonged examination with the arterial tree distended with pulsatile blood flow did not reveal other veins suitable for anastomosis. It was evident in the postoperative period that this 5 mm lumen did provide adequate drainage.

Tendon Repair

Because of their proximity to the vascular repairs, no extensor tenorrhaphies were performed. Likewise, the extensive dissection required to expose the flexor tendons in the depths of the plantar surface precluded their repair. This, with other considerations to be discussed later, caused us to leave the tendons at this point.

Skin Closure

Dermal sutures were placed medially and laterally to approximate the skin edges

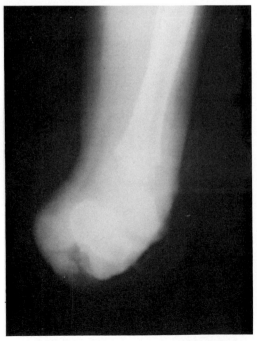

FIGURE 9-4   Roentgenogram of hindfoot.

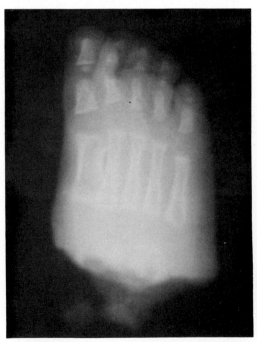

FIGURE 9-5   Roentgenogram of hindfoot.

there. The dorsal and plantar surfaces were left open to allow excess venous blood and lymph to escape from the forefoot.

Postoperative Care

Upon completion of the vascular anastomoses, low-molecular-weight dextran (40) was begun and continued for the initial twelve postoperative hours. Then intravenous anticoagulation was begun with heparin (1000 units every six hours) and continued for eight days, when it was stopped in anticipation of operative wound closure. Oral acetylsalicylic acid (480 mg daily in divided doses) was then begun and continued until the patient was discharged from the hospital.

Starting with the induction of anesthesia and continuing for the first two weeks of hospitalization, cephalothin (250 mg) was given every eight hours. During the postoperative period, sedation was also achieved with 15 mg of phenobarbital daily in divided doses.

Normal saline dressings were changed every twelve hours. Initially large stains were seen on the dressings and interpreted as representing lymphatic outflow. The size of the stains gradually diminished. On the seventh postoperative day the wound was covered with biologic dressings (porcine skin grafts, (Fig. 9-6). They were changed daily to permit reassessment of the wound

and served two major purposes.[10] The first was protection of the wound from bacterial contamination, the second to determine the "take" of subsequent autogenous skin grafts. When secretions from the wound were minimal the pigskin grafts would remain "stuck" to the wound and split-thickness skin autografts (Fig. 9-7) could probably be successfully applied.

Wound Closure

On the tenth postoperative day, the dorsal defect was closed with 4-0 nylon suture and the medial and plantar surfaces were closed with autogenous split-thickness skin grafts. Both wounds healed primarily.

Immobilization

A plaster cylinder applied over bulky padding suspended the foot free of the bed in any position and restricted knee movement during the early healing stages. The foot and ankle were free for inspection and frequent dressing changes. On the twenty-seventh day, the calcaneal-tibial pin was removed and a long leg cast applied. The remaining pins were removed at a cast change six weeks after injury. Cast immobilization was continued for three months with active weight bearing permitted during the latter days.

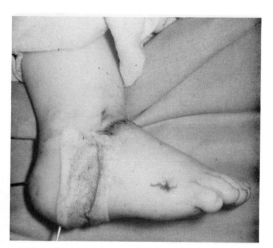

FIGURE 9-6 After application of porcine grafts.

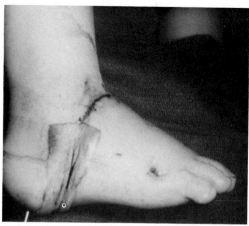

FIGURE 9-7 Split-thickness autografts were now applied.

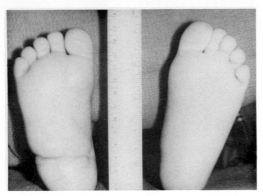

FIGURE 9–8 There was little discrepancy in sizes of feet; pictured 6 months after injury.

Ambulation and Protection

After the cast was removed the insensitive forefoot was protected with a shoe fabricated from Aliplast sheet and adhesive tape. Routine skin care was done by the patient's mother, who was instructed to report any skin changes. She closely supervised his ambulation. By six months after the injury (Fig. 9-8), he was enjoying normal outdoor activities and wearing sneakers.

Delayed Nerve Repair

Five months after the injury, the patient entered the hospital for a secondary neurorrhaphy of the medial and lateral plantar nerves. Preoperatively, a retrograde contralateral femoral arteriogram (Fig. 9-9) documented the patency of the arterial repair and the re-established collateral circulation.

The secondary neurorrhaphy was done under magnification with 9-0 nylon suture. At this level, the nerve had divided into medial and lateral plantar nerves, and separate nerve repairs were necessary.

Reconstructions

In the ensuing months, the patient's mother noticed that the boy became "pigeon-toed." Re-examination revealed no associated deformity of the forefoot and there was no clawing of the toes (Fig. 9-12). There was strong inversion of the foot (Fig. 9-11); the anterior tibial and posterior tibial tendons had undergone tenodesis at the amputation site and were functional. There was also active eversion of the foot, but this was of lesser strength, suggesting that the peroneals had also tenodesed but probably with more shortening.

Because of this, the patient was returned to the operating room nineteen months from the time of the injury for a shortening Z-plasty of the peroneus brevis and longus tendons at the level of the ankle. During the operative exploration, both tendons were found to be in continuity via scar with the distal end of the peroneus brevis tendon at the level of amputation. After surgery, the extremity was immobilized in a short leg cast. This cast was removed and mobilization started. The foot appeared to have better balance.

Measurements of the foot taken fif-

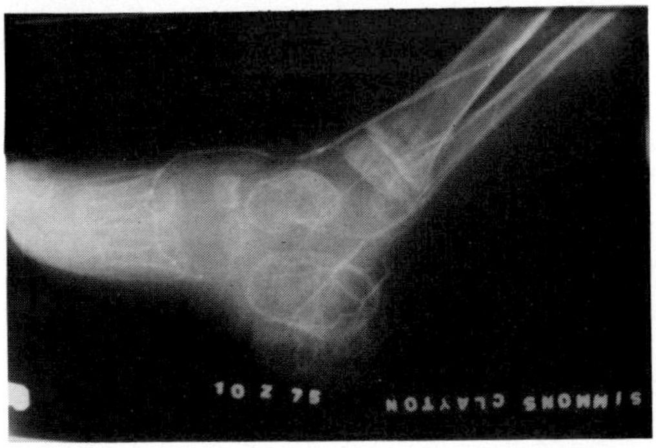

FIGURE 9–9 Arteriogram five months after injury.

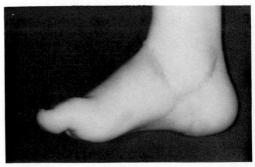

FIGURE 9–10 Multiple views of foot nine months after surgery.

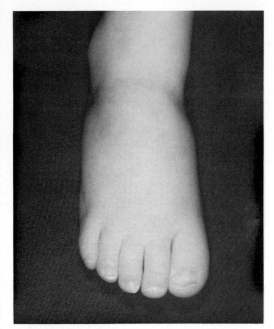

FIGURE 9-11 Note tendency toward inversion of foot, even at rest.

teen months after injury indicated progressive growth with minimal size discrepancy.

DISCUSSION

It is unfortunate that emphasis has been placed almost exclusively on upper extremity replantation. Although Harris[12] did not indicate what "very special circumstances" would be needed to warrant an attempt at replantation in a lower extremity, it may. be assumed that he considers current prosthetic rehabilitation as satisfactory functional reconstruction in most cases. Buncke[3] has also alluded to the attitude of pessimism toward lower extremity replantation in the English-speaking world.

The Chinese[3,18,20,26] have documented their success in these cases, some of which have been observed by Western physicians. McDowell[18] reported two cases seen during a visit to Shanghai. One case was a mid-thigh replantation and the other a replantation of the foot at the ankle. O'Brien[20] and Roth[26] separately reported the same case from Peking. A woman suffered bilateral lower extremity amputation; the levels were midleg on the right and through the ankle on the left. Because of severe soft-tissue injury to the right leg, this side was left as a below-knee amputation. The left foot was also severely damaged; for this reason, the undamaged right foot was replanted to the left leg. The extensor tendons were repaired. The peroneal tendons were sutured to the long toe flexors in the replanted foot. The results were said to be quite satisfactory, but the accompanying pictures show marked clawing of the toes.

Buncke[3] reported a very similar case he saw in Hangchow. In this male, no tendon repairs were done and accompanying photographs show no evidence of clawing.

O'Brien[21,23] reported his own case of successful replantation in a two-year-old boy with a through-ankle amputation. Two years after replantation, the foot is growing but is narrower than the normal foot. He anticipates future surgery because of damage to the distal tibial epiphysis.

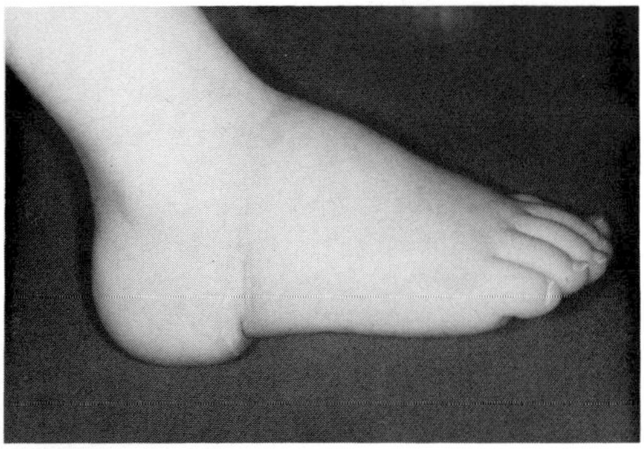

FIGURE 9-12 There is no clawing of toes. All toes have good range of passive dorsiflexion.

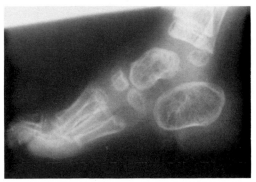

FIGURE 9-13 Lateral roentgenogram of foot eleven months after injury.

Although several cases of foot replantation have been documented and two satisfactorily described, adequate functional information is not available. Based on a comparison of our case with O'Brien's,[23] some observations are pertinent.

Apparently, as in hand replantations, the axiom that "children do better" may well apply. There seems to be no marked impairment of growth of epiphyseal plates that are not mechanically disrupted at the time of the original injury. Transient ischemia does not markedly impair future growth.

In the upper extremity replantations, all structures are repaired primarily whenever possible;[14] this is the time that repair is technically the easiest. Tendon repair in *foot* replantations may not always be desirable.

Some reasons can be advanced for this. Replanted hands usually develop intrinsic minus deformity, on the basis of both ischemic and denervation changes. The intrinsics of the foot, unlike those of the hand, are inserted only on the proximal phalanges and do not act to extend the interphalangeal joints.[15] Were it technically possible to do a perfect repair of long toe extensors and flexors at this level of amputation, it is quite likely the hyperextension deformity at the metatarsophalangeal joints would develop. This would be followed by clawing in the absence of the mediating effect of the intrinsics on flexor-extensor balance. The toes of the replanted feet, if they regularly develop clawing, would not be functional in gait. All of the problems associated with claw toes, including that of proper footwear, would need to be dealt with. Those cases where tendon repairs have been done do appear to develop this deformity. Perhaps this is a defeatist attitude, but we think that it is a reasonable conclusion, at least in the instance of through-the-foot amputations such as this one.

Based on experiences with imbalanced feet from other causes, we would have preferred to transfer the anterior tibial tendon, which was strong, laterally in our patient's foot. This would have involved surgical trauma and reaction in the exact vicinity of

the only major artery that was repaired. We considered the shortening Z-plasty of the somewhat more weak peroneals to be a less satisfactory alternative.

Some established principles of replantation surgery deserve emphasis. The mode of injury will determine replantibility. The guillotine amputation is most successful. Multiple fractures, distal bruising, or severe soft-tissue injury with or without avulsion may well be contraindications.

The method of handling of the amputated part may be decisive. The amputated part should be stored in a dry plastic bag that is surrounded by ice, and warm ischemia time should be minimized.[2,8,16]

Thorough débridement is vitally important. This includes shortening of bone to allow tension-free vascular anastomoses, as documented by the Chinese.[3,20,23]

Microsurgical background,[2,5,24] perfected by constant laboratory practice, is mandatory for active members of the replantation team. Urbaniak[29] has stressed the need for a designated team with representation from orthopaedic surgery, plastic surgery, neurosurgery, and vascular surgery, and with technical support from specialists in hematology, pediatrics, physical medicine, and others as the need arises. The written protocol for our replantation team has contributed to the efficient handling of replantation cases.

Some principles of replantation surgery remain controversial. The role of perfusion may be correlated with the tissue structure and mass in deciding whether or not to perfuse distally.[11,22] In digital replantations, intimal disruption may follow perfusions with very small pressure gradients and lead to thrombosis and failure. Blood rheologists further indicate that normal blood does not clot in normal vessels when subjected to no-flow states. However, larger tissue masses may include significant amounts of muscle. Here the use of perfusion to achieve "core cooling" would appear to be advantageous. Warm muscle is much more susceptible to ischemia. Surface cooling coupled with perfusion with cold perfusate decreases the disastrous effects of muscle ischemia and greatly prolongs the duration of ischemia which can be tolerated.

Sympathetic blockade is claimed to be of value by some authors.[7] Dermatotomy and fasciotomy can reduce cylindrical pressure in the extremity and reduce the risk of compromise[9] of vascular structures and muscles. Indiscriminate use can lead to wound infection.

There are two major causes for failure in replantation. Arterial thrombosis may occur within the first few hours and is heralded by a blanched appearance and poor digital tissue turgor. Venous thrombosis appears two to four days after replantation as a dusky, mottled, cool replant with engorgement. Both findings are indications for immediate re-exploration of the vascular repairs. If re-exploration is necessary, results are still often good. If subsequent re-explorations are needed, chances for success are much diminished.

Most authors advocate the repair of two veins for each repaired artery to improve drainage. On occasion, this cannot be done. In these instances, additional lymphatic and venous drainage can often by achieved by incomplete wound closure, or the "venous window" technique.

In our case, only one vein could be repaired and these strategies were employed. If the wound edges are not completely closed, the replanted tissue can remain decompressed by bleeding and by lymphatic drainage into the dressing[27] as was done here. A more extreme case was reported by Chunprapaph.[4] In his successful four-finger replantation there was a loss of fourteen units of blood in the postoperative period. As Corry[6] has stated, an initially good result may be compromised unless venous and lymphatic drainage can occur (an index finger was lost because the wound sealed and drainage from the wound ceased). In our patient drainage steadily decreased over a period of ten days. The wound was then completely closed by direct suture and split-thickness skin grafts. Because drainage occurred, swelling and compromise of circulation never became a problem.

Another factor that contributed to this success was the type of immobilization.[30] The foot was held in dorsiflexion by a pin placed through the heel into the distal tibia. A short cylinder cast prevented motion at the knee. This protected the vascular repair from undue movement and yet allowed the entire foot to remain free in moist soft dressings for inspection and débridement. There was no encircling cast on the foot or ankle to impede circulation if swelling occurred.

It is obvious, then, that it is technically possible to replant after lower extremity injuries. Early on, there are no difficulties that have not been previously encountered and successfully dealt with in the upper extremity. The foot is important for locomotion and stability. Since prehensility is not as important, we may reasonably anticipate even better functional results than in the hand.

The foot, however, takes the trauma of weight bearing and this is one problem not encountered in the upper extremity. Technically, this should not be an insurmountable problem. Insensitive feet caused by other causes, such as diabetes, lues, and syringomyelia can be protected and maintained from further soft tissue or bone injury.[13] The favorable difference in replantation is that we may anticipate at least partial return of protective sensation after nerve repair.

SUMMARY

An amputated forefoot was successfully replanted in a two-and-one-half-year-old boy after a guillotine-type amputation by a lawn mower. Our experiences in this case are reported and compared with other cases reported in the literature. Routine and specific details involved in the successful replantation of any amputated extremity and specifically the forefoot are discussed.

There seem to be no major reasons why the same vigorous approach used in upper-limb replantation should not be applied to the lower extremities. At the worst, failures can be converted to amputations, while successful results will allow patients to regain near normal gait with good function while avoiding a lifetime of involvement with prosthetic or orthotic appliances. Satisfactory function of this foot is maintained today more than four years postoperatively.

REFERENCES

1. Bilos, Z.J., Labinsky, H. and Khazie, H.: Forearm replantation. A case report of a two year follow-up. *Ill. Med. J.* 145:315–16, 1974.

2. Boyes, J.G.: Reimplantation of extremities by microvascular suture. *N. C. Med. J.* 35(8):479–81, 1974.

3. Buncke, H.J.: Replantation surgery in China. *Plast. Reconstr. Surg.* 52(5):476–89, 1973.

4. Chunprapaph, B.: Replantation of portions of four fingers in one hand. *New Engl. J. Med.* 291:460–61, 1974.

5. Cobbert, J.R. and Bowen, J.E.: Severed digits. *Brit. Med. J.* 3:40, 1974.

6. Corry, R.H. and Russell, P.S.: Replantation of severed fingers. *Ann. Surg.* 179:255–59, 1974.

7. Davies, K.H.: Guanethidine sympathetic blockade; its value in reimplantation surgery. *Brit. Med. J.* 1(6014):876–77, 1976.

8. Editorial: Severed fingers. *Brit. Med. J.* 2:291, 1974.

9. Editorial: Replantation of severed limbs. *Brit. Med. J.* 2:722, 1975.

10. Elliott, R.A. and Hoehn, J.G.: Use of commercial porcine skin for wound dressings. *Plast. Reconstr. Surg.* 53(4):401–05, 1973.

11. Harashina, T. and Buncke, H.J.: Study of washout solutions for microvascular replantation and transplantation. *Plast. Reconstr. Surg.* 56:542–48, 1975.

12. Harris, W.H. and Malt, R.A.: Late results of human limb replantation. *J. Trauma* 14:44–52, 1974.

13. Jacobs, R.L.: Neuropathic Foot in the diabetic patient. In *Foot Science.* Philadelphia: W.B. Saunders Co., 1976, pp. 235–53.

14. Jaffe, S., Earles, A.S., Fleegler, E.J. and Husni, E.A.: Replantation of amputated extremities: report of five cases. *Ohio State Med. J.* 381–86, 1975.

15. Kelikian, H.: *Hallux Valgus, Allied Deformities of the Forefoot and Metatarsalgia.* Philadelphia and London: W.B. Saunders Co. 1963.

16. Kleinert, H.E., Serafin, D., Juntz, J.E. and Atasoy, E.: Reimplantation of amputated digits and hands. *Ortho. Clin. North Amer.* 4(4):957–67, 1973.

17. Malt, R.A. and McKhann, C.F.: Replantation of severed arms. *JAMA* 189:716–22, 1964.

18. McDowell, F.: Get in there and replant! *Plast. Reconstr. Surg.* 52(5):562–67, 1973.

19. O'Brien, B.: Replantation surgery. *Clin. Plast. Surg.* 1(3):405–26, 1974.

20. O'Brien, B.: Replantation surgery in China. *Med. J. Australia* 2:255–59, 1974.

21. O'Brien, B.: Replantation and reconstructive microvascular surgery. *Ann. Roy. Coll. Surg.* 85:87–103, 1976.

22. O'Brien, B.M., MacLeod, Miller, G.D.H., Newing, R.K., Hayhurst, J.W. and Morrison, W.A.: Clinical replantation of digits. *Plast. Reconstr. Surg.* 52(5):490–502, 1973.

23. O'Brien, B.M.: Personal communication.

24. Owen, E.: The operating microscope isn't everything. *J. Bone Joint Surg.* 58(B):397–98, 1976.

25. Ross, P.M., Schwentker, E.P. and Bryan, H.: Mutilating lawn mower injuries in children. *JAMA* 236(5):480–81, 1976.

26. Roth, R.B.: Replantation in China. *JAMA* 1127–28, 1974.

27. Serafin, D., Kutz, J.E. and Kleinert, H.E.: Replantation of a completely amputated distal thumb without venous anastomosis. *Plast. Reconstr. Surg.* 52(5):579–82, 1973.

28. Tosatti, B.: Transplantation and reimplantation in the arts. *Surgery* 75(3):389–97, 1973.

29. Urbaniak, J.B.: Personal communication.

30. Weiland, A., Robinson, H. and Futrell, J.W.: External stabilitization of a replanted upper extremity: case report. *J. Trauma* 16(3):239–41, 1976.

Chapter Ten

ANKLE ARTHRODESIS: Long-Term Follow-Up with Gait Analysis

SHELDON R. SIMON, M. D.
JOHN MAZUR, M. D.

The best possible treatment for advanced disabling arthritis of the ankle joint remains in doubt. Fusion has been the primary surgical method for managing painful diseased ankles, but since motion is lost, some investigators have looked for an alternative procedure. With the success of the total hip-joint prosthetic replacement, many in the orthopaedic community feel they have found the solution to all joint problems. Making painful diseased joints mobile and pain free is exactly the result we would all like to obtain. However, not all joint replacements that have been tried have been as successful as the total hip replacement. For example, in total knee replacements the complication rate is 16 to 20 per cent. In the case of ankle joint replacements, there are too few and too short follow-up times to assess their value accurately.

Scholz[14] in 1976 presented a short-term follow-up of thirty-one patients with total ankle replacements. In his clinical evaluation Scholz found 20 per cent excellent results, 60 per cent good results, 13.4 per cent fair and 6.6 per cent poor results. His only complications were two patients with superficial wound necrosis.

Waugh et al.[18] presented twenty-five cases in which the Irvine ankle arthroplasty was used. The average follow-up was eight and one-half months. He had one septic case that had to be fused and another that resulted in an amputation.

In a third study, Newton[12] described thirty total ankle replacements with an average of two years' follow-up. These total ankle replacements were placed in patients with either traumatic arthritis or rheumatoid arthritis. Newton's follow-up examination showed an average non-weight-bearing motion of 5° of dorsiflexion and 20° of plantar flexion. The functional range of motion during gait was not presented. In Newton's series there were three poor results: one patient continued to have a painful unstable joint, another became septic, and a third patient had to have a B/K amputation.

In all of these studies the follow-up times were short and the reports are at best preliminary. They do not take into account the later complications of joint replacement such as component loosening, late sepsis, or component wear. The question arises: Is maintaining ankle motion, however appealing, all that necessary to warrant an unknown risk-benefit ratio of total ankle replacement?

In the literature the alternative treatment, ankle arthrodesis, has generally been accepted as yielding good long-term clinical results. Barr and Record[2] in 1953 presented a long-term follow-up of forty-three ankle fusions. Their patients had varying conditions of polio, traumatic arthritis, nerve palsies, and rheumatoid arthritis. The results were good in all except two patients, who had fair results. Barr and Record state, "Pain due to intra-articular lesions is relieved, deformity and instability are corrected, and the compensatory mobility of the subtalar and mid-tarsal joints permits a surprisingly free range of foot motion after fusion of the ankle joint. Patients with solid arthrodesis of the ankle have been found to have practically no disability and to be able to stand, walk, run or jump in normal fashion." The functional ability reported in Barr and Record's study was based on the patients' subjective opinions and not upon objective criteria.

Ratliff[13] reviewed fifty-nine patients after Charnley compression arthrodesis with one to nine years of follow-up. In his clinical assessment there were 61 per cent excellent results, 18 per cent good, 19 per cent fair and 2 per cent poor results. Of his fifty-nine patients only six walked with a limp and only two patients had persistent pain. It was felt that this pain was due to pre-existing arthritis of the subtalar joint.

More recently, Campbell et al.[4] presented a follow-up study of eighteen patients who had undergone ankle fusion for post-traumatic arthritis. The results were good, with only four complications: two superficial wound infections, one pseudarthrosis, and one peroneal nerve palsy.

There are numerous other articles in the orthopaedic literature,[1,3,5,6,7,8,9,10,17,20,21,22] which come to the conclusion that, in general, ankle arthrodesis can result in a stable, pain-free joint without serious complications. In none of these studies, however, have the criteria for the reported results been clearly defined, nor do any reports critically analyze the gaits of these patients. It is the purpose of this study to present a long-term follow-up of patients with fused ankles in such a manner as to critically assess their function in activities of daily living; to accurately analyze their gaits in the laboratory, thus determining the effect of ankle fusion on the total pattern of walking; and to correlate the results of gait analysis with functional activity. We might hope that the information gained will help define the need, if any, for the development of a total ankle replacement and possibly its future indications.

MATERIALS AND METHODS

Clinical Material

All the medical records of patients who had undergone ankle fusion between January 1965 and January 1974 at the Massachusetts General Hospital were reviewed. A total of twenty-two ankle fusions were done. It was possible to contact thirteen patients, with nine patients being lost to follow-up. Of the thirteen, twelve agreed to be studied and one refused to return for examination.

The clinical histories prior to ankle arthrodesis are summarized in Table 10-1. The patients in this group had all undergone ankle fusion for traumatic arthritis, pain being their chief complaint. The pain was severe, beginning immediately after the initial treatment. The progression of the pain was rapid in every case.

The time interval between the date of fusion and the date of follow-up examination was from two years, seven months to twelve years, nine months, with an average of eight years, three months.

The clinical evaluation consisted of a patient interview and physical examination. The patients were questioned as to the presence and severity of pain with relation to daily activities such as running and walking on a level, on hills, or on stairs. An attempt was made to determine their levels of activity both in terms of employment and in terms of recreational sports activities. The degree to which the patients could carry out these activities was investigated, especially in regard to the distance they

TABLE 10-1   Summary of Case Histories Prior to Ankle Arthrodesis

PATIENT AGE SEX	NATURE OF ORIGINAL INJURY	ORIGINAL TREATMENT	ONSET OF PAIN AFTER TREATMENT	TIME INTERVAL INJURY AND FUSION	TYPE OF FUSION
W.A. 31 M	Compound fracture, distal tibia	Débridement, cast	Immediate	4 years	Charnley compression
W.J. 35 M	Compound fracture, ankle	Débridement, cast	Immediate	3 years	Transfibular graft
J.H. 54 M	Supination external rotation ankle	ORIF*	Immediate	6 years	Charnley compression
J.L. 51 M	Compound fracture, distal tibia	Débridement, cast	Immediate	15 years	Charnley compression
D.B. 51 F	Supination external rotation fracture, ankle	ORIF	Immediate	4 years	Charnley compression
R.D. 42 F	Supination external rotation fracture, ankle	ORIF	Immediate	2 years	Charnley compression
F.G. 65 M	Supination external rotation fracture, ankle	Closed reduction, cast	1 year after treatment	3 years	Charnley compression
S.L. 58 F	Supination external rotation fracture, ankle	ORIF	Immediate	3 years	Charnley compression
A.B. 32 M	Supination external rotation fracture, ankle	Closed Reduction, cast	Immediate	3 years	Fibular graft
O.D. 53 M	Supination external rotation fracture, ankle	ORIF	2 years after treatment	4 years	Charnley compression
D.D. 41	Supination external rotation fracture, ankle	ORIF	4 months after treatment	1 year	Hatt fusion
M.W. 38 F	Pronation external rotation fracture, ankle	ORIF	Immediate	4 years	Charnley compression

*Open reduction internal fixation.

could walk or run. If they were limited, the cause of the limitation was determined. The patients were questioned as to the use of special compensatory devices such as special shoes, braces, or other means of support.

The physical examination consisted of a complete orthopaedic examination. All were evaluated in regard to stance, gait, anthropomorphic measurements, range of motion of all joints, and muscle testing. Special attention was directed toward determining the position of the fused ankle, motion in the subtalar and midtarsal joints, heel position, and the presence of callosities.

A standing lateral x-ray was obtained to measure the exact position of the ankle fusion. Two lateral views were also obtained with dorsiflexion and plantar flexion stress to measure the amount of midtarsal motion (Fig. 10-1). In addition to the lateral x-rays, A-P and mortise views were obtained. The x-rays were examined closely for any pathologic findings in the subtalar and midtarsal joints. The degenerative changes found were graded in the following way: If there was minimal joint narrowing

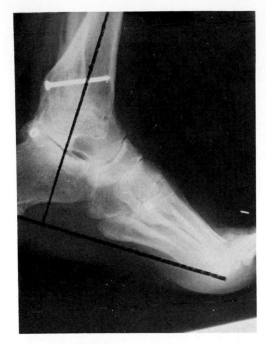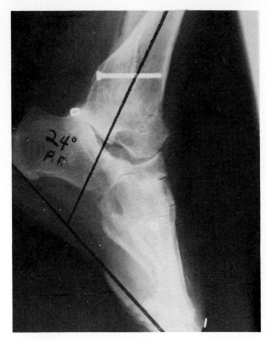

FIGURE 10–1   Lateral x-rays of the foot with dorsiflexion-plantar flexion stress.

and minimal subchondral bone sclerosis, we graded this as having minimal degenerative changes. If there was more significant narrowing, sclerosis, and the presence of small osteophytes, this was rated as having moderate changes. The patients rated as having severe changes had x-rays that showed severe narrowing, sclerosis, and significant osteophyte formation.

To evaluate objectively the results of the clinical examination, a weighted point system for grading ankle function was developed in a manner similar to the Harris Hip Rating System. This point system (Table 10–2) allows an integrated objective evaluation taking into account all major functional considerations. The main emphasis of this system has been on pain and functional activities. A normal person would score one hundred points. Because of the lack of ankle motion, our patients could score a maximum of a ninety, as ten points are given for full range of motion.

Gait Analysis

A gait analysis laboratory has been established at the Children's Hospital Medical Center in Boston. The description of the facilities has already been published.[15] For the interested reader Appendix I describes the gait analysis laboratory facilities.

The patients were prepared for the gait analysis according to the following standard protocol. One-inch black squares of tape with white dots were placed in the following positions: on the dorsum of the foot between the first and second metatarsals; just proximal to the lateral aspect of the calcaneocuboid joint; on the lateral malleolus; on the patella; on the lateral aspect of the knee; on the anterior-superior iliac spine; on the superior tip of the sternum; on the lateral aspect of the neck at approximately C6; on the tip of the acromion process at the shoulder; on the lateral epicondyle of the elbow; and on the dorsum of the wrist. Ten-inch wooden rods with red tips were then fixed snugly onto the femur and tibiae for determining internal and external rotation. An additional 10-inch wooden rod mounted on a 3 foot x 3 foot lucite base was placed on the skin overlying the midportion of the posterior aspect of the sac-

TABLE 10-2   Ankle Evaluation

Name	Diagnosis
Hospital #	Operation
Age	Date of Surgery
Date of Exam	Surgeon
Pre- or PostOp	R or L

PAIN

None or ignores	50
Slight on going up or down stairs or on prolonged walking (no compromise on activities of daily living).	45
Moderate pain when going up or down stairs or on prolonged walking. No pain in level gait. Occasional non-narcotic pain medication.	40
Pain in level gait with more pain on stairs. No rest pain. Daily pain medicine.	25
At-rest or night pain in addition to ambulatory pain. Narcotic pain medication required.	10
Continuous pain regardless of activity.	0
Disabled because of pain.	0

Total _____

FUNCTION

Limp, antalgic:

None	6
slight	4
moderate	2
marked	0

Distance walked:

unlimited	6
4-6 blocks	4
1-3 blocks	2
indoors only	1
bed-chair	0
unable	0

Support:

none	6
cane, long walks only	5
cane, full time	3
two canes or crutches	1
walker or unable	0

Hills (up):

normally	3
rotates foot or leg	2
on toes or rotates body	1
any means or unable	0

Hills (down):

normally	3
rotates foot or leg	2
rotates body	1
any means	0

Stairs (up):

normally	3
needs banister	2

TABLE 10-2 Ankle Evaluation—Continued

one stair at a time	1
any means or unable	0
Stairs (down):	
normally	3
needs banister	2
one stair at a time	1
any means or unable	0

CALF STRENGTH AND ANKLE STABILITY

Stable, able to stand on toes with 10 repetitions	5
Stable, able to stand on toes with 5 repetitions	3
Stable, able to stand on toes with 1 repetition	1
Unstable, unable to stand on toes	0

RUNNING

Able to run as much as desired	5
Able to run but limited	3
Unable to run	0

MOTION

Dorsiflexion:

40 degrees	5
30 degrees	4
20 degrees	3
10 degrees	2
5 degrees	1
0 degrees	0

MOTION

Plantar flexion:

40 degrees	5
30 degrees	4
20 degrees	3
10 degrees	2
5 degrees	1
0 degrees	0

TOTAL: _____

rum to help define the pelvis.

To record EMG activity during the gait cycle, Beckman electrodes were placed over the muscle bellies. The muscle groups studied included the gastrocsoleus, anterior tibialis, peroneals, rectus, gluteus maximus, gluteus medius, and medial hamstrings. Needle electrodes were placed in several patients to check the accuracy of the surface electrodes and to obtain a recording from the soleus.

Recording of the actual walk was then performed with the patient walking back and forth along the 50-foot walkway a minimum of twenty-four times. Twelve of the walks were performed with shoes and twelve without shoes. In order to get the most accurate measurement of midtarsal motion during gait a zoom lens was used on the side of the ankle fusion in half of the runs, while in the other half, a standard 12.5-mm lens was used. In several patients with particularly long stride lengths a wide 10-mm lens was necessary to adequately visualize an entire gait cycle from heel strike to heel strike.

After each session the EMG and force plate data were displayed and recorded for each run. The film data were computerized and the gait cycles were displayed as stick figures in three views: right, front, and left. After the two-dimensional projected coordinates of each joint were recorded, a subsequent program translated these into the true three-dimensional coordinates of each joint on the walkways. The kinematic data included: all joint motions in three planes, positions of limb segments, trunk angle, velocity of gait, stride length, and percentage of time spent in each phase of the gait cycle. A three-dimensional stick figure representation of the walk was displayed and recorded.

The force plate data were analyzed to determine the foot-floor reaction in the vertical, fore-aft, and medial-lateral directions; the resultant vector of the foot-floor reaction; and the pathway of the dynamic center of mass. The forces about the ankle, knee, and hip joints were calculated using a computer program combining the force plate and film data.

The EMG data were then correlated with the force plate and film data to determine the phasic activity of the muscle groups.

The gait analysis was done as described for each patient with and without shoes. The results were compared with normal patients and with the opposite leg. An attempt was made to correlate the information from the gait analysis with the clinical evaluation.

RESULTS

Clinical Evaluation

All the patients studied were solidly fused at the ankle, and there were no complications related to their surgery. They were all dramatically improved as a result of their ankle fusions and, in general, were able to return to their pre-injury activity levels. All the patients could walk without support with relatively normal clinical gaits. None of the patients required pain medication.

This group of patients was physically quite active. Nearly all patients were able to return to their pre-injury occupations and leisure sports (Table 10-3). One patient could not return to his former position only because of job regulations. One patient never attempted to return to her recreational sport.

The ankle evaluation scores are recorded in Table 10-4 for each patient. The average ankle evaluation score preoperatively was 40.3 with a standard deviation of 11.2. After arthrodesis, the average score was 80.8 with a standard deviation of 8.9. The improvement seen was statistically significant at the 99 per cent confidence level.

To better understand the disability created by an ankle arthrodesis, the points lost in the various categories of the ankle evaluation grading system were tabulated (Table 10-5). Nine of the twelve patients were able to walk painlessly without a significant limp for an unlimited distance. Three of the twelve developed some minor discomfort in the arch of the foot or in the midtarsal area only after prolonged walking.

All the patients stated that they could walk up stairs and hills without much difficulty. When questioned closely, a few admitted making certain minor compensations when negotiating hills. Seven found it easier to walk up and down inclines by externally rotating the foot on the fused side. One patient fused in plantarflexion found it necessary to walk up hills on her toes. Climbing stairs gave the patients little trouble. Eight could climb stairs normally, three used a banister for assistance, and one took one stair at a time.

In general, the patients scored very well in every category of the grading system with the exception of running. Only three patients felt that they could run to their satisfaction. Two patients felt their ability to run was impaired both in terms of speed and distance. Seven patients could not run at all. An attempt was made to correlate the ability to run with the various factors studied, such as position of the fusion,

TABLE 10-3   Physical Activity of Patients

PATIENT	PRE-INJURY OCCUPATION	ABILITY TO RETURN TO WORK	PRE-INJURY SPORTS	POST-FUSION SPORTS
W.A.	Paper cutter	Fully employed	Hunting, hockey, baseball	Same as pre-injury
W.J.	Telephone lineman	Fully employed	Hunting, hockey, softball	Same as pre-injury
J.H.	Salesman	Fully employed	Hunting, fishing	Same as pre-injury
I.L.	Gunner in Air Force	Fully employed as an administrative officer	Golf	Same as pre-injury
D.B.	Salesman	Fully employed	Swimming	Same as pre-injury
R.D.	Homemaker	Able to do only light housework	Bowling	None
F.G.	Vice president of a corporation	Fully employed	Golf	Same as pre-injury
S.L.	Nurse	Fully employed	Golf, ice skating	Same as pre-injury
A.B.	Truck driver	Fully employed	Hockey	Same as pre-injury
O.D.	Mail clerk	Total disability due to back pain	None	None
D.D.	Machinist	Fully employed	Bowling	Same as pre-injury
M.W.	Dental hygienist	Fully employed	Skiing, jogging	Same as pre-injury

presence of the degenerative changes on x-ray in the foot, muscle atrophy, and so on. The only correlation that could be found was in the age of the patients. All the patients under forty could run, only one of the two patients in their forties could run, and no patient over fifty could run. In terms of life-style and patient desires, however, none of the nonrunners felt this to be a major disability, as they were happy with their activity levels.

On physical examination (Table 10-6) all of the patients showed a marked degree of calf atrophy (average 1 1/3 inches) on the side of the fusion. However, contractions could be felt in the gastrocsoleus group when the patients were asked to plantar flex their feet, showing these muscles to be physiologically intact.

Leg length discrepancies (Table 10-6) were generally insignificant except in two patients, W.A. and J.H. These discrepancies were a direct result of their original injuries and not the result of the ankle arth-

TABLE 10-4   Pre- and Postfusion Ankle Evaluation Scores

PATIENT	PREOPERATIVE SCORE	POSTOPERATIVE SCORE	DIFFERENCE
W.A.	27	82	55
W.J.	53	90	37
J.H.	43	83	40
I.L.	43	81	38
D.B.	35	75	40
R.D.	13	63	50
F.G.	56	87	31
S.L.	46	83	37
A.B.	48	90	42
O.D.	44	63	19
D.D.	37	88	51
M.W.	39	84	45

TABLE 10–5 **Distribution of Points Lost in the Various Categories of the Ankle Evaluation Grading System**

PATIENT	TOTAL (100)*	PAIN (50)	LIMP (6)	DISTANCE (6)	SUPPORT (6)	HILLS (6)	STAIRS (6)	STABILITY (5)	RUNNING (5)	R.O.M. (10)
W.A.	18	0	4	0	0	2	0	0	2	10
W.J.	10	0	0	0	0	0	0	0	0	10
J.H.	17	0	0	0	0	2	0	0	5	10
I.L.	19	0	2	0	0	2	0	0	5	10
D.B.	25	5	2	0	0	2	1	0	5	10
R.D.	37	10	2	4	0	2	2	0	5	10
F.G.	13	0	0	0	0	1	0	0	5	10
S.L.	17	0	2	0	0	0	0	0	5	10
A.B.	10	0	0	0	0	0	0	0	0	10
O.D.	37	10	2	4	0	2	4	0	5	10
D.D.	12	0	0	0	0	0	0	0	2	10
M.W.	16	0	2	0	0	2	2	0	0	10
Avg.	19.2	2.1	1.3	0.6	0	1.25	0.75	0	3	10

* Numbers in parentheses represent total possible points in each category.

rodesis. Subtalar inversion-eversion (Table 10–6) was markedly diminished in every patient. The plantar flexion-dorsiflexion motion of the midfoot, however, was surprisingly large and easy to demonstrate by passive range-of-motion testing. This will be discussed later with the x-ray results.

The position of the heel was related to callus formation (Table 10–6) as the heel in either varus or valgus alters the weight-bearing surface of the foot. In this particular group of patients none of the calluses was clinically significant, as none was painful.

The orthopaedic examinations of these patients were otherwise unremarkable. There were no other clinically significant abnormalities, and there was no evidence of any untoward effects of the ankle arthrodesis upon the remainder of the musculoskeletal system.

On lateral standing x-rays we found the position of the ankle fusion to be quite varied (Table 10–7). Two patients, W.A. and J.H., were positioned in plantar flexion because of ther marked leg length discrepancies. In general, the positions were near neutral or in a few degrees of plantar flexion. All patients fused in plantar flexion felt that they were significantly limited in walking barefoot. These patients found it necessary to pay close attention to the size heel they wore. Patients fused close to neutral found that they could walk

TABLE 10–6 **Positive Physical Examination Findings**

PATIENT	CALF ATROPHY (INCHES)	LEG LENGTH DISCREPANCY (INCHES)	SUBTALAR MOTION (INVERSION/EVERSION DEGREES)	POSITION OF HEEL	CALLUSES
W.A.	2 1/2	1″ short	0/10	10° valgus	1st metatarsal head
W.J.	1/2	Equal	10/10	Neutral	None
J.H.	1 3/4	1/8″ short	0/0	5° varus	5th metatarsal head
I.L.	3	2 1/4″ short	0/0	Neutral	None
D.B.	1	Equal	5/5	Neutral	None
R.D.	3/4	1/2″ short	10/10	Neutral	None
F.G.	1 1/2	Equal	0/0	5° varus	5th metatarsal head
S.L.	1	Equal	0/0	Neutral	None
A.B.	3/4	Equal	0/0	Neutral	None
O.D.	1	Equal	0/0	Neutral	None
D.D.	3/4	1/2″ short	0/10	10° valgus	1st metatarsal head
M.W.	1	1/2″ short	0/0	5° varus	5th metatarsal head

TABLE 10–7   Position of Ankle Fusion, Midtarsal Motion and X-ray Changes of Degenerative Arthritis in Subtalar and Midtarsal Joints

PATIENT	POSITION OF FUSION	DEGREES DF/PF IN SUBTALAR AND MIDTARSAL JOINTS	X-RAY EVIDENCE OF DJD IN SUBTALAR AND MIDTARSAL JOINTS
W.A.	24° PF	−24° DF/29° PF	Severe
W.J.	2° PF	−2° DF/30° PF	Minimal
J.H.	1° DF	+1° DF/12° PF	Moderate
I.L.	19° PF	−19° DF/27° PF	Severe
D.B.	8° PF	−8° DF/38° PF	Moderate
R.D.	6° PF	6° DF/24° PF	Moderate
F.G.	7° PF	−7° DF/15° PF	Moderate
S.L.	4° PF	−4° DF/28° PF	Minimal
A.B.	5° PF	−5° DF/30° PF	Minimal
O.D.	7° PF	−7° DF/15° PF	Moderate
D.D.	1° DF	1° DF/24° PF	Minimal
M.W.	5° PF	−5° DF/32° PF	Minimal

equally well with or without shoes and they did not have to concern themselves about shoe heel size.

X-ray examinations (Table 10–7) show that all of the patients had evidence of some degenerative changes in the subtalar and midtarsal joints. The degree of the changes varied among patients, but no correlation could be found between symptoms and the x-ray appearance of the joints.

The x-ray measurements of the plantar flexion-dorsiflexion motion of the midtarsal and metatarsal joints were large (Table 10–7). The average arc of motion was 16° with a standard deviation of 8.4°. There was a trend for the patients with severe subtalar, midtarsal, and metatarsal joint narrowing to have smaller arcs of motion in the midfoot. However, there was no statistically significant correlation between the degree of x-ray changes and the arcs of motion.

Walking Speed, Stride Dimensions and Temporal Components of Gait with Shoes

Gait analysis of patients with unilateral ankle arthrodesis strongly supports the results of the clinical evaluation. Under normal circumstances and while wearing shoes, these patients are able to achieve very useful gaits with only minor altera-

tions from the normal. Despite the variation in fusion positions, the group of patients was very homogeneous with respect to their gaits, and therefore, the gait analysis data were averaged and the standard deviations given.

In patients with fused ankles, a decreased free walking speed was consistently noted (Table 10–8). Their mean free walking velocities was found to be 223±35 ft/min, with the normal velocity being 297±40 ft/min.[6] The main reason for the slower velocities was shorter stride length. These patients had an average stride length of 4.28±.51 feet as compared with the normal 5.12±.43 feet.[16] No attempt was made to maintain a normal walking speed by increasing their cadences. The cadence remained essentially unchanged or slightly slower, being 104 steps/min with a cycle duration time of 1.16±.10, as compared with a normal average cadence of 113 steps/min with an average cycle duration time of 1.06±.09 sec.

It should be pointed out that these differences in stride length and free walking velocity are relatively small. In fact, we were not able to show a statistically significant difference in the stride lengths and velocities between normal subjects and patients with fused ankles.

Within a given gait cycle the temporal components and stride dimensions of each leg (step length) in this group of patients

TABLE 10-8   Comparison of the Temporal Components of Gait and Stride Dimensions Between Patients with an Ankle Fusion and Normal Patients*

	NORMALS** WITH SHOES	PATIENTS WITH ANKLE FUSIONS WITH SHOES
Free walking velocity (ft/min)	297±40	223±35
Cycle duration	1.06±.09	1.16±.10
Cadence (steps/min)	113	104
Stride length (ft)	5.12±.43	4.28±.51
Weight acceptance phase % of cycle duration (sec)	12%±4 .13±.04	15.3%±2 .18±.04
Single limb stance % of cycle duration (sec)	38%±4 .40±.04	32.8%±2 .38±.04
Weight release % of cycle duration (sec)	12%±4 .13±.04	15.1%±2.0 .18±.04
Swing phase % of cycle duration (sec)	38%±4 .40±.04	36.8%±3 .42±.04

*Means ± one standard deviation
**Data taken from Gore, D.R. and Murray, M.P.: *J. Bone Joint Surg.* 57A:760, 1975.

were symmetrical and similar to a normal subject. Single limb stance on the fused side was only slightly shorter (32.8 per cent of the cycle) than single limb stance on the sound side (36.8 per cent of the cycle). Swing phase on the fused side was slightly longer than on the normal side. The amount of time spent in double limb stance was minimally longer than normal for both legs. In double limb stance patients spent an equal amount of time in both weight acceptance and weight release. The step lengths were approximately equal for both sides—26 inches for the fused side and 25 inches for the sound side.

Rotations of the Pelvis, Hips, Knees, and Ankles with Shoes

During gait, the range of motion and rotational patterns for all the joints above the tibia appeared no different in these patients than similar data derived from normal subjects. Figures 10-2 through 10-14 display the movements of the limb segments about the pelvis, hips, and knees in the sagittal, coronal, and transverse

planes. Each figure shows that the motion about each point in all three planes was symmetrical with respect to both the fused and the sound sides. In addition, it is difficult to distinguish our fused patients' joint rotations from the normal patients'.[16]

The sagittal patterns of rotation in the joints below the tibia were slightly altered from the normal. During gait, 23±10° of dorsiflexion-plantar flexion motion were recorded between the tibia and the metatarsal heads on the side of the fused ankle (Fig. 10-15). In normal subjects with full ankle and midtarsal motion, the total excursion of motion between the metatarsal heads and tibia during gait has been reported to be 32±9°.[11] Of the total arc of motion, "dorsiflexion" was limited to the maximum of midtarsal motion noted on the stress x-rays. The degree of plantar flexion found during gait, however, showed an even greater arc of motion than that found by the x-ray measurements. The *pattern* of tibia-foot motion was also strikingly similar to what one sees in normal subjects with the following differences. During weight acceptance, (0 to 15 per cent of the cycle) the foot remains in greater

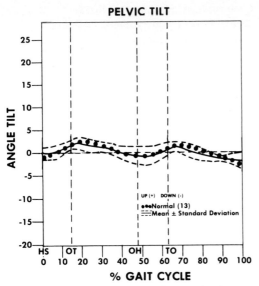

FIGURE 10-2   Pelvic tilt. All figures with shoes.

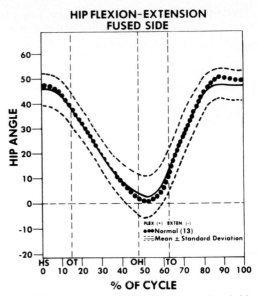

FIGURE 10-3.   Hip flexion-extension on fused side. All figures with shoes.

than normal plantar flexion. A slower than normal rise to the maximum dorsiflexion is seen in single limb stance (15 to 48 per cent of the cycle). Plantar flexion motion is not reversed at toe-off as in the normal subjects (63 per cent of the cycle) but is reversed later in swing phase at 75 per cent of the cycle.

Despite the presence of a normal ankle on the opposite side, an altered rotational pattern was also observed (Fig. 10-16). In fact the dorsiflexion-plantar flexion motion between the tibia and foot on the sound side more clearly resembled that seen on the fused side than that seen in normal

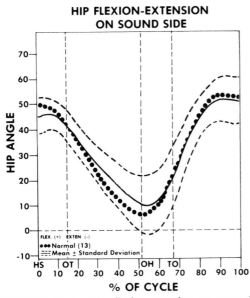

FIGURE 10-4.   Hip flexion-extension on normal side. All figures with shoes.

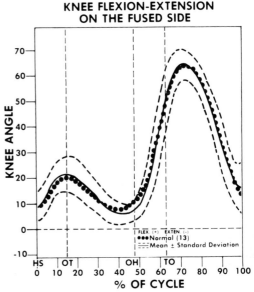

FIGURE 10-5.   Knee flexion-extension on fused side.

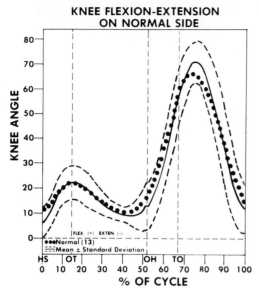

FIGURE 10-6. Knee flexion-extension on normal side.

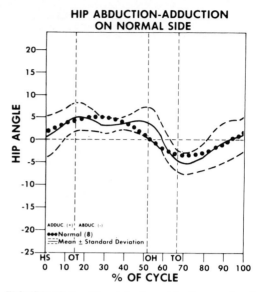

FIGURE 10-7. Hip abduction-adduction on fused side.

subjects. During weight acceptance, the foot was positioned in marked plantar flexion. In single limb stance a lower than normal rise to maximum dorsiflexion was also seen, and in swing phase there was little if any dorsiflexion noted. The similarities in the sagittal rotational patterns between the tibia and foot held true for each patient

and were not just an artifact of averaging the data.

EMG and Force Plate Recordings with Shoes

In every patient, despite the ankle

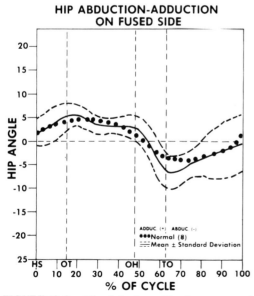

FIGURE 10-8. Hip abduction-adduction on normal side.

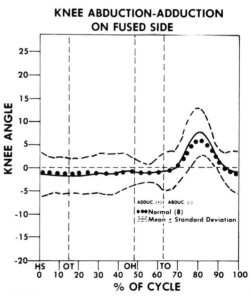

FIGURE 10-9. Knee abduction-adduction on fused side.

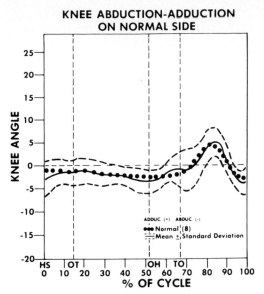

FIGURE 10–10. Knee abduction-adduction on normal side.

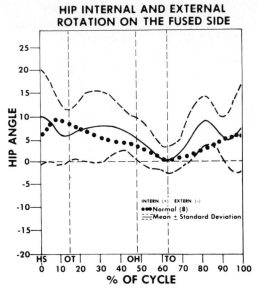

FIGURE 10–11. Hip internal and external rotation on fused side.

fusion, EMG activity was recorded from every muscle about the ankle examined (Fig. 10-17). This activity in these muscles was phasic, but not phasic in a normal fashion. For example, the anterior tibial muscle was electrically active not only during swing, but at specific times during the stance phase. The plantar flexors of the

foot not only fired in stance but also in swing. These findings were consistent in all patients during all walks recorded.

The medial hamstring showed the normal EMG activity both at the end of swing and during weight acceptance. All twelve of these patients showed additional hamstring activity during midstance, a clearly

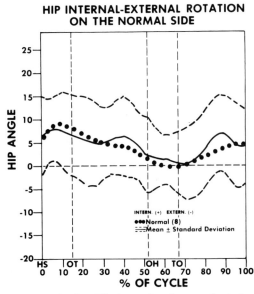

FIGURE 10–12. Hip internal and external rotation on normal side.

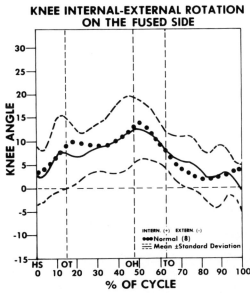

FIGURE 10–13. Knee internal-external rotation on fused side.

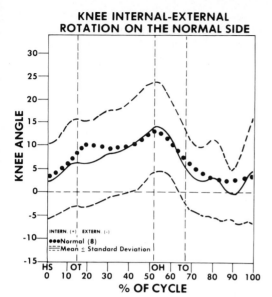

FIGURE 10–14.   Knee internal-external rotation on normal side.

abnormal finding.

It was easy to determine when the anterior tibial, peroneal, gastrocsoleus, and medial hamstring muscles were firing. It was difficult, however, to determine when the other muscles of the thigh and buttocks were active in all patients. For this reason

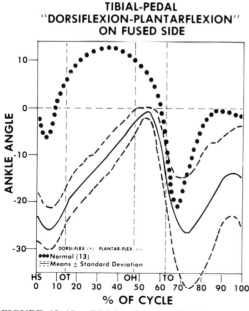

FIGURE 10–15.   Tibial-pedal "dorsiflexion-plantar flexion" on fused side.

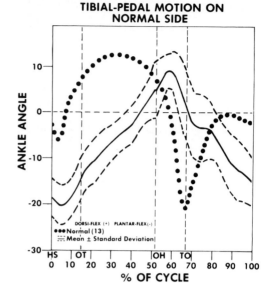

FIGURE 10–16.   Tibial-pedal motion on normal side. All figures with shoes.

no interpretation of the rectus, gluteus medius, or gluteus maximus muscles is given.

The force plate recordings (Fig. 10-18) in the vertical, forward, and lateral directions were normal for all our fused-ankle patients. This is strong evidence for these patients having close to normal gaits.

Figure 10-19 shows the force vector calculated from the force plate data. It is simultaneously recorded with a stick figure representation of a typical patient walking through a complete gait cycle. At heel strike the force vector is through the heel. The force vector then traveled normally from the heel through the midfoot to the toe during the stance phase. The force vector-body relationships were normal for each patient in each phase of the walking cycle.

Effect of Walking Barefoot on the Gait Analysis

The gaits of these patients were adversely affected by walking barefoot. Without shoes, the stride lengths and gait velocities were both decreased (Table 10-9). Pairing the data showed a mean difference in velocity of 18.4 ± 4.5 ft/min and a mean

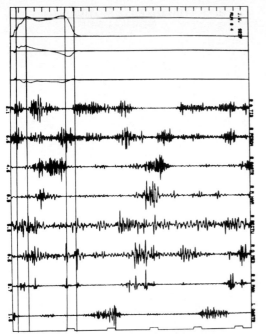

FIGURE 10–17. Foot floor reaction forces for a single stance period and EMG activity of eight muscles for three seconds of a representative gait cycle of a patient having ankle arthrodesis. The three top horizontal graphs represent the vertical, fore-aft, and medial-lateral foot floor reactions lasting approximately one-half second and appearing very similar to normal individuals. The EMG recordings below illustrate relatively normal phasic activity in all muscles including those which normally control the ankle.

difference in stride length of .47±.07 ft. The patients therefore walk with a statistically significant lower velocity and a shorter stride length barefoot than they could with shoes.

One patient fused in severe plantar flexion hyperextended his knee at midstance while walking barefoot. Shoes with a heel to compensate for the plantar-flexed position corrected this, and he no longer hyperextended his knee.

Another patient fused in severe plantar flexion walked on his toes barefoot. Figure 10-20 is the force vector and stick figure representation of his gait without shoes. At foot strike the force vector is seen to pass through the toes. By wearing shoes with an appropriate heel he then walked normally heel to toe with normal force vectors.

DISCUSSION AND CONCLUSIONS

The patients with solid ankle fusions who were studied function very well in normal daily living. All of the patients studied could walk reasonable distances on level ground without pain. The fusion permitted these patients to return to their occupations and recreational activities. On this basis we

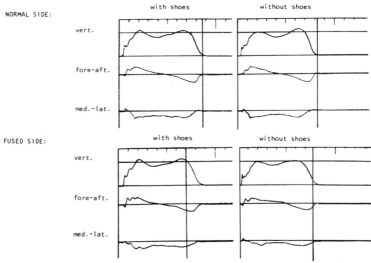

FIGURE 10-18. The stance phase foot-floor reaction forces while walking, of an individual having an ankle arthrodesis. The top group of graphs represents the stance phase in the leg having a normal ankle, the bottom graphs represent those of the leg having an ankle arthrodesis. Note the similarity in all vertical, fore-aft, or medial-lateral tracings regardless of which leg was monitored or whether the individual wore shoes.

TABLE 10–9   Stride Lengths and Velocities of Gait in Patients with Ankle Fusions Barefoot and Wearing Shoes

PATIENT	STRIDE LENGTH WITH SHOES (FT)	STRIDE LENGTH BAREFOOT (FT)	DIFFERENCE WITH SHOES-BAREFOOT (FT)	VELOCITY WITH SHOES (FT/MIN)	VELOCITY BAREFOOT (FT/MIN)	DIFFERENCES WITH SHOES-BAREFOOT (FT/MIN)
W.A.	4.27	3.83	.44	203.1	194.7	8.4
W.J.	4.03	4.18	—0.15	188.7	202.2	—13.5
J.H.	4.60	4.30	0.30	260.4	252.9	7.5
I.L.	4.94	4.17	0.77	251.4	227.3	24.1
D.B.	3.48	2.93	0.55	189.5	176.0	13.5
R.D.	3.76	3.30	0.46	194.4	173.3	21.5
F.G.	4.52	4.01	0.51	255.0	231.3	24.5
S.L.	4.35	4.05	0.30	233.0	220.9	12.1
A.B.	4.94	4.12	0.82	264.4	213.0	51.4
O.D.	3.49	2.95	0.54	158.8	145.1	13.7
D.D.	4.79	4.12	0.67	228.2	199.2	29.0
M.W.	4.22	3.78	0.44	243.3	214.2	29.0

feel that all of these patients could be classified as having excellent results.

According to our clinical evaluation grading system, these patients did show some limitations. It should be noted that our evaluation system is extensive and critically assesses the patients' abilities not only under normal conditions but also under the increased stress conditions of walking long distances, negotiating stairs and hills, and running. Nine of the twelve patients could not run. Three had some minor discomfort after walking for long distances, and eight had to make some minor compensations when negotiating hills and stairs. Scoring the patients with the grading system, we found nine of twelve (75 percent) excellent, one (8.6 percent) good, and two (16.5 percent) fair results.

The gait studies on these patients explain why such normal activity is possible after an ankle fusion. The gait analysis studies objectively examined the patients during the normal condition of free, level walking. The normal findings in their gaits were the most important aspects of this report. While wearing shoes all of the patients could walk with a relatively good

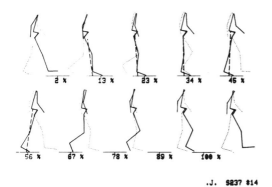

.J. S237 S14

FIGURE 10-19. Representative sagittal plane stick figures and the vectors of foot-floor reaction forces (heavy dotted line) of a typical patient having an ankle arthrodesis during representative samples of the walking cycle. Both motions and vector quantities for each interval of the gait cycle are similar to those for normal individuals. Note the tibia-foot is schematically drawn from lines connecting dots located at the knee, ankle, and first metatarsal head of the foot.

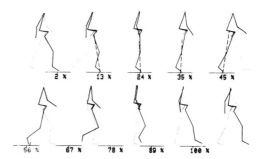

.L. S239 S33

FIGURE 10-20. Similar graphic representation as noted in Figure 10-19 of a individual with a right ankle arthrodesis fused in 19° of plantarflexion walking barefoot. Note the initial foot-floor contact occurs with the toes and the relative change in leg and vector alignment in the first three-fourths of the stance phase is different than in a normal individual wolking.

free-walking velocity and with a consistently rhythmic gait. There were no unusual movements of the trunk and limbs above the ankle. The rotational patterns of the pelvis, hips, and knees were remarkably normal. There were no gross abnormalities in the force plate recordings, and the force vectors maintained a normal relationship to the body.

The patients have very normal gaits, yet they all had ankle fusions. To produce the normal gaits it appears that there are three compensatory mechanisms that work: (1) utilization of the arc of motion available in the small joints of the foot, (2) the altered pattern of tibial-metatarsal rotation on the normal side; and (3) more appropriate position of the tibia with shoes. The important aspects of these compensatory mechanisms are that they all occur below the tibia, do not involve grossly abnormal movements of the limb segments, and do not require added muscle activity.

The first compensatory mechanism is the utilization of the normal arc of motion available in the midtarsal and metatarsal joints. What is normally considered to be ankle motion is, in fact, the motion of the ankle itself coupled with the motion of the small joints of the foot. The normal available arc of motion found in the small joints of the foot has been previously reported to be 13° to 15°.[26] By x-ray stress films we found a very similar arc of motion in the patients studied. We found dorsiflexion to be limited to the position of the ankle fusion, but could easily demonstrate an average of 16° of plantar flexion. During gait, we found an even greater degree of plantar flexion (23±10°). The patient with a fused ankle uses this midtarsal motion to simulate the total ankle-foot motion of the normal subject.

The second compensatory mechanism is the altered tibial-foot rotational pattern on the side of the normal ankle. This rotational pattern mimicked the "dorsiflexion-plantar flexion" motion of the fused side. This ability of the normal side to adjust in such a manner, though producing a slightly abnormal pattern, allows the patient to maintain a symmetric gait.

The third compensatory mechanism is the effect of shoes upon gait. By wearing shoes with a heel, the tibia is placed in a more forward position during stance. This is advantageous, as the tibia must advance to allow the body to advance. In normal subjects the tibia is allowed to come forward by means of dorsiflexion of the foot and ankle. Dorsiflexion in all these patients is limited, but in all patients fused in less than 10° of plantar flexion, dorsiflexion is apparently sufficient as to not require other compensatory mechanisms. Yet even here the use of shoes did improve the stride length and velocity with heel heights that the patient individually adjusted. One can only wonder if this adjusting is made on the criterion of putting the tibia as far forward as possible to increase stride length but still maintain stability. Patients fused in marked plantar flexion (greater than 10°) have an even greater limitation of dorsiflexion. In this situation the patients must either hyperextend at the knee if the leg is long and the foot is flat on the ground, as did patient W.A., or walk on the toes if the leg is short, as did I.L. Both patients were able to correct their abnormal gait patterns by wearing shoes.

The clinical and gait analysis results for this group of patients were better than expected. We therefore searched the literature to see if these results could be supported by other authors. Most long-term follow-up studies of ankle arthrodeses[2,4,5,8,9,13,17,21,22] did support our results, as they also concluded that patients with ankle arthrodesis function very well under normal conditions. There are a few articles, whose authors found poorer clinical results than those we present.[6,7,16] These poorer results, however, can be explained. Fuller and Mackell [6] studied twenty-eight ankles with only 50 percent clinically acceptable results. Twenty-five of their patients were fused in 10° of plantar flexion. We have shown that severe plantar flexion is detrimental, as it does not allow the tibia to come forward normally in stance, causing patients to "back-knee" or to toe-walk. In fact, this is exactly what Fuller and Mackell found. Thus we agree with these authors that better clinical results can be obtained by fusing in a more neutral position.

Johnson and Boseker[7] studied one hundred and forty ankles that had undergone fusion and found only 53 percent good results. In this study a third of the patients had fusions not only of the ankle but also of the subtalar and midtarsal joints. We have shown that the motion in the small joints of the foot is necessary for these patients to compensate for the fused ankle. Therefore, we feel that Johnson's poorer results were due to the more extensive fusion.

Our conclusion is that, subjectively and objectively, patients with ankle fusions function quite well in activities of daily living provided they meet the following criteria: (1) They must have enough compensatory motion in the midtarsal and metatarsal joints of the foot, (2) their other ankle should have a normal range of motion, and (3) they must wear shoes with appropriately sized heels. On the other hand, if a total ankle replacement were to be considered as an alternative to arthrodesis, it would have to improve upon results presented here without adding any disadvantages. A total ankle procedure would need to: (1) still provide a pain-free and stable joint, (2) allow enough dorsiflexion in stance to permit the forward progress of the tibia, (3) allow a faster walking velocity than is seen in fused ankle patients, (4) allow the patients to run, and (5) have an acceptable complication rate.

The rheumatoid patient with an involved ankle may not meet the criteria for recommending an ankle arthrodesis. Many times they have involvement not only of the ankle but also of the small joints of the foot. They then would not be able to compensate for a fused ankle and other compensatory mechanisms would be needed. Therefore, the rheumatoid patient may be a candidate for a total ankle replacement. The use of a total ankle prosthesis and ankle arthrodesis in rheumatoid patients warrants further investigation.

Special Note: This paper received the 1978 Klinkicht Award at the meeting of the American Orthopaedic Foot Society.

ACKNOWLEDGEMENT

The authors wish to acknowledge the support of Mr. Evan Schwartz, without whose assistance the work could not have been done. This work was also supported in part by the Orthopaedic Research and Education Fund Grant No. 249.

REFERENCES

1. Baker, O.L.: SACH heel improves results of ankle fusion. *J. Bone Joint Surg.* 52A: 1485-1486, 1970.
2. Barr, J.S. and Record, E.E.: Arthrodesis of the ankle joint. *New Engl. J. Med.* 248: 53-56, 1953.
3. Boyd, H: Indications for fusion of the ankle. *Ortho. Clin. North Amer. 5:* 191-192, 1974.
4. Campbell, C.J., Rinehart, W.T. and Wienak, A.: Arthrodesis of the ankle. Deep autogenous inlay grafts with maximum cancellous bone opposition. *J. Bone Joint Surg.* 56A: 63-70, 1974.
5. Guinard, E.G. and Peterson, R.E.: Distraction-compression bone graft arthrodesis of the ankle, a method especially applicable in children. *J. Bone Joint Surg.* 45A: 481-490, 1963.
6. Fuller, A.E. and Mackell, J.: Ankle arthrodesis—a clinical review. *J. Bone Joint Surg.* 56B: 587, 1974.
7. Johnson, E.W. Jr., and Boseker, E.: Arthrodesis of the ankle. *Arch. Surg.* 97:766-773, 1968.
8. Kennedy, J.C.: Arthrodesis of the ankle with particular reference to the Gallie procedure: a review of 50 cases. *J. Bone Joint Surg.* 42A: 1308-1316, 1960.
9. Lance, J., Pavel, T., Patterson, R., Frier, B. and Larsen, L: Ankle arthrodesis. *J. Bone Joint Surg.* 53A: 1031, 1971.
10. Milgram, JE.: Relief of the painful foot. *J. Bone Joint Surg.* 46A: 1111, 1964.
11. Murray, M.P., Gore, D.R., Sepic, S.B. and Gardner, G.M.: Walking patterns of men with unilateral surgical hip fusion. *J. Bone Joint Surg.* 57A: 761, 1975.
12. Newton, E.: Total ankle replacement arthroplasty: an alternative to ankle fusion. *J. Bone Joint Surg.* 57A: 1033, 1975.
13. Ratliff, A.H.C.: Compression arthrodesis of the ankle. *J. Bone Joint Surg.* 41B: 524, 1959.
14. Scholz, K.C.: Total ankle replacement arthroplasty. III. In Bateman, J.E. (Ed.): *Foot Science.* Philadelphia: W.B. Saunders, 1976.
15. Simon, S.R. Deutsch S.D., Nuzzo, R.M. Mansour, J.M., Jackson, J.L. and Rosenthal, R.K.: Genu recurvatum in spastic cerebral palsy. *J. Bone Joint Surgery.* 60-A: 882-894, 1978.
16. Stauffer, R.N.: Total ankle joint replacement as

an alternative to arthrodesis. *Geriatrics* 31: 79-82, 1976.

17. Thomas, F.B.: Arthrodesis of the ankle. *J. Bone Joint Surg.* 51B: 53, 1969.

18. Waugh, T. R. Evanski, P. and McMaster, W.: Irvine ankle arthroplasty: design, operative technique and preliminary results. *J. Bone Joint Surg.* 58A: 115, 1976.

19. Wesley, H.S., Kavat, R. and Kleigner, B.: Roentgen measurement of ankle flexion extension. *Clin. Ortho.* 85: 167, 1969.

20. White, A.: A precision posterior ankle fusion. *Clin. Ortho.* 98: 239-250, 1974.

21. Wilson, H.J.: Arthrodesis of ankles. *J. Bone Joint Surg.* 51A: 275, 1969.

22. Verkelst, M., Muller, J., Hoogmartens, M. and Spaar, F.: Arthrodesis of the ankle joint with complete removal of the distal part of the fibula. *Clin. Ortho.* 118: 93-99, 1976.

APPENDIX

Gait Analysis Laboratory Facilities

A gait analysis laboratory has been established at the Children's Hospital in Boston. The laboratory consists of a walkway of over 50 feet in length with a force plate midway along the walkway length. Three 16-mm cameras set at fifty frames per second are positioned to examine the patient as he crosses the force plate. The force plate is transparent, which allows a camera to be set underneath it in order to photograph the contacting area of the foot and the floor during stance phase. The force plate consists of seven piezoelectric load cells that allow force measurements to be obtained of the foot-floor contact in the vertical, fore-aft, and medial-lateral directions as well as obtaining torque and the center of pressure readings of the foot during the entire stance phase.

The film, after being developed, is analyzed on a Vanguard Motion Analyzer. Screening of each frame is made on the motion analyzer. An observer using an electronic pen can obtain the desired data points from the film. The pen is electronically on line to a PDP 11/34 Computer, and the desired information is recorded, analyzed, and plotted on an X-Y Plotter. The results of the limb displacements over the walk cycles can thus be evaluated and recorded.

Muscle activity can be simultaneously obtained from either surface or needle electrodes using lightweight EMG recording equipment. Muscular activity obtained is directly relayed to the computer and processed in a manner similar to that obtained from the force plate.

Chapter Eleven

QUADRUPLE ARTHRODESIS with ILIAC BONE GRAFT

MELVIN H. JAHSS, M.D.
PETER A. GODSICK, M.D.
HOWARD LEVIN, M.D.

We intend to present a simple, atraumatic technique of arthrodesing the subtalar complex which, to date, has given a 100 per cent success rate. The operation was performed on ninety four patients comprising one hundred and five feet (eleven had bilateral fusions). It was undertaken for subtalar disability due to varying underlying primary etiologic findings (Tables 11-1, 11-2). All but two procedures were either performed by the senior author or supervised by him, spanning a period of nineteen years.

The majority of patients were between twenty five and forty five years, surgery in the youngest age groups was usually for pain secondary to tarsal coalition, or for "spastic flat foot" where conservative therapy had failed. The most frequent primary etiologic factor was fibrous ankylosis of the subtalar complex secondary to fractures of the os calcis.

The majority of patients had fractures of the os calcis with painful limited sub-

TABLE 11-1   General Statistics

Number of patients: 94	Male: 65
Number of feet: 105	Female: 40
Pantalar (included in above): 3	Age: 13–62 years
Bilateral: 11	Follow-up: 1–19 years
Left (only): 49; Right (only): 34	

TABLE 11-2   Etiology

Fracture of os calcis (one bilateral): 34, including 3 primary arthrodeses
Spastic flat foot (includes subtalar fibrous ankylosis): 20
Tarsal coalition (15):
  a) Talocalcaneal: 11 (8 males)
  b) Calcaneonavicular: 3
  c) Talonavicular synostosis: 1
Osteoarthritis subtalar complex: 9
Poliomyelitis: 6
Rheumatoid arthritis: 5
Aseptic necrosis of adult tarsal navicular: 3
Cerebral palsy, pes cavus, failed prior triple arthrodesis: 2 each
Pes planus, arthrogryposis, bullet in posterior subtalar joint, subtalar dislocation, fracture of talus, compound fracture of ankle, crush injury: 1 each

talar motion of over one year's duration. Primary quadruple arthrodesis was done on three patients in whom the subtalar joints were severely comminuted.

"Spastic flat feet" included cases of suspected tarsal coalition such as an oblique medial facet seen on posterior tangential os calcis views. They did not include cases of hypermobile pes planus. All these patients had considerable painful restriction of subtalar motion which remained the same or moved only slightly more under general anesthesia.

93

The osteoarthritic group included cases of spastic flat feet where secondary arthritic changes were more evident on x-rays.

It is interesting to note that the vast majority of tarsal coalitions (talocalcaneal) were males. The number of calcaneonavicular bars treated was limited, owing to the fact that they were usually treated by the pediatric orthopaedic service.

Prior experience with aseptic necrosis of the adult tarsal navicular revealed that symptoms were not relieved by local fusions. Quadruple arthrodesis was necessary, as was extending the fusion to the adjacent lateral and middle cuneiforms (see fig. 11-12).

Autogenous ipsilateral iliac bone grafts were used in most cases except where large wedges of bone were removed to correct deformity (Table 11-3). In these cases the wedges of bone were used for grafting. In two patients freeze-dried bone was used. In one case "boplant" was used, with considerable soft tissue reaction occuring within a few days. More recently, sufficient bone has been obtained for grafting from the outer table and underlying cancellous portion of the distal third of the os calcis where there has been considerable lateral spread of the os calcis secondary to an old fracture. This technique relieves the tension under the peroneals, decreases the chances of the lateral abutment syndrome, and also permits soft-tissue closure without tension.

Operative Indications and Contraindications

Operative indications consisted of persistent or recurrent disabling pain in the subtalar complex which was unrelieved by conservative treatment such as shoe corrections, orthoses, anti-inflammatory medication, non-weight bearing, and sinus tarsus injections. All patients had either secondary degenerative changes noted on x-rays or painful fibrous ankylosis, in two cases due to prolonged immobilization for orthopaedic problems elsewhere in the same limb. The only patients usually without subtalar pain were those with a neurologic

TABLE 11-3   Operative Statistics

BONE GRAFTS
  a) Autogenous: 93
  b) Navy: 2
  c) "Boplant": 1 (severe reaction)
  d) None: 9

IMMOBILIZATION
  a) Long leg cast, 2 weeks, then
  b) Short leg cast
  c) Weight bearing: 6 weeks
  d) Total immobilization: 3½ months

COMPLICATIONS
  a) Infection/iliac wound: 3 (transitory)

deficit such as poliomyelitis, where gross deformity or muscle imbalance necessitated the arthrodesis followed, when indicated, by appropriate tendon transplant.

Contraindications included being over sixty two years of age, vascular impairment, diabetes, systemic problems, and poor local soft tissue, including prior infection. Forefoot equinus (including cavus) or equinovarus (e.g., compartment syndrome) was usually corrected by tarsometatarsal arthrodesis, except when the subtalar complex was painful, already fixed, or when the heel was in significant varus or valgus.

Anatomic Considerations

The standard triple arthrodesis aside from the calcaneocuboid and talonavicular joints usually includes fusion of both the posterior and medial facets of the talocalcaneal joint, the latter often through a separate medial incision. Fusion of the posterior facet requires opening the peroneal retinaculum, retracting the peroneal tendons, and cutting part of the fibular collateral ligament. This may result in some ankle instability. Excess stripping or removal of too much of the talus may cause aseptic necrosis of the talus.[2,3]

To obviate these problems, simplify the operation, and lessen the extent of soft-tissue and bone surgery, the posterior and medial facets need not be disturbed. Instead, a careful extra-articular fusion is performed in the sinus tarsus, supplemented by autogenous iliac bone. In the uncommonly seen cases of relatively marked fixed heel varus or valgus, the posterior facet will have to be exposed and an appropriate wedge resected.

An even more significant problem encountered in triple arthrodesis is the inconstant fusion of the talar head to the usually quite sclerotic adjacent navicular, resulting in approximately a 15 per cent rate of nonunion, of which 50 per cent are painful and require refusion.[1,3,4,5] Anatomic dissection reveals a ½-inch flat oval facet between the inferior lateral end of the navicular which overlaps a similar area on the upper surface of the cuboid (Fig. 11-1). This should be considered as the fourth joint of the subtalar complex. Of equal importance, one should note that there is an intersection where the anterior ends of the talus and calcaneus meet the posterior surfaces of the navicular and cuboid (Fig. 11-1). By carefully denuding this intersection as well as the naviculocuboid joint (Fig. 11-2), solid fusion is invariably obtained as well as "cross-fusions" between each of these bones (Figs. 11-3, 11-4). Thus if nonunion occurs between the talus and navicular, painless stability is assured by a plantar-based, "U"-shaped fusion between the naviculocuboid, cuboid-calcaneus, and cal-

caneotalar joints (Figs. 11-5; su Fig. 11-8)). It should be noted that the standard fusion is simply a proximally based "U"-shaped fusion (Fig. 11-6). If the talonavicular as well as the calcaneocuboid joints fail to fuse, stabilization is still assured by a cross-fusion of the navicular to the calcaneus in the form of a "Z"-fusion (Fig. 11-7) or by a calcaneotalocuboid-navicular "Z"-fusion (see Fig. 11-9).

Since 5 to 10 per cent of the calcaneo-cuboid and talocalcaneal joints may not fuse,[1,3,4,5] cross-fusions between the calcaneus and navicular (Figs. 11-7, 11-8) or talus and cuboid (Fig. 11-9) negate this problem. Aside from four possible "U"- and four "Z"-fusions, other types of fusions may occur, such as an "E"-fusion (Fig. 11-10) or combinations of U-, Z-, and E- fusions (Fig. 11-11), affording further stability as well as approaching a mathematical zero percentage of surgical failures.

Roentgenographic evaluation of cross-fusions should include routine lateral as well as overexposed anterior tangential (Figs. 11-4, 11-12) and medial oblique views of the foot. For the purpose of this study x-rays were also taken of the ankle to determine if any late degenerative changes occured in this area.

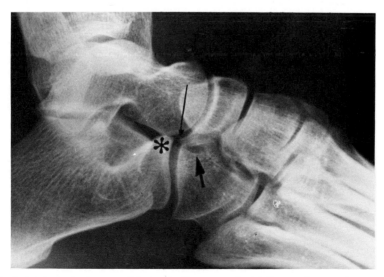

FIGURE 11-1 Lateral roentgenogram of foot revealing anatomic details: anterior-superior process of os calcis (*); naviculocuboid joint joint (heavy arrow); intersection of talus, calcaneus, navicular, and cuboid (fine arrow).

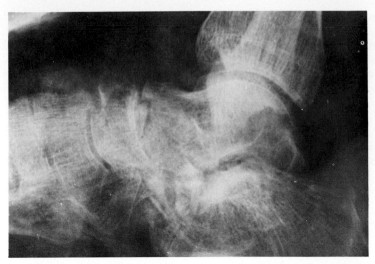

FIGURE 11-2 Postoperative appearance of quadruple arthrodesis supplemented with iliac bone. Normally, a section of outer iliac table is also laid down over fusion site. Note packing of intersection and sinus tarsus, plus denudation of all four joints.

Operative Technique

The patient is intubated and placed partially on the side opposite the surgery with the ipsilateral arm over a padded Mayo stand that is on the opposite side of the table. Sandbags are placed above the pelvis with or without a kidney rest. Pillows and blankets are placed between the legs, especially the knees, and firm blankets behind the foot and ankle for countersup-

port. Both hips and knees are kept partially flexed. No tourniquet is used—this results in minimal postoperative swelling and pain.

The main palpable landmark is the anterior-superior tubercle of the os calcis (Fig. 11-1), which marks the center of the incision. The incision starts posterior-inferiorly from the peroneal tendons just inferior and distal to the lateral malleolus, curves slightly forward and distally across

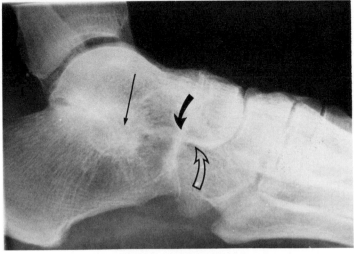

FIGURE 11-3 Lateral view revealing fusion of all elements including sinus tarsus, intersection, and naviculocuboid joint.

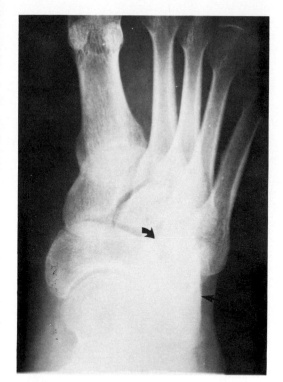

FIGURE 11-4 Anterior tangential view revealing solid lateral fusion incorporating iliac graft with lateral aspect of calcaneus, talus, navicular, and cuboid.

the anterior calcaneal tubercle, and continues to the long extensor tendons superiorly-distally. The posterior arm of this incision

should not run back any further posteriorly, as it is not only unnecessary but increases the tendency for wound slough.[3,5]

Inferiorly, just under the skin and lying on a thin layer of subcutaneous fat, may be seen one or two branches of the sural nerve, and similarly there may be found dorsally one or two branches of the superficial peroneal nerve. These cutaneous sensory branches should, if possible, be spared, especially the sural branches, as painful neuroma may occur.[3] The thin layer of subcutaneous fat and fascia is cut in line with the skin incision without retracting or undermining the skin. At this point, the peroneal retinaculum will be seen inferiorly overlying the peroneal tendons, peroneus tertius and the lateral long toe extensors will be seen superiorly. The muscle belly of the extensor digitorum brevis extends from the peroneal tendons to just under the lateral extensor tendons. A curved clamp is run under the entire muscle belly hugging bone, and the muscle is cut across and reflected to either side with the skin and subcutaneous tissue, thus creating two good vascular soft tissue flaps that permit sound skin healing. Occasionally, brisk bleeding may be encountered at this point superiorly from a branch of the lateral tarsal artery which may be tied off or controlled by pressure packing.

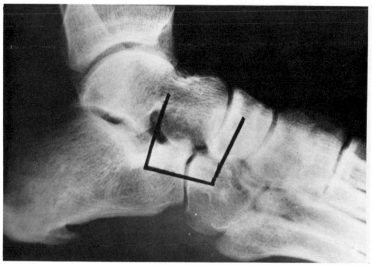

FIGURE 11-5 Plantar-based "U"-shaped fusion of naviculorcuboid, calcaneocuboid, and talocalcaneal joints. Foot is stable in spite of nonunion of talonavicular joint.

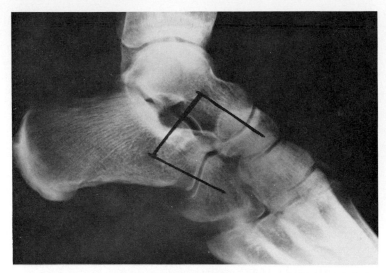

FIGURE 11–6   Standard triple arthrodesis, which is a proximally based "U"-fusion.

All further dissection is now performed with #15 blades rather than periosteal elevators, which are ineffective. In the usual fashion the capsule between the calcaneocuboid joint is excised; then the talonavicular joint, which lies superiorly in the same vertical line as the calcaneocuboid joint, is similarly excised. The sinus tarsus is cleaned out, starting under the neck of the talus and working backward toward the posterior facet, removing capsule, sinus tarsus fat pad, and interosseus ligament. The calceneocuboid and talonavicular joints are denuded of a thin layer of cortical and subchondral bone using thin flat osteotomes and curved gouges. Since most of these feet are in spastic valgus and abduction, one should avoid the tendency to remove wedges of bone wider laterally than medially, which further increases the valgus deformity. Any equinus is corrected by taking an appropriate dorsal wedge from

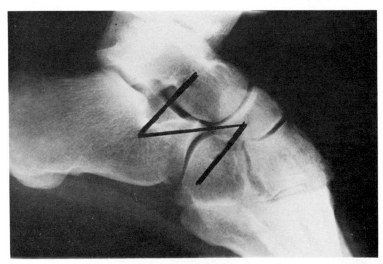

FIGURE 11–7   Transverse "Z"-fusion through intersection; it involves cuboid-navicular, naviculocalcaneal, and talocalcaneal joints. The four bones are stabilized even if nonunion occurs between the talonavicular and calcaneocuboid joints.

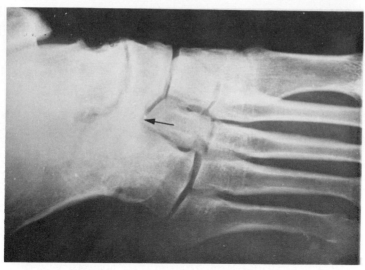

FIGURE 11-8 View illustrating nonunion of talonavicular joint, but navicular is stabilized by heavy cross-fusion to calcaneus as well as to cuboid.

the talonavicular joint and adjacent surface of the calcaneocuboid joint.

Avoid taking an excessive dorsal wedge over the lateral column of the foot for fear of creating a rocker bottom,[3] which usually occurs under the cuboid or base of the fifth metatarsal. Similarly, even a small dorsal wedge, inadvertently taken while performing a triple arthrodesis for pes planus, may cause a rocker bottom. Excess valgus is corrected by packing the joints laterally with bone graft. Occasionally, fixed contracture of the peroneus ter-

tius partially prevents the valgus correction and may be simply tenotomized. The ultimate aim is to make the foot plantigrade with the ankle at 90°, the hindfoot in neutral to 5° valgus, and, most important, all the metatarsals level. The slightest bit of forefoot varus is disastrous, since these patients no longer have compensatory subtalar motion and develop painful calluses under the fifth ray.

The sinus tarsus is now denuded of cortical bone, with interlocking strips of bone being gouged out from the inferior

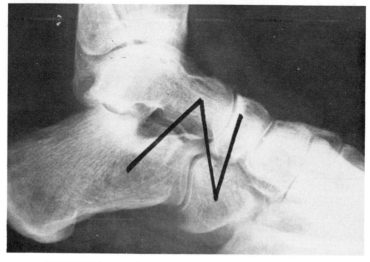

FIGURE 11-9 Calcaneotalocuboid-navicular "Z"-fusion.

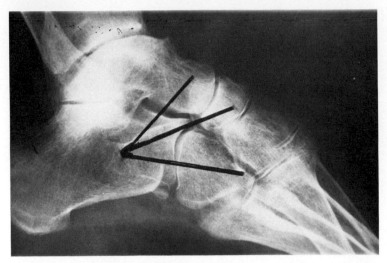

FIGURE 11–10 "E"-fusion based in cuboid.

surface of the neck of the talus and the opposing superior surface of the calcaneus. If desired, the posterior facet may be partially destroyed with small gouges or chisels at the posterior aspect of the sinus tarsus even though visualization is limited. The medial facet is left undisturbed. The *naviculocuboid* joint is now excised. The *intersection* where the talus, navicular, calcaneus, and cuboid bones join is carefully decorticated.

The lateral surface of the calcaneus is exposed posteriorly as far as the peroneal tendons and denuded of its lateral cortex using a small gouge. The strips of bone are turned down into the adjacent interesection, sinus tarsus and calcaneocuboid joint. Enough cancellous bone is also removed from the calcaneus to narrow the heel sufficiently to make room for the bone graft and also to permit lax closure of the soft-tissue flaps. In cases of prior fractures of the os calcis, the widened heel requires even further narrowing, including behind the stretched-out peroneal tendons.

Through a generous iliac incision a

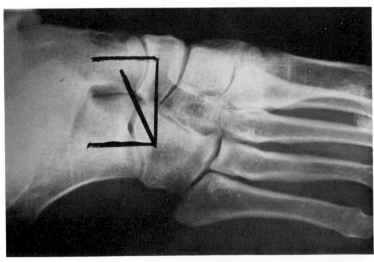

FIGURE 11–11 Distal "U" cuboid "E", plus vertical "Z"-fusion (calcaneocuboid-talonavicular). Since all bones are stabilized, nonuion between the talus and calcaneus is of no clinical significance.

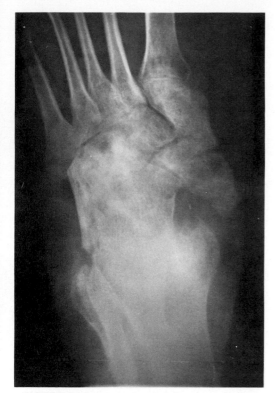

FIGURE 11-12 Anterior tangential view revealing solid lateral fusion mass. Fusion was extended to lateral and middle cuneiforms in this case of aseptic necrosis of adult tarsal navicular.

large piece (minimum, 2 in x 3 in) of outer table of ilium is removed along with as much cancellous bone as possible. The cancellous bone is packed into all the denuded joints, the sinus tarsus, and the intersection area while the foot is held in the plantigrade position. If needed, extra bone may be obtained by nicking off pieces from the removed outer table. Finally, a section of the outer table is fashioned to fit and lie over the entire raw surface of the fusion site with the smooth outer surface of the table facing laterally. As previously noted, when significant wedges of bone are removed to correct gross deformity, they are used in place of the iliac graft. In two cases, freeze-dried bone was used as graft with success and without any soft-tissue reaction. It is not necessary or advisable to use internal fixation such as staples, which were used twice.

The iliac wound is closed in the usual way using closed suction. The foot wound is closed with two mattress sutures across the muscle flaps, followed by OOO interrupted Dermalon skin sutures. Vessels are not tied but clamped and then released at the time of closure. No skin retraction is used nor are pickups on the skin used.

The foot is wrapped in sterile sheet wadding and a long leg cast is applied with the forefoot in a plantigrade position, the ankle at 90°, while the external rotation deformity that is frequently present is minimized. The knee is held in 15° to 20° of flexion. Other types of casts such as short leg casts and long leg casts with the knee in more flexion were found to be more uncomfortable postoperatively. In only one case was it necessary to split the cast owing to moderate postoperative swelling. The absence of tourniquet, avoidance of ties or coagulation currents, minimal dissection, and careful soft-tissue management result in minimal postoperative swelling and discomfort. No slough occurred except in the case in which beef bone was used as a graft.

The leg is kept elevated for four to five days. Non-weight-bearing crutch walking is permitted in seven to ten days, and short a leg cast is applied on the fourteenth day, at which time the foot and iliac sutures are removed.

Full weight bearing in a plaster boot is permitted and encouraged six weeks postoperatively, and the cast is removed three and one-half months postoperatively, irrespective of the x-ray appearance at this time, which usually reveals partial fusion. As noted, postoperative x-rays should include slightly overexposed anterior tangential and medial oblique views of the foot along with the standard lateral view. Upon removal of the final cast further support is discouraged, and the patients are taught to exercise their ankle joints, which are usually already quite supple if they have been walking in their casts. No special shoes are worn when the cast is removed.

Results

With regard to the iliac wound, there were three cases of mild infection with associated discomfort. They responded to antibiotics within a week. The use of closed suction appeared to make no difference in postoperative iliac wound discomfort or morbidity.

There were no cases of wound slough or infection in the foot, except for the one previously mentioned case where beef bone graft was used. There was no immediate postoperative morbidity, except for one case of transitory dermatitis secondary to betadine allergy. There were no cases of subcutaneous neuroma formation. One patient complained of tenderness over a buried staple.

All feet were clinically fused in three and one-half months, except for one patient for whom a further six weeks period of immobilization was necessary because of discomfort and suspected fusion failure. This patient had a severe flexible type of vertical talus with most of the talus being displaced medially, making the talonavicular and sinus tarsus fusion difficult. An accessory medial fusion probably should have been performed.

Follow-up examination revealed an average 6° to 8° loss of ankle motion (plantar flexion) compared with the normal side. However, since dorsiplantar motion occurs in the subtalar complex, the true amount of loss of ankle motion is minimal if there is any at all. No patients revealed evidence of surgically created rocker-bottom feet.

Follow-up x-rays revealed approximately 15 per cent nonunions between the navicular and talus, but in every instance fusion occurred between the navicular and cuboid or in a cross-union union to the anterior calcaneus (Fig. 11–8); the feet were free of pain and clinically solid. No nonunions occurred elsewhere. The solid mass of lateral fusion is most often discernible on the anterior tangential view. There were no cases of aseptic necrosis of the talus. Late osteoarthritis was not observed in the ankle.

SUMMARY

A technique has been described for fusing the subtalar complex which has been performed on one hundred and five feet over a period of nineteen years without one case of failure or significant postoperative morbidity. The anatomic basis and surgical technique responsible for the success rate have been carefully detailed.

REFERENCES

1. Friedenberg, Z.B.: Arthrodesis of the tarsal bones. A study of failure of fusions. *Arch. Surg.* 57:162, 1948.
2. Marek, F. M. and Schein, A. J.: Aseptic necrosis of the astragalus following arthrodesing procedures of the tarsus. *J. Bone Jont Surg.* 27: 587, 1945.
3. Patterson, R.L., Jr., Parrish, F.F. and Hathaway, E.N.: Stabilizing operations on the foot. A study of the indications, techniques used and end results. *J. Bone Joint Surg.* 32A:1, 1950.
4. Williams, P.F. and Menelaus, M.B.: Triple arthrodesis by inlay grafting—a method suitable for the undeformed or valgus foot. *J. Bone Joint Surg.* 598: 333, 1977.
5. Wilson, F.C., Jr., Gardner, F., Lamotte, P. and Williams, J.C.: Triple arthrodesis. A study of the factors affecting fusion after three hundred and one procedures. *J. Bone Joint Surg.* 47A:340, 1965.

Chapter Twelve

POST-TRAUMATIC PERONEAL TENDINITIS

Robert H. Fitzgerald, Jr., M.D.
Mark B. Coventry, M.D.

Limitation of normal excursion of the peroneal tendons at the level of the peroneal trochlea after trauma is a cause of lateral tarsal pain. It has been ascribed to traumatic arthritis of the subtalar joint, to lateral ligamentous sprain, or to involvement of the sinus tarsi. In 1927, Hackenbroch[4] described stenosing tenosynovitis of the peroneal tendon sheaths that occurred after ankle sprains in two patients as "rigid fibrous thickening of the retinaculum musculorum peronaeorum inferius." Kashiwagi and Inamatsu[7] described pain over the inferior peroneal retinaculum when callus or adhesions (or both) about the peroneal tendons followed calcaneal fractures and inhibited the normal excursion of these tendons. We wish to discuss the clinical history, physical findings, diagnostic procedures, and treatment of this syndrome.

NORMAL ANATOMY

The tendons of the peroneus longus and brevis enter a common sheath 4 cm proximal to the lateral malleolus. They pass through the superior retinaculum and behind the lateral malleolus within this common sheath. Proximal to the peroneal trochlea of the calcaneus, the tendons enter separate sheaths. Each sheath is covered by the inferior retinaculum, an extension of the cruciate crural ligament, at the level of the peroneal trochlea. The sheath about the peroneus brevis extends to within 1 cm of the insertion of the tendon into the tuberosity at the base of the fifth metatarsal. The other sheath, enveloping the tendon of the peroneus longus as it passes from the plantar aspect of the peroneal trochlea, ends as it glides to the undersurface of the cuboid. A second sheath envelops the peroneus longus as it emerges from a canal formed by the long plantar ligament and cuboid groove. In 46 percent of the specimens examined by Grant,[3] the two sheaths were in continuity on the plantar aspect of the tendon.

CLINICAL MATERIAL

Nineteen patients with pain localized to the lateral aspect of the heel after injury were studied (Table 12-1). Eleven had calcaneal fractures, six had ankle sprains, one had a medial malleolus fracture, and one had a subtalar fracture. All patients noted accentuation of the pain when walking barefoot or on rough terrain. Physical examination revealed an antalgic gait, limitation of motion of the subtalar joint, and point tenderness over the peroneal tendons at the inferior peroneal retinaculum. Forced plantar flexion and inversion accentuated the symptoms.

The diagnosis of post-traumatic peroneal tendinitis is strongly suggested if the pain is relieved by the injection of 1 to 2 ml of a local anesthetic into the tendon sheath. Peroneal tenography was performed in

TABLE 12–1   Nineteen Patients With Post-traumatic Peroneal Tendinitis

CASE	SEX AND AGE	TYPE OF TRAUMA	SYMPTOMS	DURATION	CLINICAL FINDINGS	ROENTGENO-GRAPHIC FINDINGS	TENOGRAPHIC FINDINGS	INJECTIONS Lidocaine (% Pain Relief)	Steroid	SURGICAL PATHOLOGIC FINDINGS	RESULT AND FOLLOW-UP
1	F, 49	Calcaneal fracture	Lateral heel pain	18 months	Point tenderness at inferior peroneal retinaculum; no subtalar motion; limp	Widened calcaneus; heterotopic bone	Blockage at inferior peroneal retinaculum	No injection	No	Adhesions of peroneus longus; bony prominence of lateral calcaneal wall	Good; return of subtalar motion (18 months)
2	M, 27	Calcaneal fracture	Lateral heel pain on rough terrain	3 years	Pain with inversion (limited to 5°); limp	Subtalar arthrosis	Constriction at inferior peroneal retinaculum	No injection	No	Adhesions of peroneus longus and brevis	Good (3 years)
3	F, 52	Calcaneal fracture	Lateral heel pain	12 months	Point tenderness at inferior peroneal retinaculum	Widened calcaneus	Constriction of peroneal tendon sheath	100	Yes	Constriction of both tendon sheaths at inferior peroneal retinaculum; bony prominence of lateral wall	Good (5 years)
4	M, 22	Calcaneal fracture	Lateral heel pain; inability to ambulate on rough terrain	10 months	Point tenderness at inferior peroneal retinaculum; no subtalar motion; limp	Widened calcaneus	Blockage at inferior peroneal retinaculum	85	Yes	Adhesions of peroneus longus; bony prominence	Good; return of subtalar motion (3 years)
5	F, 55	Calcaneal fracture	Lateral heel pain	12 months	No subtalar motion	Subtalar arthrosis; widened calcaneus	Attenuation of sheath of peroneus brevis	80	Yes	Frayed peroneus brevis; bony prominence	Good for 1 year; then required triple arthrodesis
6	F, 46	Calcaneal fracture	Lateral heel pain	12 months	Point tenderness at inferior peroneal retinaculum	Subtalar arthrosis; widened calcaneus	Lateral displacement of peroneal tendon sheath	50	Yes	Extensive adhesions and subluxation of peroneus brevis and longus	Good (1 year)
7	M, 24	Calcaneal fracture	Lateral heel pain	8 months	Point tenderness at inferior peroneal retinaculum; limp	Widened calcaneus with hypertrophic bone	Blockage of dye at inferior peroneal retinaculum	90	No	Extensive adhesions of both peroneus longus and brevis; bony prominence	Good (3 years)
8	M, 51	Calcaneal fracture	Lateral heel pain	11 years	No subtalar motion	Subtalar arthrosis	Not performed	70	Yes	Adhesions of peroneus longus and brevis	Good (2 years)
9	M, 53	Calcaneal fracture	Lateral heel pain	5 years	No subtalar motion; point tenderness at inferior peroneal retinaculum; forced inversion—painful	Subtalar arthrosis	Not performed	No injection	No	Adhesions of peroneus longus and brevis; bony prominence	Good; return of subtalar motion (3 years)
10	M, 63	Calcaneal fracture	Lateral heel pain	12 months	Tenderness over peroneal tendons	Widened calcaneus; subtalar arthrosis	Blockage at inferior peroneal retinaculum	No injection	No	Adhesions of peroneus longus and brevis; pseudoderms form	Good for 5 years; then a triple arthrodesis was performed
11	F, 65	Calcaneal fracture	Lateral heel pain	6 years	Tenderness of peroneal tendons	Widened calcaneus	Not performed	100	Yes	No surgery	75% relief of pain (3 years)
12	M, 33	Subtalar fracture	Lateral ankle pain, "giving away"	10 months	Point tenderness at inferior peroneal retinaculum; no subtalar motion; limp	Subtalar incongruity	Constriction at inferior peroneal retinaculum	50	Yes	Adhesions of peroneus longus and brevis	Good, but has mild pain on medial aspect of ankle (2 years)
13	M, 47	Medial malleolar fracture	Lateral heel fracture with radiation into peroneal muscles	2 years	Point tenderness at inferior peroneal retinaculum; 5° inversion	Mild arthrosis of ankle	Attenuation of tendon sheath of peroneus longus or brevis at inferior retinaculum	75	Yes	Adhesions of peroneus longus with pseudotumor formation; old avulsion of inferior peroneal retinaculum	Good (2 years)
14	M, 51	Inversion ankle sprain	Lateral heel pain on rough terrain	11 months	Tenderness over inferior peroneal retinaculum	Heterotopic bone in soft tissues laterally	Blockage of dye at inferior peroneal retinaculum	90	Yes	Pseudotumor formation of peroneus longus; heterotopic bone within substance of peroneus longus	Continued pain but not incapacitating; neuroma of sural nerve (2 years)
15	F, 20	Inversion ankle sprain	Lateral heel pain	12 months	Tenderness over inferior peroneal retinaculum	Normal	Not performed	100	Yes	Constriction of peroneus longus; heterotopic bone within substance of peroneus longus	Good (10 years)
16	M, 41	Inversion ankle sprain	Lateral heel pain	12 months	Point tenderness over inferior peroneal retinaculum	Normal	Constriction of peroneal tendon sheaths at inferior peroneal retinaculum	100	Yes	Constriction of peroneus longus and brevis at the back of the inferior peroneal retinaculum	No improvement (medically retired)
17	F, 18	Inversion ankle sprain	Lateral heel pain	7 months	Restriction (50%) of subtalar motion; limp; tenderness over inferior peroneal retinaculum	Normal	Not performed	100	Yes	No surgery	Good; return of full subtalar motion (2 years)
18	F, 57	Inversion ankle sprain	Lateral heel pain	6 months	Tenderness over inferior peroneal retinaculum	Normal	Not performed	95	Yes	No surgery	Good (3 years)
19	M, 32	Inversion ankle sprain	Lateral heel pain	3 years	Forced plantar flexion with inversion recreated pain	Normal	Not performed	100	Yes	No surgery	Good (2 years)

twelve patients by the intrasynovial injection of Hypaque 60 into the common peroneal tendon sheath proximal to the ankle.[1] The procedures were performed under roentgenographic control with an image intensifier. In all twelve patients, either complete block or construction of the peroneal tendon sheath(s) at the level of the inferior peroneal retinaculum was demonstrated. In those patients with incomplete block on tenography, a pseudotumor formation of the peroneus longus was noted at the level of the inferior peroneal retinaculum (Fig. 12–1).

Four patients did not undergo surgery: three with ankle sprain and one with a calcaneal fracture. In these four, the injection of a steroid, in addition to the local anes-

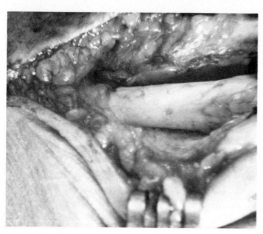

FIGURE 12-1. Pseudotumor formation of peroneal tendon just proximal to inferior peroneal retinaculum.

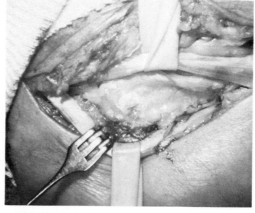

FIGURE 12-2. Bony prominence of lateral calcaneal wall beneath peroneus longus tendon.

thetic, resulted in complete relief of symptoms. During twenty-four months of follow-up, none has required further treatment. The other ten who received an intrasynovial injection of steroid experienced only temporary pain relief of from two to seven days.

Fifteen patients (ten with os calcis fracture, three with ankle sprain, one with a subtalar fracture, and one with a medial malleolar fracture) underwent surgical exploration of the peroneal tendon sheaths. All fifteen were found to have fibrosis and scarring of the peroneal tendons. Release of the retinaculum and tenolysis of the peroneus longus and brevis (leaving the sheaths open) were performed in all the patients. Of the fifteen, six (all with old calcaneal fractures) had excision of bony prominences of the lateral calcaneal wall beneath the peroneal tendon sheaths (Fig. 12-2). One patient with the residual of an inversion sprain had heterotopic bone within the substance of the peroneus longus tendon; the heterotopic bone was excised, in addition to decompression of the peroneal tendons. These procedures afforded relief of pain that varied by patient estimate from 80 to 100 percent in twelve of the fifteen patients.

Of the fifteen surgical patients, two who were unrelieved after surgery had had inversion ankle sprains that occurred at work. Neither patient had roentgeno-

graphic evidence of injury to the subtalar joint. One of these patients without subtalar motion either before or after operation had sufficient improvement (50 to 60 percent) to begin farming, but he found that ambulation on rough terrain was difficult. The other patient whose occupation required extensive ambulation was forced to seek medical retirement. Two other patients noted significant improvement for one to five years after surgery. Both patients had roentgenographic evidence of incongruity and early degenerative changes of the subtalar joint. However, both patients have had triple arthrodesis for degenerative arthrosis of the subtalar joint one and five years after tenolysis of the peroneal tendons. The remaining eleven patients (os calcis fracture in eight, ankle sprain in one, subtalar fracture in one, medial malleolar fracture in one) returned to their previous occupations, which were varied in their physical requirements.

ILLUSTRATIVE CASE REPORTS

Case 4 (Table 12-1). A 22-year-old man fell 40 feet from a roof, sustaining compression fractures of T11 and L1 and comminuted fracture of the calcaneus (Fig. 12-3). Closed reduction using a Steinmann pin, as described by Essex-Lopresti,[2] partially restored the subtalar joint, but the lateral calcaneal wall remained

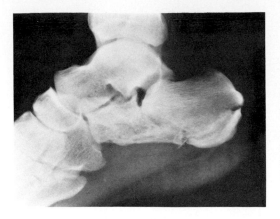

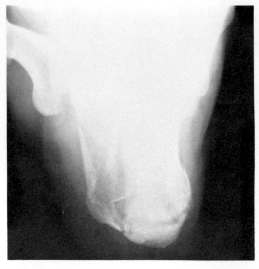

FIGURE 12–3. Comminuted calcaneal fracture with loss of tuber joint angle and displacement of lateral wall of calcaneus (case 4).

displaced and bulging (Fig. 12-4). After six weeks of cast immobilization, partial weight bearing was begun. With resumption of full weight bearing, he noted pain over the lateral aspect of the ankle.

Ten months after his injury, he could walk only one block with shoes and only short distances barefoot because of pain in the lateral ankle and heel region (Fig. 12-5). Walking on uneven surfaces precipitated exquisite pain. Examination revealed no eversion or inversion motion at the subtalar region. Pressure over the peroneal tendons opposite the os calcis and forced plantar flexion reproduced his pain. An injection of 2 ml of 1 percent lidocaine into the

common peroneal tendon sheath afforded the patient significant relief of pain. Peroneal tenography demonstrated stenosis of the tendon sheaths at the level of the inferior peroneal retinaculum (Fig. 12-6). Surgery revealed that the peroneus longus was adherent to its tendon sheaths at the level of the inferior peroneal retrophic bone. Release of the inferior peroneal retinaculum, tenolysis, and excision of the hypertrophic bone relieved the symptoms. Three years after the procedure, the patient was employed full time as a dispatcher and could walk considerable distances without pain.

Case 13. (Table 12-1). A 47-year-old man fell from a flatbed truck, sustaining a medial

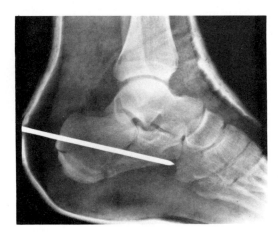

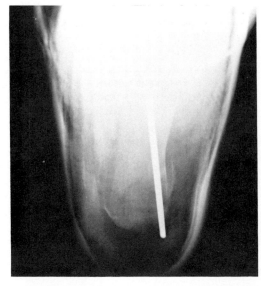

FIGURE 12–4. Closed reduction was performed with a Steinmann pin, using method of Essex-Lopresti. Lateral wall remained displaced (case 4).

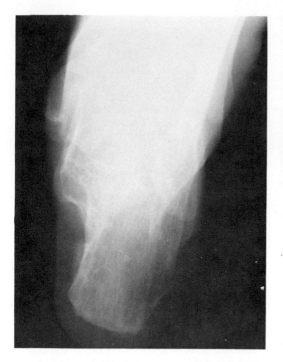

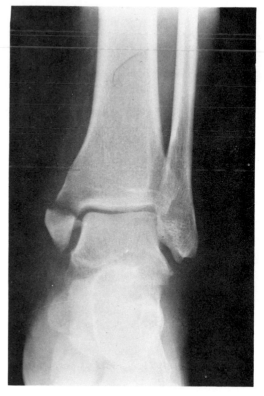

FIGURE 12–5. Distortion of subtalar joint and widening of lateral calcaneal wall one year after fracture (case 4).

malleolar fracture that was treated with open reduction and internal fixation in 1973 (Fig. 12–7). With removal of the cast and resump-

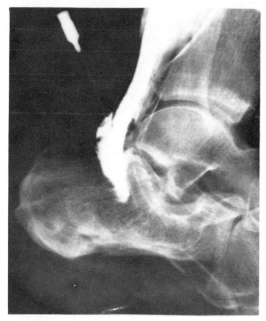

FIGURE 12–6. Partial filling of peroneus brevis tendon sheath and complete blockage of dye in peroneus longus tendon sheath proximal to inferior peroneal retinaculum (case 4).

FIGURE 12–7. Medial malleolar fracture sustained in a fall (case 13).

tion of weight bearing, the patient noted persistent lateral ankle pain. The medial malleolar screws were removed eight months postoperatively, without relief of his pain.

When first seen at the Mayo Clinic, the patient complained of lateral ankle and heel pain with extension into the peroneal musculature (Fig. 12-8). He had an antalgic, flatfooted gait. There was diffuse tenderness over the calcaneofibular ligament and peroneal tendons, with loss of subtalar motion. Initially, he was treated with a patellar-tendon-bearing brace and obtained partial relief of his symptoms for one year. At that time, the tenderness was localized to the peroneal tendons at the level of the inferior peroneal retinaculum. An intrasynovial injection of 2 ml of 1 percent lidocaine and 0.5 ml of betamethasone relieved 75 percent of the discomfort. A peroneal tenogram demonstrated constriction of the peroneus longus at the level of the inferior peroneal retinaculum (Fig. 12-9). At surgery, the peroneus longus was firmly scarred to adjacent soft-tissue structures, beginning just proximal to the peroneal trochlea and the inferior peroneal retinaculum and continuing distally for approximately 2 cm. There was pseudotumorous enlargement of the tendon proximal to the constriction by scar tissue. Once the tendon had been freed of adhesions and the inferior peroneal retinaculum released, a small (0.5 x 0.5 x 0.5 cm) cartilaginous

nodule could be palpated within the substance of the tendon. The peroneus brevis had a normal excursion.

The patient has been followed for two years after tenolysis. He has returned to his occupation as an automobile mechanic, working eight to ten hours a day. He has had 90 percent of his pain relieved. He avoids walking on rough terrain (no subtalar motion was restored by surgery).

DISCUSSION

Although Hackenbroch[4] credited Hildebrand[5] with the initial description of this syndrome, Hildebrand actually described luxation of the peroneal tendons at the level of the fibula after injury to the superior peroneal retinaculum and used the term "tendovaginitis chronica deformans." The increased mobility and dislocation of the tendons distinguish it from the post-traumatic peroneal tendinitis that Hackenbroch so clearly described.

Parvin and Ford[8] discussed the gross thickening of the common peroneal tendon sheath and constriction of the peroneal tendons proximal to the peroneal tubercle within the common sheath behind the lateral malleolus. The similarity of this syn-

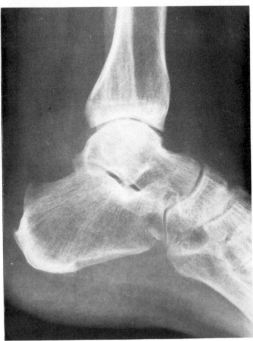
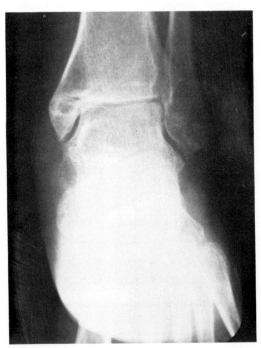

FIGURE 12-8.   Roentgenographic appearance after removal of internal malleolar screws (case 13).

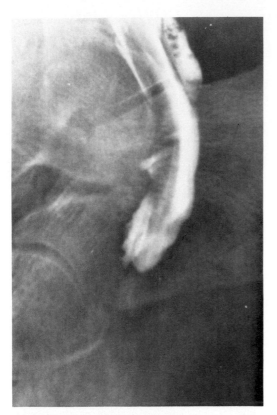

FIGURE 12-9. Peroneal tenogram. Blockage of dye about both tendons and constriction of peroneus longus tendon sheath (case 13).

drome to de Quervain's disease resulted in their use of "stenosing tenosynovitis" of the common peroneal tendon sheaths to describe the syndrome. Neither of the two patients described by Parvin and Ford had a history of trauma, and neither had difficulty in walking on rough terrain. The pathologic changes noted were similar but were located about the superior peroneal retinaculum.

In describing calcaneofibular abutment after crush fracture of the calcaneus, Isbister[6] noted compression of the peroneal tendons in two of five patients. He advocated excision of the tip of the fibula for relief of symptoms.

Subtalar or triple arthrodesis has often been the treatment for residual pain after calcaneal fractures, on the assumption that the pain is caused by arthritis. Some pa-

tients have peroneal tendinitis that is amenable to a more limited procedure. As demonstrated by the two patients who subsequently underwent triple arthrodesis, peroneal tenolysis does not preclude further surgery if the derangement of the subtalar joint requires it at a future date. Although many of our patients did not obtain complete relief of pain, all but two noted alleviation of 80 to 100 percent of preoperative discomfort. The two patients who failed to achieve satisfactory results after peroneal tenolysis achieved temporary relief with an intrasynovial steroid and lidocaine injection and had evidence of abnormality on peroneal tenograms. Although neither patient had roentgenographic evidence of an injury to the subtalar joint, no motion of the subtalar joint was present after an apparent inversion ankle sprain. We cannot identify any factors that explain these failures.

One should suspect this syndrome in all patients who have persistent pain after calcaneal fracture, or after any ankle injury, if the pain is in the region of the peroneal tendons distal to the lateral malleolus.

REFERENCES

1. Deyerle, W. M.: Long term follow-up of fractures of the os calcis: diagnostic peroneal synoviagram. *Ortho. Clin. North Amer.* 4:213-27, 1973.
2. Essex-Lopresti, P.: The mechanism, reduction technique, and results in fractures of the os calcis. *Brit. J. Surg.* 39:395-419, 1952.
3. Grant, J. C. B.: *An Atlas of Anatomy.* (4 th Ed.). Baltimore: Williams & Wilkins Company, 1956, Figure 287.
4. Hackenbroch, M.: Eine seltene Lokalisation der stenosierenden Tendovaginitis (an der Sehnenscheide bei Peroneen). *Munch. Med. Wochenschr.* 1: 932, 1927.
5. Hildebrand, O.: Tendovaginitis chronica deformans und Luxation der Peronealsehnen. *Dtsch. Z. Chir.* 86:526-31, 1907.
6. Isbister, J. F. S. C.: Calcaneo-fibular abutment following crush fracture of the calcaneus. *J. Bone Joint Surg.* 56B:274-78, 1974.
7. Kashiwagi, D. and Inamatsu, N.: Diagnosis and treatment of fractures of the os calcis. *Kobe J. Med. Sci.* 11 Suppl: 21-26, 1965.
8. Parvin, R. W. and Ford, L. T.: Stenosing tenosynovitis of the common peroneal tendon sheath. *J. Bone Joint Surg.* 38A:1352-57, 1956.

Chapter Thirteen

RECURRENT DISLOCATION OF THE PERONEAL TENDONS

A. A. Savastano, M.D.

Traumatic dislocation of the peroneal tendons was first described by Monteggia in a ballet dancer. Since then a number of articles have appeared in the literature. The most common cause of traumatic dislocation of the peroneal tendons is skiing, although other sports such as football, soccer, basketball, and ice skating produce their quota of such injuries. An article by Mounier-Kuhn and Marsann[1] indicates that twenty-two of their cases occurred in males and twenty-two in females in their series of forty-four, but ten of our eleven cases occurred in males and one in a young woman. The youngest in our series was a twelve-year-old girl and the oldest was a thirty-three year-old male.

ANATOMY OF THE PERONEAL MECHANISM

The peroneal muscles arise from the lateral surface of the fibula, the intermuscular septa, and the crural fascia.[2] They extend obliquely downward into tendons that pass behind the fibular malleolus, applying themselves closely to a shallow groove in the posterior portion of the fibular malleolus. Slightly beyond the tip of the fibula, they separate and continue to their insertion. The peroneus longus inserts into the lateral side of the base of the first metatarsal and the lateral side of the first cuneiform, the peroneus brevis inserts into the tuberosity at the base of the fifth metatarsal bone. A common sheath encloses them as they pass behind the fibula. A thickened portion of the sheath lying about 1 cm above the fibular tip is known as the superior retinaculum. In effect, these tendons are contained in a fibro-osseous tunnel as they pass behind the fibula, the medial border of which is formed by strong fibers of the posterior talofibular and calcaneofibular ligaments.[2] The anterior wall is made up of the bony ridge of the fibular groove and the retinaculum which arises from it. The retinaculum and calcaneofibular ligament inserting into the os calcis form the posterior wall of the tunnel. The peroneals are active evertors of the foot; however, they also act in synergism with other flexor and extensor tendons. They contribute to the final pronation and push off in the second stage of walking. They also contribute considerably to the stability of the ankle joint.[2]

The peroneus longus and brevis are supplied by a branch of the superficial peroneal nerve containing fibers from the 4th and 5th lumbar and 1st sacral nerves. The sural nerve, which is formed by the junction of the medial sural cutaneous with the peroneal anastamotic branch, is an important nerve on the lateral aspect of the ankle.[2]

Anatomic variance may contribute to dislocations. A shallow depression on the posterior aspect of the distal fibula may be responsible for some of the dislocations

Edwards found that the groove was

absent in 11 per cent of his cases and that actual convexity was found in 7 per cent. The retinaculum may also be subject to considerable variation, since it may be totally absent or may be lax, as is found in cases of polio. People who are subjected to habitual pronation may also have a lax retinaculum; this occurs in jockeys.

Regarding the mechanism of injury, as previously stated, the ankle goes into a sudden forceful dorsiflexion with the foot slightly inverted, followed by a violent reflex contraction of the peroneals. For the dislocation to take place, the peroneals must go into a violent reflex action. When these accidents occur during skiing, the usual course is that the ski tip dives into the snow, becomes fixed there, and the patient is thrown forward, causing a dorsiflexion of the ankle. Other injuries that may be present include rupture of the Achilles tendon, transverse fracture of the tibia, and transverse fracture of the fibula.

ETIOLOGY

Although trauma is the predominant cause of these lesions, some authors indicate that there are associated causative factors. Among these are a congenitally shallow retromalleolar groove and underdeveloped fibrous sheaths. The most frequent congenital anomaly found in the series of Mounier-Kuhn and Marsan[1] was a congenital subluxation or dislocation of the peroneal tendon.

Acquired lesions,[3] such as fractures of the external malleolus, can also result in displacement of the tendons, either from callus formation or from an ununited marginal fragment.

Some of the lesions may primarily involve the fibrous portion of the sheath and may represent either a rupture of the sheath from the posterior edge of the malleolus or an actual avulsion of its bony attachment.

DIAGNOSIS

It must be repeated that it is very important to be careful in making a diag-nosis when there is a history of an injury to the outer aspect of the ankle. In taking x-rays, stress films of the ankle are advised when there is any question of the integrity of the mortise. A diagnosis of traumatic dislocation of the peroneal tendons may be obscured by spontaneous reduction or by swelling and edema with hemorrhage. The swelling and ecchymosis, whether complete or partial, are usually present in the region of the superior peroneal retinaculum in the early stages. Sharp tenderness in the sulcus as well as along the distal fibula is characteristic. The pain is usually increased by eversion of the foot against resistance. X-rays should be taken which may indicate an avulsion fracture, stress films, as stated, occasionally are necessary. The x-rays may reveal a rim type of fracture.

In chronic cases this condition is often misdiagnosed as a chronic ankle sprain. The clinical aspects of this syndrome can present different pictures. The syndrome may be characterized by intermittent swelling over the peroneal tendons as they loop around the external malleolus following a traumatic incident during which the ankle dorsiflexes and inverts. In this type of lesion, the patient usually does not seek medical attention until several months or even years after the initial injury.

Another form of the peroneal tendon syndrome is characterized by the tendons slipping practically with each step or by the tendons remaining always displaced. These patients, too, generally visit a physician long after the initial cause.

In another situation, the tendons will dislocate and remain irreducibly dislocated.

Peroneal tenosynovitis can be found following injuries and is characterized by swelling and pain behind the external malleolus.

In the usual case the patient will give a history of acute trauma. In most cases the injury will result from the ankle being forcibly dorsiflexed and inverted. Soon after the incident the patient will present with tenderness over the external malleolar area associated with swelling and ecchymosis. X-rays are usually negative, although they may show a fracture of the distal tip of the fibula or an osteoperiosteal tear at the distal end of the fibula. In most of these cases, a clinical diagnosis of sprain of the lateral ligament of the ankle joint is made. If a very careful examination of the ankle is made at this time, one may or may not be able to dislocate the peroneal tendon by having the patient dorsiflex and invert the foot at the ankle, at the same time grasping the peroneal tendons and pushing them up over the external malleolar area. In these instances it is the superior retinaculum that ruptures. These cases will present moderate swelling around the external fibular malleolus together with moderate tenderness along the posterior border of the fibula. If an attempt is made to feel the tendons one can feel two round, thin ropes rolling underneath the fingers. X-rays should be taken to rule out fractures.

The peroneus longus and brevis may dislocate at the same time; if only one of the tendons dislocates, it is usually the peroneus brevis. At surgery one may find the tendons to be frayed, roughened, or even split into two or more strips.

TREATMENT

Initial treatment should always be conservative. The usual conservative treatment should consist of strapping, compression, elevation, and ice applications. If one is sure of the diagnosis, the application of a plaster boot with the foot in slight equinus and eversion is important, and this should be left in place from four to six weeks. If a recurrence takes place, the treatment of choice is surgery. Among the types of repairs that have been used are:

1. Deepening of the fibular sulcus.

2. Simple suture of the retinaculum.

3. A periosteal flap may be raised from the external malleolus and rotated to reinforce the posterior portion of the tendon sheath.

4. The sheath may be reattached to the external malleolus by using a Bankhart type of repair, attaching it through drill holes.

5. Plication of fibrous sheaths into the malleolar periosteum.

6. Bone block operation of DuVries.[5]

7. The use of slings. Either a slip of the tendo achillis[4] or the plantaris tendon may be used.[6] All of our cases were treated with a tendo achillis sling.

OPERATIVE TECHNIQUE (ELLIS JONES)

A longitudinal incision, about 3. in long, is made along the posterior margin of the lateral malleolus (Fig. 13-1). The sural nerve is identified and retracted with a Penrose rubber drain (Fig. 13-2). The stretched or detached superior retinaculum is freed from its malleolar attachment and the peroneal tendons exposed. The tendo achillis is exposed and a flap is dissected from its lateral border for a distance of 5 in. in length and 1/4 in. in width, leaving it attached to the calcaneus (Fig. 13-3).

The lateral malleolus is exposed and a

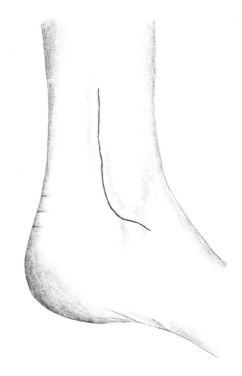

FIGURE 13-1. Line of incision, about 3 in. in length, made along posterior margin of lateral malleolus.

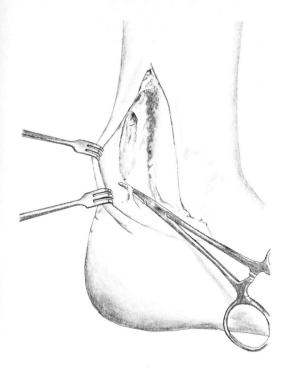

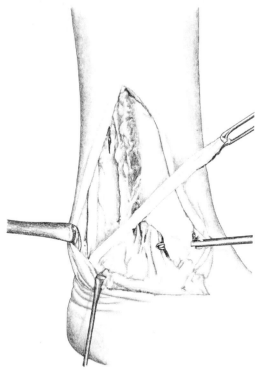

FIGURE 13-2. Sural nerve exposed and retracted Posteriorly with Penrose rubber drain.

FIGURE 13-3. Flap of tendo achillis dissected free from its lateral border, a distance of 5 in. in length and 1/4 in. in width, leaving it attached to calcaneus. A 3/8 in. drill hole is made in tip of external malleolus.

drill hole 3/8 in. in circumference is made through it in an anteroposterior direction.

The free end of the tendo achillis flap is drawn through the hole from posterior to anterior and sutured upon itself and to the periosteum (Fig. 13-4). The superior retinaculum is repaired whenever possible. The subcutaneous layer and skin are closed in the usual manner and a plaster boot is applied with the ankle at right angle.

POST-OPERATIVE CARE

This has consisted of keeping the patient in a plaster boot for four to six weeks. Crutches with weight bearing is the rule during the plaster boot phase. Following the removal of the plaster boot a cane is used and gradual exercises are started.

Case Report

This is the case of a twenty-three-year-old varsity basketball player who collided with an opponent in an intercollegiate basketball game in December 1968, sustaining an injury to his left ankle. Immediately following the injury he could not walk; he hopped off the basketball court and was immediately examined. At the time he had extreme tenderness over both the internal and external malleolar areas and had difficulty in everting, inverting, dorsiflexing, and plantar flexing his ankle. Immediate compression bandages were applied together with ice applications and elevation, in spite of which the ankle became moderately swollen and remained quite tender. Repeat x-rays in multiple views, as well as stress films, were negative. A few days later a plaster boot was applied because of the persistence of the pain. The plaster boot was left in place for approximately three weeks. The pain subsided; however, as the

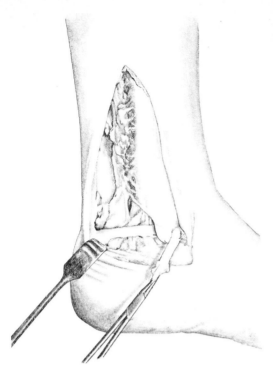

FIGURE 13–4. Free end of tendo achillis flap drawn through hole in distal tip of lateral malleolus, suturing it upon itself and thus maintaining peroneal tendons in the fibular sulcus.

patient resumed practice sessions he felt something repeatedly slip in his ankle, causing him to stop practice. A diagnosis of chronic dislocation of the peroneal tendons was made, as we could manually dislocate the tendons. An attempt was made to keep him playing by strapping his ankle with a compression felt pad over the external malleolar area. This failed; consequently, he underwent a tendon achillis sling surgical repair in April 1969 with an excellent result. He gradually resumed basketball practice and did play the following two seasons without any problems whatsoever. He regained full and complete eversion, inversion, dorsiflexion and plantar flexion and has offered no complaints whatever to date, even after strenuous workouts or intercollegiate basketball games.

In summary, the operation was done on eleven different patients, ten of whom were males and one was a female. The youngest was twelve years of age and the oldest thirty-three years of age. The left ankle was affected seven times and the right ankle four times. Three were injured while playing basketball, two during football, three during track, one during soccer, one fell off a ladder, and another tripped over a stone (Table 13-1). The final results were excellent in every case. None of our patients had any appreciable problem with their feet before injury.

RESULTS

The results in our cases have been excellent, as all of our patients have returned to their previous sport or activity with full and complete participation. In particular, we have had no problems with the tendo achillis and there has been no

TABLE 13–1   Statistics*

PATIENT	SEX	OPERATION DATE	SIDE AFFECTED	PHYSICAL ENDEAVOR	FINAL RESULT
WB	M	6-2-72	Left	Basketball	Excellent
GB	M	11-1-71	Left	Baseball	Excellent
JM	M	6-8-73	Right	Track	Excellent
LL	m	6-2-72	Left	Basketball	Excellent
EM	M	4-23-69	Left	Basketball	Excellent
LEB	M	3-16-70	Left	Soccer	Excellent
LB	M	2-4-72	Left	Football	Excellent
CEA	M	5-4-72	Right	Track	Excellent
CA	M	9-10-71	Right	Tripped on stone	Excellent
GHR	M	1-19-72	Left	Football	Excellent
CG	F	2-1-78	Left	Track	Excellent

*The longest follow-up is nine years, the shortest is four months, the mean being six years.

weakness of dorsiflexion or eversion of the ankle.

CONCLUSIONS

1. Take a careful history of the mechanics of injury.

2. X-rays, including stress films, are essential.

3. Treat early cases conservatively.

4. Recurrent cases should be treated surgically.

REFERENCES

1. Mounier-Kuhn, A. and Marsan, C. L.: Peroneal tendon syndrome. *Ann. de Chirurgie* 22:641–49, 1967.
2. Gray, H. F.R.S., Lewis, W. H.: *Anatomy of the Human Body*. Pliladelphia: Lea & Febiger.
3. Murr, S.J.: Dislocation of the peroneal tendons with marginal fracture of the lateral malleolus. *J. Bone Joint Surg.* 43B:563–65, 1961.
4. Jones, E.: Operative treatment of chronic dislocation of peroneal tendons. *J. Bone Joint Surg.* 14:574, 1932.
5. Du Vries, H. L.: *Surgery of the Foot*. St. Louis: C.V. Mosby Co., 1959.
6. Miller, J.W.: Dislocation of peroneal tendons—a new operative procedure. *Am. J. Ortho.* 9:136–37, 1967.

Chapter Fourteen

GRICE ARTHRODESIS IN NONPARALYTIC FLEXIBLE FLAT FEET

Nicholas J. Giannestras, M.D.
Ronald W. Smith, M.D.

Subtalar arthrodesis has been used for almost seventy-five years to correct the valgus foot deformity.[12] This stabilization procedure has been used for paralytic, rigid, and flexible flat-foot deformities.[6,8,16] In 1952 Grice reported an extra-articular method of fusing the subtalar joint for correction of paralytic valgus deformities. The extra-articular operation did not interfere with growth of the tarsal bones of children and precluded the loss of height in the hind foot that occurred with other techniques of talocalcaneal arthrodesis.

Most evaluations of the Grice procedure have been done in patients with paralytic deformities. The few studies that have dealt with nonparalytic flat feet have offered conflicting conclusions about the usefulness of the operation.

Our study of fifty-three feet, all nonparalytic flexible flat feet, is a roentgenographic and in-depth clinical evaluation of patients who have had a Grice procedure at least five years prior to re-examination.

Our pre-study questions included:

1. Did the Grice procedure provide demonstrable lasting correction of the longitudinal arch?
2. Did an adjunct anterior tibial tendon transfer improve the result?
3. Did the use of distal fibular graft cause ankle valgus?
4. Were there resultant secondary changes in the peritalar joints?

MATERIALS AND METHODS

The operations reviewed were performed between 1959 and 1971 by Dr. Giannestras. Indications for surgery were the presence of symptomatic flat feet that did not respond to treatment with shoe corrections and arch supports. "Symptomatic" referred to foot or leg pain.

The surgical technique followed closely that described by Grice and is as follows:

The incision was centered over the sinus tarsi, extending from the border of the peroneus tertius medially to the level of the peroneal tendon sheath laterally. The exposure was enhanced by partially reflecting the origin of the extensor digitorum brevis. The soft tissue in the sinus tarsi was removed. The calcaneus was reduced under the talus, correcting the excessive heel valgus. With the talocalcaneal relationship reduced, an osteotome was placed vertically in the sinus tarsi to act as a temporary buttress. The proper width of the osteotome was selected to maintain the talocalcaneal relationship. Slots were fashioned in the superior surface of the anterior calcaneus and the inferior surface of the neck of the talus. Since 1963 the graft has been taken from the distal fibula, at least 10 cm above the tip of the lateral malleolus. A full thickness of fibula has been used. The ends of the graft were cut obliquely to be fashioned as pegs, which fit into the slots in the talus and calcaneus. The graft was impacted into place.

Cases treated before 1963 were performed with bone graft from the proximal tibia as originally described by Grice.

Thirteen patients (twenty-four feet) received a transfer of the tibialis anterior tendon as an adjunct to the subtalar arthrodesis. The technique involved dividing the tendon from its insertion and passing it from plantar to dorsal through a hole drilled in the medial tuberosity of the navicular. The tendon was then reflected on itself and sutured.

Closure was made with a synthetic absorbable suture or subcuticular wire. A short leg cast was well molded under the medial arch. Weight bearing was not permitted. The cast was removed when the graft appeared on roentgenogram to be incorporated, usually two to three months after surgery.

A total of thirty-two patients were sought for review, but four patients were lost to follow-up. Of the twenty-eight patients located, all but three of them were examined recently by the authors. The other three patients had moved away and were examined by orthopaedic surgeons in their area according to a protocol.

Twenty-five of the patients had bilateral Grice procedures; a total of fifty-three feet were evaluated. Thirteen of the twenty-eight patients were male. The mean age of all patients (both sexes) at the time of surgery was twelve years and ranged from five to thirty years. At follow-up the mean age was twenty-three years and ranged from fifteen to forty-five years. The average follow-up was eleven years and ranged from five years to seventeen years.

The evaluations included a history of pre- and postoperative symptoms, physical examination, photographs to show the arch and hindfoot posture, and standing roentgenograms of the feet and ankles. Preoperative standing x-rays of the feet were available for review in twenty-one patients.

Symptoms

The patients were asked about pain or fatigue in the feet or legs before operation and at the time of follow-up. A query was made about shoe wear before and after surgical correction.

Medial Longitudinal Arch

The medial longitudinal arch was considered satisfactory if, upon examination of the feet on a glass-top footstool, one third or more of the arch was free of weight-bearing contact. The footstool allowed visualization of the plantar surface of the feet while they were in a weight-bearing posture.

Subtalar Motion

The restriction of subtalar motion was classified as severe, moderate, mild, or unrestricted. "Severe" restriction meant that there was almost no movement as the hind foot was passively abducted or adducted. "Mild" restriction was applied to patients who had minimal or no restriction of adduction, though abduction was limited to the neutral position.

Ankle Motion

Ankle motion was measured goniometrically with the patient prone and the knee flexed 90°. The angle was measured between the distal fibula and the plane of the plantar aspect of the lateral midfoot.

Hindfoot Position

The presence of heel varus or valgus was assessed by observing the posterior aspect of the hind foot with the patient standing. Where present, the impression of heel varus was confirmed by the photographs or by excessive lateral heel wear on the shoes.

Roentgenographic Evaluation

The roentgenographic examinations studied included the standing anterior-posterior and lateral views of the feet and the standing anterior-posterior and lateral views of the ankle. Roentgenographic arch measurements studied on the lateral view of the foot included the talar flexion angle,[5] the lateral talocalcaneal angle, the calcaneal-first metatarsal angle, the naviculo-cuneiform angle,[3] and the arch ratio.[2] The calcaneal pitch (the longitudinal axis of the calcaneus relative to the plantar surface of the foot) was also measured but was not considered an index of the medial longitudinal arch (Fig.14-1).

Measurements made on the anterior-posterior view of the foot were not empha-

sized. They were diffi assess in the mature foo ping shadows of the tar tibia. Articulations adja joint were closely exam tive changes, particula spur formation. Standin examined for angular de otalar joint and pseudar fibula graft donor site.

RESULT

Clinical Asse

Relief of Symptoms

Twenty-one patients or almost complete relief leg symptoms after ope tients felt that, though symptomatic relief, some still present, at least durin

Two patients would they had to make the cho these patients had a varu was bothered by abnorm other patient was a danc

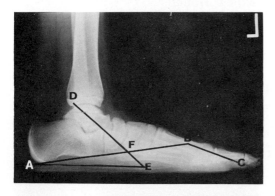

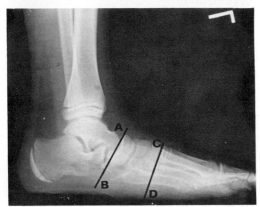

FIGURE 14-1 (A) AB passes through posterior and anterior plantar prominences of calcaneus. DE passes through long axis of talus. AE is parallell to weight-bearing surface. BC passes parallel to long axis of first metatarsal.

BAE is calcaneal pitch; DEA is talar flexion angle. ABC is calcaneal-first metatarsal angle; DFA is lateral talocalcaneal angle. Note preoperative talar beak in case 1.

(B) AB is skeletal length of foot, except the toes, along a line extending between plantar aspect of posterior calcaneus and first metatarsal head. CD is height of arch, the perpendicular distance between dorsal articular surface of talar head and line AB. CD/AB is arch ratio (case 1).

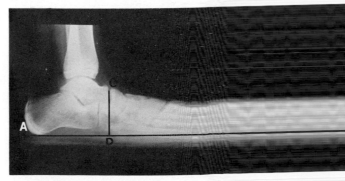

(C) AB passes through dors of proximal articular surface of allel to cuneiform-first metatar tween two lines is naviculocune gence of two lines plantarly is number and correlates with a fla gence of the two lines is given a the more negative numbers tend posture (case 22).

Thirteen patients (twenty-four feet) received a transfer of the tibialis anterior tendon as an adjunct to the subtalar arthrodesis. The technique involved dividing the tendon from its insertion and passing it from plantar to dorsal through a hole drilled in the medial tuberosity of the navicular. The tendon was then reflected on itself and sutured.

Closure was made with a synthetic absorbable suture or subcuticular wire. A short leg cast was well molded under the medial arch. Weight bearing was not permitted. The cast was removed when the graft appeared on roentgenogram to be incorporated, usually two to three months after surgery.

A total of thirty-two patients were sought for review, but four patients were lost to follow-up. Of the twenty-eight patients located, all but three of them were examined recently by the authors. The other three patients had moved away and were examined by orthopaedic surgeons in their area according to a protocol.

Twenty-five of the patients had bilateral Grice procedures; a total of fifty-three feet were evaluated. Thirteen of the twenty-eight patients were male. The mean age of all patients (both sexes) at the time of surgery was twelve years and ranged from five to thirty years. At follow-up the mean age was twenty-three years and ranged from fifteen to forty-five years. The average follow-up was eleven years and ranged from five years to seventeen years.

The evaluations included a history of pre- and postoperative symptoms, physical examination, photographs to show the arch and hindfoot posture, and standing roentgenograms of the feet and ankles. Preoperative standing x-rays of the feet were available for review in twenty-one patients.

Symptoms

The patients were asked about pain or fatigue in the feet or legs before operation and at the time of follow-up. A query was made about shoe wear before and after surgical correction.

Medial Longitudinal Arch

The medial longitudinal arch was considered satisfactory if, upon examination of the feet on a glass-top footstool, one third or more of the arch was free of weight-bearing contact. The footstool allowed visualization of the plantar surface of the feet while they were in a weight-bearing posture.

Subtalar Motion

The restriction of subtalar motion was classified as severe, moderate, mild, or unrestricted. "Severe" restriction meant that there was almost no movement as the hind foot was passively abducted or adducted. "Mild" restriction was applied to patients who had minimal or no restriction of adduction, though abduction was limited to the neutral position.

Ankle Motion

Ankle motion was measured goniometrically with the patient prone and the knee flexed 90°. The angle was measured between the distal fibula and the plane of the plantar aspect of the lateral midfoot.

Hindfoot Position

The presence of heel varus or valgus was assessed by observing the posterior aspect of the hind foot with the patient standing. Where present, the impression of heel varus was confirmed by the photographs or by excessive lateral heel wear on the shoes.

Roentgenographic Evaluation

The roentgenographic examinations studied included the standing anterior-posterior and lateral views of the feet and the standing anterior-posterior and lateral views of the ankle. Roentgenographic arch measurements studied on the lateral view of the foot included the talar flexion angle,[5] the lateral talocalcaneal angle, the calcaneal-first metatarsal angle, the naviculo-cuneiform angle,[3] and the arch ratio.[2] The calcaneal pitch (the longitudinal axis of the calcaneus relative to the plantar surface of the foot) was also measured but was not considered an index of the medial longitudinal arch (Fig. 14-1).

Measurements made on the anterior-posterior view of the foot were not empha-

sized. They were difficult to accurately assess in the mature foot, owing to overlapping shadows of the tarsal bones and distal tibia. Articulations adjacent to the subtalar joint were closely examined for degenerative changes, particularly narrowing and spur formation. Standing ankle x-rays were examined for angular deformity at the tibiotalar joint and pseudarthrosis at the distal fibula graft donor site.

RESULTS

Clinical Assessment

Relief of Symptoms

Twenty-one patients received complete or almost complete relief of their foot and leg symptoms after operation. Seven patients felt that, though they had partial symptomatic relief, some discomfort was still present, at least during activity.

Two patients would refuse surgery if they had to make the choice again. One of these patients had a varus deformity and was bothered by abnormal shoe wear. The other patient was a dancer who regretted

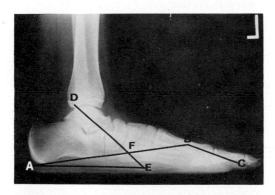

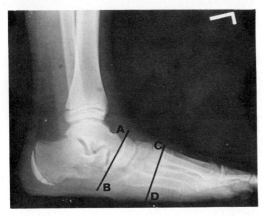

FIGURE 14-1 (A) AB passes through posterior and anterior plantar prominences of calcaneus. DE passes through long axis of talus. AE is parallell to weight-bearing surface. BC passes parallel to long axis of first metatarsal.

BAE is calcaneal pitch; DEA is talar flexion angle. ABC is calcaneal-first metatarsal angle; DFA is lateral talocalcaneal angle. Note preoperative talar beak in case 1.

(B) AB is skeletal length of foot, except the toes, along a line extending between plantar aspect of posterior calcaneus and first metatarsal head. CD is height of arch, the perpendicular distance between dorsal articular surface of talar head and line AB. CD/AB is arch ratio (case 1).

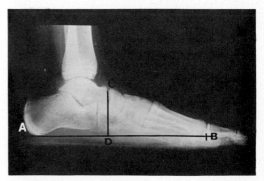

(C) AB passes through dorsal and plantar points of proximal articular surface of navicular. CD is parallel to cuneiform-first metatarsal joint. Angle between two lines is naviculocuneiforn angle. Divergence of two lines plantarly is given as a positive number and correlates with a flat foot. Dorsal divergence of the two lines is given as a negative number, the more negative numbers tending toward a cavus posture (case 22).

the subtalar restriction and a feeling of weak ankles that were "easily sprained." Twenty-one patients stated they would request their operation if given the choice again. Three patients were not sure retrospectively, if they would have surgery, and two patients were not asked.

Improvement of Shoe Wear

Eight patients recalled having excessive or abnormal shoe wear preoperatively and stated they had relief of the problem postoperatively. Four patients who didn't recall the presence or absence of preoperative shoe wear problems had "excessive" heel wear at the time of follow-up.

Arch Appearance

All but four of the fifty-three feet assessed for arch appearance had a clinically satisfactory arch (Fig. 14–2).

Ankle Range of Motion

Forty-seven feet were evaluated for clinical range of motion. The mean extension capacity was 12°; the range was from -2° to 23°. Despite relatively good extension, most patients had difficulty lifting the forefoot off the floor when they were asked to walk on their heels. The mean flexion capacity was 46°; the range was 14° to 64°.

Subtalar Range of Motion

In the forty-nine feet evaluated for subtalar motion, the results were as follows: no restriction, three; mild restriction, ninteen; moderate restriction, eighteen; and severe restriction, nine. Of seven patients tested and found to have severe restrictions of subtalar motion, in five the ankle flexion was restricted to less than 40°. There was no correlation between subtalar restriction and ankle extension. Two patients complained of stiff feet vulnerable to frequent ankle sprains. Two patients with severe subtalar restriction did not have ankle motion measurements.

Roentgenologic Assessment

Pre- and postoperative roentgenographic arch measurements are summarized in Table 14–1. The postoperative change in all five parameters was statistically highly significant ($P < 0.01$) as determined by Student's t tests. The most demonstrative postoperative changes occurred in the talar flexion angle and the lateral talocalcaneal angle. The postoperative reduction in the lateral talocalcaneal angle was due primarily to the change in the position of the talus, not to a lessening of the calcaneal pitch. The mean pre- and postoperative calcaneal pitch angles were 13° and 14°, respectively.

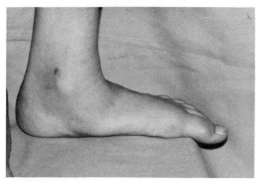 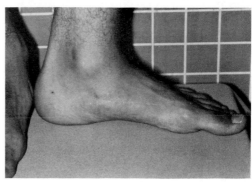

FIGURE 14–2 Clinical appearance of medial longitudinal arch was improved by surgery (case 2).(a) Preoperative. (b) Six years postoperative Grice and anterior tibial tendon transfer.

TABLE 14-1   Roetgenographic Measurements

	PRE-OPERATIVE MEAN	POST-OPERATIVE MEAN	PRE-OPERATIVE RANGE	POST-OPERATIVE RANGE	FEET MEASURED	t*
Talar flexion	36°	21°	20°–52°	9°–33°	39	12.83**
Lateral talocalcaneal angle	49°	36°	35°–69°	19°–48°	39	11.45**
Calcaneal-first metatarsal angle	148°	141°	135°–165°	129°–157°	39	7.71**
Naviculocuneiform angle	4°	−2°	(−7°)–17°	(−21°)–7°	37	7.67**
Arch ratio	.24°	.30°	.17°–.30°	.25°–.36°	27	7.57**

*t = Student's *t* score.
** P < 0.01

Associated Procedures

The talar flexion angle was used to compare the correction gained in ten feet treated with an adjunctive anterior tibial tendon transfer, and in twenty-one feet in which a Grice operation without additional procedures was performed. The preoperative roentgenograms were not available for an additional nine patients with an anterior tibial tendon transfer and for four patients treated with "Grice-only." The tendon transfer group had a mean correction in the talar flexion angle of 19° compared with 11° in the "Grice-only" group; this difference was statistically significant (P<0.05). This was not an age-associated difference, however, since the age composition of the two groups was similar. The preoperative mean talar flexion angle was 32.7° in the "Grice-only" patients, compared with 38.5° for the group with tendon transfer, but this difference did not quite reach significance (at the 0.05 probability level).

A varus deformity developed in six of nineteen feet in which the anterior tibial tendon transfer was used, and in two of the twenty-five feet operated on without adjunctive tendon surgery.

Nine feet were treated with other modifications such as a first metatarsal-cuneiform capsulotomy and posterior tibial tendon transfer to the plantar aspect of the navicular. The subgroups were too small to evaluate separately.

Patient Age

There was a significant (P<0.05) negative correlation (-0.50) between the patient's age at the time of surgery and the degrees of correction in the talar flexion angle, implying that younger patients tended to have a greater correction with the Grice procedure than older patients.

Consequences of Fibular Graft on Ankle Valgus

Patients with a pseudarthrosis at the fibular donor site were asymptomatic. It was difficult to elicit tenderness in this area even with the knowledge that a pseudarthrosis was present (Fig. 14-3).

Fibular graft was used in thirty-six

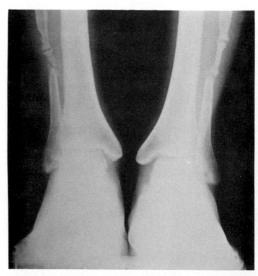

FIGURE 14-3 Bilateral pseudarthrosis developed at fibular graft donor site. Standing roentgenogram eleven years after operation showed ankle valgus of 5° on right and 6° on left (case 9).

TABLE 14-2   Ankle Angle on Standing Roentgenogram

FIBULAR GRAFT, DONOR SITE PSEUDARTHROSIS (7 FEET)	FIBULAR GRAFT, DONOR SITE HEALED (29 FEET)	TIBIAL GRAFT OR NONOPERATED FOOT (15 FEET)
Mean 6.7° Range 4°–12°	Mean 4.5° Range (—3°)–10°	Mean 3.1° Range 0°–8°

feet. In the large majority of these patients, the graft donor site was centered 11 to 13 cm above the inferior tip of the lateral malleolus (as measured on the follow-up ankle x-rays).

There was a mean ankle angle of 7° among patients who developed pseudarthrosis at the fibular donor site. This was significantly greater ($P>0.05$) than the angle among another group of patients who had fibular grafts and healed donor sites (Table 14–2). There was no significant difference ($P>0.05$) in the ankle angle between patients who had normal healing of the fibular donor site and patients who had an undisturbed fibula.

There was no significant association (correlation coefficient was not significantly different from 0) between the development of ankle valgus and the age at which surgery was performed.

Adverse Developments

Graft Absorption

Absorption of the bone graft developed in thirteen of the fifty-three feet (Fig. 14-4). The incidence of graft dissolution was 25 per cent in the thirty-six feet in which fibula was used. Correction of the talar flexion angle was maintained in all but one patient with a failed graft union.

The angle of the graft placement did not appear to influence the development of graft absorption. The angle of the graft was defined as zero when the axis of the graft was perpendicular to the plantar surface of the foot on weight-bearing roentgenograms, and it was given a positive value when the talar portion of the graft was anterior to the calcaneal portion. Many patients developed complete bony incorporation, and thus for these individuals it was not possible to measure the graft axis on the late follow-up x-rays.

In twenty-two of the twenty-six feet in which the graft angle was measurable, the graft lay with the talar portion anterior to the calcaneal portion. The mean graft angle was the same, 19°, in the twenty feet with an intact graft and in the six feet which developed graft absorption.

The mean age at the time of surgery was eleven years in the twelve feet that developed a graft defect and twelve years in the forty feet with an intact graft.

Three patients required further surgery because of graft defects.

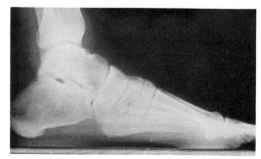

FIGURE 14–4   Graft absorption. Grice procedure was performed with anterior tibial tendon transfer at age nine years, using a fibular graft. Significant improvement in ultimate talar flexion angle was accomplished despite pseudarthrosis. Patient also had graft defect in right foot. There was pain in feet bilaterally with prolonged standing (case 12).

(a) Nine months after operation, showing early graft absorption at calcaneus. (b) Eleven years postoperative.

One patient developed bilateral subtalar pseudarthroses following bilateral Grice procedures done elsewhere. Only this patient's right foot was included in our series. It was reoperated on, and the remnant of the original graft was used. After the second operation healing was complete. The left foot was not reoperated on because it was asymptomatic. One of our patients was reoperated on for subtalar pseudarthrosis three years following the original surgery. The subsequent surgery resulted in complete graft incorporation. Another patient severely twisted her ankle three months following the Grice procedure. A fracture through the graft was diagnosed. The fracture did not heal over the subsequent six months, and she required re-operation.

Varus Deformity

Five patients had clinical evidence of a unilateral hindfoot varus at follow-up. Two other patients, one with bilateral varus overcorrection, had been treated with a calcaneal osteotomy which successfully remedied the varus appearance. Six of the eight feet with overcorrection had a supplementary anterior tibial tendon transfer with the initial surgery. The talar flexion angle had been corrected to less than 20° in all but one foot (Table 14–3).

The five patients with a varus hindfoot posture at follow-up were generally unaware of the deformity and were without complaints.

Changes in Adjacent Joints

Thirty-four feet showed both changes of enlargement and beaking in the talar head (Fig. 14–5). In some cases there was early beaking on the dorsal head of the talus preoperatively. In twenty-three feet there was a suggestion of impingement between the dorsal talar neck and the anterior lip of the tibia. This was indicated by spur formation, notching, or sclerosis on the dorsal talar neck (Fig. 14-6). Five feet revealed some arthropathy at the talonavicular joint with spur formation or joint narrowing. There was a wide variation in the amount of narrowing at the subtalar joint. None of the patients developed a "ball and socket ankle joint."

Metatarsal Calluses

Significant calluses on the plantar surface of the metatarsal heads developed in

TABLE 14–3   Summary of Patients with Postoperative Varus Deformity

PATIENT NO.	SIDE	AGE AT SURGERY (YEARS, MONTHS)	ASSOCIATED PROCEDURE	PREOPERATIVE TALAR FLEXION ANGLE	POSTOPERATIVE TALAR FLEXION ANGLE	PERCENT CORRECTION	REMEDIAL SURGERY
6	Right	13, 3	Tibialis anterior transfer	39°	9°	77	
10	Left	11, 7	Tibialis anterior transfer	40°	18°	55	
11	Right	11, 11	Tibialis anterior transfer	34°	19°	44	
15	Right	8, 9	None	42°	14°	67	
17	Right	10, 0	Tibialis anterior transfer	—	*15°	—	Bilateral calcaneal osteotomies performed 8 months after original surgery
	Left	10, 0	Tibialis anterior transfer	—	*16°	—	
18	Right	14, 4	Tibialis anterior transfer	40°	21°	48	
28	Right	13, 4	None	29°	19°	34	Calcaneal osteotomy 3 years after original surgery

*Only data following revision was available.

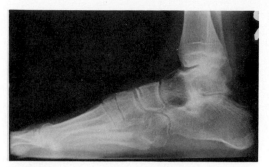

FIGURE 14-5 Changes in talar head developed postoperatively, particularly on superior surface. Note correction of flexed talus (case 16).

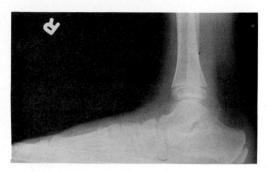

(A) Three years before operation.
(B) Twelve years after operation.

nineteen feet. Most of the calluses were under the fifth metatarsal head, but calluses under the third and fourth heads were also common.

DISCUSSION

Most reviews of the Grice procedure involve paralytic deformities. However, in addition to our series, Haraldsson[5] and Ross[13] have studied patients with neurologically normal, flexible flat feet. Their con-

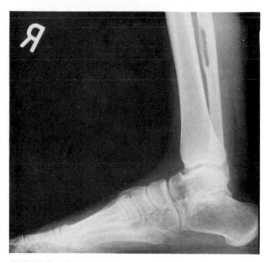

FIGURE 14-6 Impingement at anterior talotibial joint is demonstrated in patient eleven years after Grice procedure. Sclerosis is present at adjacent surfaces of anterior tibia and talar neck. Interposed ossicle is visible. Preoperative roentgenograms were normal in tibiotalar area.

clusions differed; Haraldsson advocated the procedure and Ross condemned it.

Haraldsson's study involved fifty-four feet. The mean age at the time of surgery was 6.3 years, and the follow-up in thirty-four feet was over two years, the longest being seven years. The parameters evaluated included an instrumented measurement of heel valgus and footprints, and roentgenographic measurements of the talar flexion angle. Homogenous bone was used for the graft, and only the calcaneal site of the graft was notched into bone. By not engaging the graft into the substance of the talus, it was suggested that a greater excursion of inversion could be preserved. Clinically, the arch was "completely corrected" in forty-two of the fifty-four feet. The mean talar flexion angle of these "completely corrected" feet was 22°. A completely depressed arch persisted in three feet and the mean roentgenographic talar flexion angle in those was 36°. The graft was absorbed in five feet and the correction was lost in three of the five. In twenty-four of the feet reviewed by Haraldsson, the anterior tibialis tendon was transferred to the plantar surface of the navicular. There was no additional benefit gained from the tendon transfer. Haraldsson concluded that the extra-articular subtalar arthrodesis was a satisfactory procedure for "pes-plano-valgus staticus juvenilis" which doesn't respond to conservative treatment.

Ross reported on one hundred thirteen Grice procedures, twenty-eight of which were done for "relaxed flat feet." The mean age of the patients at the time of surgery in the total series was 6.6 years, ranging from four to twelve years. The follow-up ranged from four to twenty years, the mean being over eleven years. Standing x-rays, photos, and footprints were studied. Delayed or nonunion of the graft occurred in nine of the twenty-eight feet (32 per cent). Ross calculated an 86 per cent unsatisfactory rate for the "relaxed flat feet" treated by the Grice procedure. This included cases with delayed or nonunion of the graft and recurrence or incomplete correction of the deformity.

In our series based on the patients' impressions and roentgenologic measurements, there were significant benefits from the procedure. Twenty-one of our twenty-eight patients had complete or almost complete relief of pain, fatigue, or both in their feet and legs. Eight patients had a notable improvement in the problem of wearing out their shoes. Dramatic roentgenographic changes were demonstrated by measuring the talar flexion angle and lateral talocalcaneal angle in pre- and postoperative films.

Adverse developments included symptomatic restriction of subtalar motion with the sensation of an unstable ankle. Arthropathic changes at the talonavicular joint were present in five feet. There were changes in the shape of the talar head in some feet, though the changes were often mild, and in several cases abnormalities in the talar head were seen on preoperative roentgenograms. The longstanding flexed talus may have the capacity to develop beaking without coalition or arthrodesis. Tomograms were not available to rule out an occult anterior coalition. There were roentgenographic changes suggesting anterior tibiotalar impingement in some patients, and metatarsal calluses were more common than expected in this age group. Varus deformity was usually subtle but was present in eight feet. The graft was partially or completely reabsorbed in thirteen feet; however, correction was usually maintained.

The incidence of graft absorption was identical whether fibular grafts or tibial grafts were used. The overall incidence of graft absorption in our study was within the range reported in the literature. Reviewing the literature with regard to failed graft union, no cases were found of graft absorption in the two hundred eighty-six paralytic feet reviewed by Tohen and others.[14] Herold[6] reported a 40 per cent graft absorption rate using homogenous bone in Grice operations for deformities resulting from poliomyelitis. In most of Herold's cases, correction was maintained despite partial or complete graft absorption. Haraldsson's graft absorption rate using bank bone was 9 per cent, and Ross reported a graft absorption rate of 32 per cent using tibial graft.

The correction of the talar flexion angle was the most dramatic of the roentgenographic parameters measured. It would appear that the flat-foot deformity with a flexed talus is the one best suited for the Grice operation. Other roentgenographic patterns of flat-foot deformity have been described by the senior author; they are the naviculocuneiform sag and the dorsoplantar talonavicular sag.[3] The anterior-posterior talonavicular angle is a measurement related to the dorsoplantar talonavicular sag and is difficult to measure in the mature foot, since the overlying tibia obscures the measurable axis of the talus. Because of this difficulty it was not presented as data in our patients. However, from the gross appearance of the roentgenograms, the plantar-flexed talus was often associated with a dorsoplantar talonavicular sag.

There is appropriate concern by many orthopaedists about the loss of subtalar motion with the Grice procedure. Le Lievre and Chambers[1,10] have reported procedures that were designed to stabilize the subtalar joint while minimizing the loss of motion. Le Lievre corrected and stabilized the subtalar joint in a series of eighty patients, fifty-three of whom had nonparalytic flat-foot deformities. Le Lievre's operation consisted of reducing the calcaneus into a neutral position, and, in children under six, stabilizing the reduction with a staple across the sinus tarsi. The staple was routinely removed two years later. In patients over six he stabilized the reduction by impacting a conical bone wedge into the sinus tarsi without denuding bone at the talar or calcaneal surfaces.

Chambers elevated the lateral portion of the posterior calcaneal facet and adjacent sinus tarsi and supported it with a wedge of bone. In 1977 a series of patients was presented in which eighty-two hypermobile feet were operated on with the Chambers procedure.[11] Sixty-three feet were rated excellent—having adequate correction of the arch and maintenance of the "normal" range of motion.

The metatarsal calluses may be the result of an enhancement of forces on the forefoot caused by the loss of flexibility in the hindfoot.

The development of ankle valgus was not a significant problem in our patients despite the extensive use of fibular grafts. However, Wiltse, Hsu, and others have reported cases of ankle valgus following resection of the fibula. Hsu and colleagues[8] reviewed thirty-two patients for whom fibula graft was used for a Batchelor subtalar arthrodesis in paralytic foot deformities. They found that pseudarthrosis in the donor site was much more likely when the graft was taken from the distal third of the fibula instead of the middle third. Their patients with a pseudarthrosis usually developed a proximal migration of the distal fibular epiphysis, wedging of the distal tibial epiphysis, and a valgus tilt of the talus.

Wiltse[15] described seven cases of ankle valgus following resection of the fibula for various reasons. Five of his seven patients were two years old at the time of surgery, a much younger age group than our patients.

The lack of ankle valgus problems in our patients with fibular graft was probably owing to the fact that, in general, they were not very young children, all of them being at least five years old.

Varus overcorrection was severe enough in two of our patients to warrant further surgery. It is urged that the surgeon take a simulated weight-bearing lateral view roentgenogram at the time of operation to ensure that the talar flexion angle is not corrected to an angle less than 20°.

SUMMARY

In summary, we found that (1) the nonparalytic flat foot with a flexed talus could be corrected and the correction maintained for at least five years with the Grice procedure, (2) that the transfer of the tibialis anterior tendon to the navicular appeared to augment correction but also predisposed to varus overcorrection, (3) that the use of the fibular graft taken in older children did not cause significant ankle valgus, and (4) that because of restricted hindfoot motion and the development of attritional changes around the talus, the Grice procedure was indicated in nonparalytic flat feet only when the feet or legs were truly symptomatic.

The authors suggest that the ideal age for this procedure is ten to twelve years old in girls and twelve to fourteen years old in boys. In these age groups the foot is relatively mature but still maintains some flexibility that allows correction.

Further data on the procedures advocated by Chambers and Le Lievre may show that their procedures are more desirable if they truly maintain more motion. Hindfoot correction and stabilization together with maximum preservation of subtalar motion should be the goal.

REFERENCES

1. Chambers, E.F.S.: An operation for the correction of flexible flat feet of adolescents. *West. J. Surg. Obstet. Gynecol.* 54:77–86, 1946.
2. Cobey, J. C. and Sella, E.J.: Toward a definition of a flat foot. Paper presented at Yale Orthopaedic Conference, June 1976.
3. Giannestras, N.J.: Foot Disorders. In *Medical and Surgical Management.* Philadelphia: Lea & Febiger, 1973.
4. Grice, D.S.: An extra-articular arthrodesis of the subastragalar joint for correction of paralytic flat feet in children. *J. Bone Joint Surg.* 34A: 927–40, 1952.
5. Haraldsson, S.: Pes plano-valgus staticus juvenilis and its operative treatment. *Acta. Ortho. Scand.* 35:234–56, 1965.
6. Herold, H.Z.: Extra-articular subtalar arthrodesis of Grice. *J. Bone Joint Surg.* 47B:199, 1965.
7. Hoke, M.: An operation for stabilizing paralytic feet. *J. Ortho. Surg.* 3:494, 1965.
8. Hsu, L.C.S., Yau, A.C.M.C., O'Brien, J.P. and

Hodgson, A.R.: Valgus deformity of the ankle resulting from fibular resection for a graft in subtalar fusion in children. *J. Bone Joint Surg.* 54A: 585–94, 1972.

9. Leavitt, D.G.: Subastragaloid arthrodesis for the os calcis type of flatfoot. *Am. J. Surg.* 59:501–08, 1943.

10. Le Lievre, J.: Current concepts and correction in the valgus foot. *Clin. Ortho. Rel. Res.* 70:43–55, 1970.

11. Miller, G.R.: The operative treatment of hypermobile flat feet in the young child. *Clin. Ortho.* 122:95–101, 1977.

12. Nieny, K.: Zur Behandlung der Fussdeformitaten bei ausgedehnten Lahmungen. *Arch. Ortho. U. Unfall-Chir.* 3:60–64, 1905.

13. Ross, P.M. and dure. A longter the annual me of Orthopaedic February 1976

14. Tohen, A., Carn J.: Extra-artic review of 286 51B:45–52, 196

15. Wiltse, L.L.: Val sequel to acquir of the fibur 54A:595–606,

16. Zadek, I.: Trans relief of pain *Surg.* 17:453–6

over six he stabilized the reduction by impacting a conical bone wedge into the sinus tarsi without denuding bone at the talar or calcaneal surfaces.

Chambers elevated the lateral portion of the posterior calcaneal facet and adjacent sinus tarsi and supported it with a wedge of bone. In 1977 a series of patients was presented in which eighty-two hypermobile feet were operated on with the Chambers procedure.[11] Sixty-three feet were rated excellent—having adequate correction of the arch and maintenance of the "normal" range of motion.

The metatarsal calluses may be the result of an enhancement of forces on the forefoot caused by the loss of flexibility in the hindfoot.

The development of ankle valgus was not a significant problem in our patients despite the extensive use of fibular grafts. However, Wiltse, Hsu, and others have reported cases of ankle valgus following resection of the fibula. Hsu and colleagues[8] reviewed thirty-two patients for whom fibula graft was used for a Batchelor subtalar arthrodesis in paralytic foot deformities. They found that pseudarthrosis in the donor site was much more likely when the graft was taken from the distal third of the fibula instead of the middle third. Their patients with a pseudarthrosis usually developed a proximal migration of the distal fibular epiphysis, wedging of the distal tibial epiphysis, and a valgus tilt of the talus.

Wiltse[15] described seven cases of ankle valgus following resection of the fibula for various reasons. Five of his seven patients were two years old at the time of surgery, a much younger age group than our patients.

The lack of ankle valgus problems in our patients with fibular graft was probably owing to the fact that, in general, they were not very young children, all of them being at least five years old.

Varus overcorrection was severe enough in two of our patients to warrant further surgery. It is urged that the surgeon take a simulated weight-bearing lateral view roentgenogram at the time of operation to ensure that the talar flexion angle is not corrected to an angle less than 20°.

SUMMARY

In summary, we found that (1) the nonparalytic flat foot with a flexed talus could be corrected and the correction maintained for at least five years with the Grice procedure, (2) that the transfer of the tibialis anterior tendon to the navicular appeared to augment correction but also predisposed to varus overcorrection, (3) that the use of the fibular graft taken in older children did not cause significant ankle valgus, and (4) that because of restricted hindfoot motion and the development of attritional changes around the talus, the Grice procedure was indicated in nonparalytic flat feet only when the feet or legs were truly symptomatic.

The authors suggest that the ideal age for this procedure is ten to twelve years old in girls and twelve to fourteen years old in boys. In these age groups the foot is relatively mature but still maintains some flexibility that allows correction.

Further data on the procedures advocated by Chambers and Le Lievre may show that their procedures are more desirable if they truly maintain more motion. Hindfoot correction and stabilization together with maximum preservation of subtalar motion should be the goal.

REFERENCES

1. Chambers, E.F.S.: An operation for the correction of flexible flat feet of adolescents. *West. J. Surg. Obstet. Gynecol.* 54:77–86, 1946.
2. Cobey, J. C. and Sella, E.J.: Toward a definition of a flat foot. Paper presented at Yale Orthopaedic Conference, June 1976.
3. Giannestras, N.J.: Foot Disorders. In *Medical and Surgical Management.* Philadelphia: Lea & Febiger, 1973.
4. Grice, D.S.: An extra-articular arthrodesis of the subastragalar joint for correction of paralytic flat feet in children. *J. Bone Joint Surg.* 34A: 927–40, 1952.
5. Haraldsson, S.: Pes plano-valgus staticus juvenilis and its operative treatment. *Acta. Ortho. Scand.* 35:234–56, 1965.
6. Herold, H.Z.: Extra-articular subtalar arthrodesis of Grice. *J. Bone Joint Surg.* 47B:199, 1965.
7. Hoke, M.: An operation for stabilizing paralytic feet. *J. Ortho. Surg.* 3:494, 1965.
8. Hsu, L.C.S., Yau, A.C.M.C., O'Brien, J.P. and

Hodgson, A.R.: Valgus deformity of the ankle resulting from fibular resection for a graft in subtalar fusion in children. *J. Bone Joint Surg.* 54A: 585–94, 1972.

9. Leavitt, D.G.: Subastragaloid arthrodesis for the os calcis type of flatfoot. *Am. J. Surg.* 59:501–08, 1943.

10. Le Lievre, J.: Current concepts and correction in the valgus foot. *Clin. Ortho. Rel. Res.* 70:43–55, 1970.

11. Miller, G.R.: The operative treatment of hypermobile flat feet in the young child. *Clin. Ortho.* 122:95–101, 1977.

12. Nieny, K.: Zur Behandlung der Fussdeformitaten bei ausgedehnten Lahmungen. *Arch. Ortho. U. Unfall-Chir.* 3:60–64, 1905.

13. Ross, P.M. and Lyne, E.D.: The Grice procedure. A longterm evaluation. Read in part at the annual meeting of the American Academy of Orthopaedic Surgeons, Las Vegas, Nevada, February 1976.

14. Tohen, A., Carnoma, J., Chow, L. and Rosas, J.: Extra-articular subtalar arthrodesis—a review of 286 operations. *J. Bone Joint Surg.* 51B:45–52, 1969.

15. Wiltse, L.L.: Valgus deformity of the ankle—a sequel to acquired or congenital abnormalities of the fibula. *J. Bone Joint Surg.* 54A:595–606, 1972.

16. Zadek, I.: Transverse-wedge arthrodesis for the relief of pain in rigid flat-foot. *J. Bone Joint Surg.* 17:453–67, 1935.

Chapter Fifteen

SYME'S AMPUTATION OF THE DIABETIC FOOT: RESULTS UTILIZING PREOPERATIVE DOPPLER EVALUATION

F. WILLIAM WAGNER, JR., M.D.
JAMES RUSSO, M.D.
JOHN WEBB, F.R.C.S.
HILTON BUGGS, M.A.

Amputation is frequently necessary when treating diabetic patients with ischemic, infectious, or gangrenous lesions of the feet. The primary problem is selection of the amputation level. Major articles on amputation surgery are divided on clinical and laboratory assessment of level selections. Romano and Burgess stated, "Articles on amputation surgery are quite contradictory and leave the reader confused on the determination of amputation level."[6]

Since the diabetic is at increased risk in the opposite limb once amputation has become necessary, it becomes increasingly important to keep the primary amputation at the lowest level possible.[4]

Prediction of healing at the Syme's level has not been as reliable as at the below-knee level. In addition, Syme's amputation in the dysvascular patient is reported infrequently.[7,10] Dale[3] reported on twenty-two Syme's amputations, of which six required amputation to a higher level. Mazet[5] reported failure of six of eleven cases with diabetics. Sarmiento[8] reported a 50 per cent revision rate in Syme's amputations in diabetics. On the other hand, Burgess and associates[1] reported healing in below-knee amputees of ninety-four per cent in diabetics and ninety-two per cent in nondiabetics.

"It is apparent that the current problem of the geriatric amputee is not one of the prosthetic components, prosthetic design, fitting and alignment, or gait training. The current problem of the geriatric amputee is preservation of the knee joint." We feel this quote by Peterson accurately states the present problem of determining level of amputation. Recent gait studies directed by Dr. Jacquelin Perry at the Pathokinesiology Laboratory of Rancho Los Amigos Hospital have clearly established the superiority of the Syme's amputation in dysvascular patients over the below-knee and above-knee levels.[12]

MATERIALS AND METHODS

Selection of the amputation level has been determined in the past by arteriography and oscillometry coupled with clinical criteria such as presence of pulses, skin warmth, hair and nail growth, degree of neuropathy, presence or absence of necrotic tissue, and infection at the level of amputation. Intraoperative assessment of bleeding in skin and muscle has also been helpful.

Between September 1969 and March 1975, 183 Syme's amputations were performed in a two-stage method with an average success rate of 62.3 per cent. The success rate was 50 per cent for the first two years and gradually improved to 70 per cent with increased experience. When the post-tourniquet bleeding time was used for selection, 80 per cent healed. The Syme's level was abandoned if bleeding did not occur in the skin within three minutes following release of tourniquet.

Since March 1975, all patients have been evaluated using a transcutaneous Doppler flow meter to map the vascular tree, assess the pulsatility, and record the systolic pressures in the lower extremity. A Piezzo-Electric Crystal produces an ultrasonic signal, which is directed at an angle through the skin and tissues to the arterial tree. A second crystal detects the retransmitted or reflected sound beam, which is conducted through circuitry that analyzes the difference between the transmitted and reflected signals. Stationary tissues reflect the same frequency and are not heard. Moving objects such as blood vessel walls and blood cells change the reflected frequency in proportion to their velocity. Low-velocity motion of the vessel wall can be filtered out. Flow velocities of the bloodstream produce signals that are converted to an audible range.

Instruments can be added that will produce a graphic record (Fig. 15–1). In addition to mapping the flow, the probe can be used to detect systolic blood pressures below sphygmomanometer cuffs whose width is 120 per cent of the diameter of the limb at the level being measured. Pressures are measured at proximal and midthigh, above-knee, calf, ankle, midtarsal, and toe levels. Information is obtained which is pertinent both for vascular reconstruction and amputation level. The mapping obtained with the Doppler probe is frequently as accurate as that obtained by arteriography. The wave forms and pressure gradients suggest the quality of flow (Fig. 15–2). Systolic drops of 20 mm between levels are within normal range, but gradients larger than this suggest obstruction. Nonpulsatile wave forms indicate occlusion and poor collateralization. Blood pressure in the upper extremity at the antecubital fossa can be considered the "normal" pressure unless some proximal block is present. When taken with the patient supine, the leg blood pressure is little different from the arm pressure. It is known that more blood flows through the leg than is necessary for nutrition of the tissues. Up to ten times this volume can be used for cooling purposes. It is also known that it takes more blood to heal an infection and ulcer or a surgical wound than it does to maintain the tissues. Carter[2] published data in 1973 that documented poor healing of foot lesions if the ankle pressure was less than 55 mm of mercury and showed that healing was good if a pressure over 70 mm

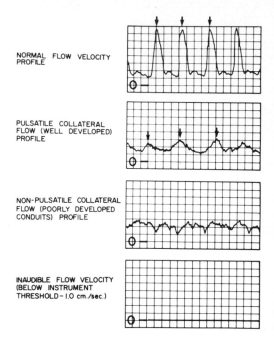

FIGURE 15–1   Tracing produced by ultrasound signals. Most pulsatile flow is above 70 mm Hg pressure and produces an ischemic index above 0.45.

ISCHEMIC INDEX

	RIGHT	LEFT
BRACHIAL ARTERY PRESSURE	140	140
ARM/CALF RATIO	1.0	.50
PULSATILE FLOW	Yes	Yes

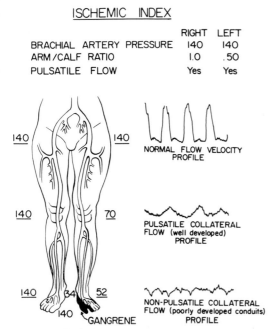

NORMAL FLOW VELOCITY PROFILE

PULSATILE COLLATERAL FLOW (well developed) PROFILE

NON-PULSATILE COLLATERAL FLOW (poorly developed conduits) PROFILE

GANGRENE

FIGURE 15-2 Ischemic index is 0.5 at calf and indicates suitable healing level there. Posterior tibial is 34 mm at ankle. Ischemic index is 34mm/140mm = 0.24, which is insufficient for healing, and a Syme amputation is not indicated.

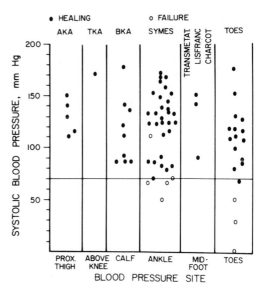

FIGURE 15-3 Syme's level showed no healing if systolic pressure was below 70 mm at ankle.

the lesions leading to amputation. Roentgenographic evidence of osteomyelitis was present in 45.2 per cent of patients, and 25.8 per cent had soft-tissue gas. Bacterial cultures showed a wide variety of organ-

of mercury was present. The results were not as predictable in diabetics.

It was felt that some method could be evolved to determine the percentage of blood flow necessary to heal a diabetic lesion. After March 1975, thirty-five diabetic patients considered for Syme's amputation were assessed by Doppler ultrasound, but the amputations were carried out on clinical criteria previously used. Every patient in whom the systolic pressure was under 70 mm of mercury did not heal at the Syme's level (Fig. 15-3, Syme's column). In addition, it was found that the ratio or index obtained by dividing the ankle pressure by the brachial artery pressure was above 0.45 in all cases that were successful (Fig. 15-4, Syme's column).

Since this first early success, all diabetic patients have been assessed by Doppler ultrasound. Treatment level is determined by the ischemic index. Vascular reconstruction is considered in patients whose index is below 0.45. Cellulitis, gangrene, deep ulceration, and abscess were

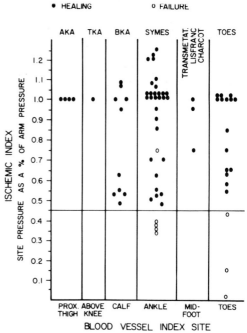

FIGURE 15-4 Syme's level showed no healing if ischemic index was below 0.45.

isms. All patients had at least two and some as many as five different bacteria. Several of the failures had postoperative infections. It appears that during a portion of their postoperative recovery period, the blood pressure may have dropped below a level sufficient to give them an index of 0.45. One of the failures also had rheumatoid arthritis and had been on high doses of corticosteroids for severe vasculitis. All failed Syme's amputations were successfully revised to below-knee levels, except one patient whose below-knee amputation failed and who required an above-knee amputation.

The surgical technique is a modification of the two-stage procedure described by Spittler.[9,11] Patients are given preoperative antibiotics and incision and drainage procedures as indicated. The circulation is evaluated intraoperatively by timing the reappearance of skin bleeding following release of tourniquet. Postoperatively, the cavity is lavaged with antibiotic solution.

RESULTS

Seventy-two Syme's amputations have been performed with a healing rate of 91.7 per cent. The average age was 60.5 years. There were thirty-eight males and thirty-four females. Fifty-one were Caucasian and twenty-one were black. The average duration of diabetes was 10.1 years with a range of one to thirty-five years. Forty per cent were insulin dependent. All patients except three became at least household ambulators.

CONCLUSIONS

Transcutaneous Doppler ultrasound has been valuable in obtaining systolic pressures and mapping arterial flow in the diabetic dysvascular lower limb. An ischemic index can be calculated from leg sys-tolic pressure divided by brachial artery systolic pressure. Use of this index in addition to clinical criteria in diabetics has raised the success rate in Syme's amputations from 62.3 per cent to 91.7 per cent in cases in which the index is over 0.45. It must be stressed that appropriate preoperative parenteral antibiotics, the two-stage surgical procedure, intraoperative evaluation of circulation, and postoperative antibiotic wound irrigation are also elements in the high success rate with Syme's amputations in the diabetic.

REFERENCES

1. Burgess, E.M., Romano, R.L., Zettl, J.H. and Shrock, R.D., Jr.: Amputation of the leg for peripheral vascular insufficiency. J. Bone Joint Surg. 53A:874,1971.
2. Carter, S.A.: The relationship of distal systolic pressures to healing of skin lesions with arterial occlusive disease with special reference to diabetes mellitus. Scan. J. Clin. Lab. Invest., Suppl 128 31:239, 1973.
3. Dale, G.M.: Syme's amputation for gangrene for peripheral vascular disease. Artif. Limbs 6:44, 1961.
4. Goldner, M.: The fate of the second leg in diabetic amputees. Diabetes 9:100, 1960.
5. Mazet, R.R.: Syme's amputation. J. Bone Joint Surg. 50A:1549, 1968.
6. Romano, R.L. and Burgess, E.M.: Level selection in lower extremity amputations. Clin. Ortho. 74:177, 1971.
7. Rosenman, L.D.: Syme amputation for ischemic disease in the foot. Am. J. Surg. 118:194, 1969.
8. Sarmiento, A. and Warren, W.D.: Re-evaluation of lower extremity amputations. Surg. Gynecol. Obstet. 129:799, 1969.
9. Spittler, A.W., Brennan, J.J. and Payne, J.W.: Syme amputation performed in two stages. J. Bone Joint Surg. 36A:37, 1954.
10. Warren, R., Thayer, T.R., Achenbach, H. and Kendall, L.G.: The Syme amputation in peripheral arterial disease. A report of six cases. Surgery 37:156, 1955.
11. Wagner, F.W.: Amputations of the foot and ankle: current status. Clin Ortho. 122:62–69, 1977.
12. Waters, R.L., Perry, J., Antonelli, D. and Hislop, H.: Energy costs of walking of amputees: the influence of level of amputation. J. Bone Joint Surg. 58A: 42, 1976.

Chapter Sixteen

ANKLE FUSIONS: A CURRENT STUDY

E. SAID, M.D. F.R.C.S. (C)
L. HUNKA, M.D. F.R.C.S. (C)
T. N. SILLER, M.D. F.R.C.S. (C)

Many methods of ankle fusion have been reported. Most of these are concerned with evaluating the results by a specific surgical technique.

Adams[1] reviewed the results of fusion by the transfibular approach. In 93 per cent of thirty ankles, fusion occurred in an average of thirteen weeks. Ratliff[2] reviewed the results of the Charnley compression arthrodesis, in which bony fusion occurred in 91 per cent of fifty-five cases, and 88 per cent had good or excellent results.

As we all know, fusion of the hip or the knee joint leaves the patient with considerable disability. With the great achievements in recent years in joint arthroplasty, we see fewer fusions of these joints being done. Whether fusion solves the problem of the painful arthritic ankle, or whether we have to wait for the perfection of arthroplasty of this joint, is one of the main concerns of this review.

MATERIALS AND METHODS

The material for this study is based on thirty-seven procedures, of which one was bilateral, in thirty-six patients treated in the hospitals shown in Table 16-1. All the charts and x-rays were reviewed. There were seven females and twenty-nine males; the average age at the time of operation was forty-five years, with a range between nineteen and sixty-seven (Fig. 16-1).

TABLE 16-1. Number and Distribution of Patients Reviewed

HOSPITAL		NO. OF PATIENTS
Queen Mary Veterans	1955–1974	15
Montreal General	1970–1974	18
Reddy Memorial	1970–1974	3
TOTAL		36

The conditions for which ankle fusion was performed (Table 16-2) were as follows: twenty-seven for post-traumatic arthritis, three for equinus deformity in spastic paraplegia, two for nonunited or malunited fractures of the ankle with instability, one as the primary treatment for severely comminuted fracture, one for tuberculous arthritis, and one for gouty arthritis. Two oper-

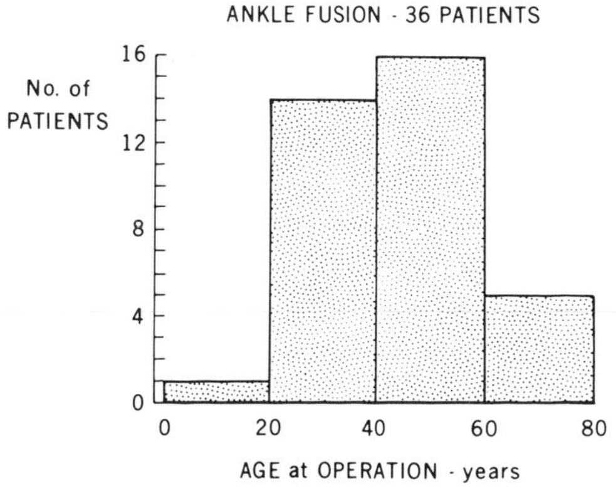

FIGURE 16-1.

131

TABLE 16–2.　Conditions for Which Ankle Fusions Were Performed

37 ANKLES	
Arthritis (post-traumatic)	27
Spastic paraplegia	3
Non-united or malunited ankle fractures	2
Severely comminuted ankle fracture	1
Tuberculous arthritis	1
Gouty arthritis	1
Miscellaneous	2

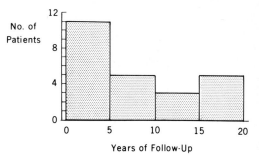

FOLLOW-UP PERIOD · 24 PATIENTS

FIGURE 16–3.

ations were performed for miscellaneous conditions, including one for chronic nonspecific synovitis and another for old post-traumatic drop-foot deformity.

In the group of patients with post-traumatic arthritis, the injury to fusion period varied from six months to thirty-five years, with an average of nine years, nine months. In 48 per cent of cases the injury to fusion period was less than five years (Fig. 16–2.

Of the thirty-six patients in the review, twenty-four could be traced. The twenty-four available for follow-up had twenty-five procedures (one was bilateral).

Of the twelve patients not included in the follow-up, two died from causes unrelated to the operative procedure. Therefore, twenty-four out of thirty-four living persons (70 per cent) participated in the follow-up interview and examination. The follow-up period (Fig. 16–3) varied from one and one-half to seventeen years with an average of seven years, five months. Fifty-four percent of the patients were followed for more than five years.

Methods of Fusion

Out of thirty-seven fusions (Table

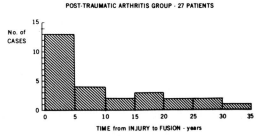

POST-TRAUMATIC ARTHRITIS GROUP · 27 PATIENTS

FIGURE 16–2.

16–3), fourteen were by the Charnley compression technique; thirteen by the Crawford Adams (R.A.F.) method, using the transfibular approach and fibular strut graft laterally; seven were fused utilizing a tibial sliding graft as an onlay, inlay, or the Hatt modification. Three ankles were fused by other methods, including one by simple cast immobilization alone, and the other two with local bone chips and staple fixation. Out of the fourteen by Charnley compression arthrodesis, five were through the classic transverse incision, and the rest through other standard anterior approaches.

Results

Fusion Rate

Bony fusion occurred in thirty-one ankles out of thirty-seven (84 per cent). Failure occurred in six (16 per cent). In the six failures, three ankles were done by Crawford Adams (R.A.F.) method, two by the Charnley compression method, and one by a tibial sliding graft. Five patients with failed fusions were refused successfully at a

TABLE 16–3.　Method of Fusion and Number of Operations

Charnley compression arthrodesis	14
—5 transverse	
—9 anterior approach	
Crawford Adams arthrodesis (R.A.F.)	13
Tibial sliding graft or Hatt modification	7
Other	3

later date, and one with an infected pseudoarthrosis had a below-knee amputation. All those with failed fusion had considerable symptoms to justify a refusion attempt.

The total period of cast immobilization after surgery (Table 16-4) varied from twelve to twenty-eight weeks, with an average of 17.5. The fusion time was studied in the thirty-one ankles in which fusion occurred successfully. Because the clinical evaluation was difficult, and in many instances impossible, the time for fusion was determined on a radiologic basis by the demonstration of bone trabeculae crossing the joint.

Fusion time (Table 16-5) varied between eleven weeks and eighteen months, with an average of 19.4 weeks. In eighteen out of thirty-one (58 per cent) fusion occurred between eleven and sixteen weeks. In the one case in which fusion occurred after eighteen months, osteomyelitis developed, and drainage was still present at the time of the review.

CLINICAL EVALUATION

The evaluation of the results was both subjective and objective with regard to (1) pain; (2) residual deformity (heel varus or valgus or rotational deformity of the foot); (3) gait (in patients in whom the ability to walk was not affected for reasons other than the fusion of the ankle); and (4) patient's own evaluation. Results were rated excellent, good, fair, or poor, according to the criteria shown in Table 16-6.

There were eleven excellent results, seven good (with one having a bilateral fusion), two fair, and four poor (Table

TABLE 16-5. Time From Operation to Fusion

31 SUCCESSFUL FUSIONS	
Less than 13 weeks	3 }58%
13 to 16 weeks	15
17 to 20 weeks	5
21 to 24 weeks	3
25 to 28 weeks	4
18 months	1

16-7). Eighteen out of twenty-four patients had excellent or good results (75 per cent). In the two who had fair results, one had internal rotation deformity of the foot and marked limp, the other had pain and swelling of his fused ankle and considerable limp. Both, however, were satisfied with the result.

In the four poor results, one had 20° of heel valgus, marked limp, and mild pain (her result was rated poor even though she was happy with it). Another had a below-knee amputation for infected pseudoarthrosis. The remaining two with poor results had chronic osteomyelitis with solid fusion, and both complained of pain.

GAIT AND ITS RELATION TO MOTION AT THE SUBTALAR AND MIDTARSAL JOINTS

Gait was studied in nineteen patients who were fused for monarticular lesions (Table 16-8). Their ability to walk was not affected for reasons other than the fusion.

Eleven showed no limp, or only minimal limp on close inspection. Five showed a mild, and three a marked limp. Out of these nineteen cases in which gait was studied, eighteen had no known preoperative lesion or stiffness of the subtalar or the midtarsal joints. In this group the mobility of these joints was clinically assessed.

Subtalar stiffness was found clinically and radiologically in sixteen out of eighteen patients, as compared with the normal foot. In eleven patients, the midtarsal joint was hypermobile, and the gait in this group was classified as excellent. Midtarsal joint motion was normal in two and less than normal in five patients. Those with normal

TABLE 16-4.

IMMOBILIZATION PERIOD	NO. OF ANKLES
12-14 weeks	12
15-17 weeks	10
18-20 weeks	6
21-23 weeks	4
24-26 weeks	4
Over 26 weeks	1

TABLE 16–6   Rating Scale of Results of Ankle Fusion

EXCELLENT:	FAIR:
no pain or minimal pain in cold weather	mild pain on regular activity
no deformity	heel valgus 10° or moderate rotation deformity of foot
no limp, or minimal limp, on close inspection	considerable limp
patient happy with result	some subjective improvement
GOOD:	**POOR:**
mild pain on excessive activity	considerable pain on regular activity
heel valgus 5° or mild rotation deformity of foot	heel valgus >10°, heel varus or considerable rotation deformity of foot
mild limp	
patient happy with result	no subjective improvement

or less than normal midtarsal joint motion showed a limp.

It would seem that fusion of the ankle has a detrimental effect on the subtalar joint. The same conclusion was reported by Ratliff.[23]

We could further conclude that compensatory hypermobility frequently occurs at the midtarsal joint in the fused ankles, resulting in an excellent gait. However, subtalar stiffness following ankle fusion does not necessarily have a detrimental effect on gait. This may be because the axis of the compensatory motion of the midtarsal joint is now parallel to the ankle, while that of the subtalar is perpendicular to it.

In patients with excellent gait, the range of pseudomovement at the midtarsal joint varied from 5° to 10° of dorsiflexion and 20° to 35° of plantar flexion.

King and colleagues[19] found that no dorsiflexion was present in twenty-five fused ankles, while midtarsal motion of 10° in the plantar direction was compatible with satisfactory gait when the ankle is fused in neutral position.

We feel that more than 10° of pseudo-plantar flexion at the midtarsal joint is needed for excellent gait and function, especially if the patient with a fused ankle is walking on a rough surface or climbing uphill.

TABLE 16–7   Results of Ankle Fusion in 24 Patients

Excellent	11 patients	—46%	⎫ 75%
Good	7 "	—29%	⎭
Fair	2 "	— 8.3%	
Poor	4 "	—16.7%	

POSITION OF FUSION

There are many statements in the literature concerning the best position of fusion.

Barr and Record[4] preferred a position of 5° of equinus; Knight recommended the right angle as the best position for men; Watson-Jones recommended 15° of equinus; Ratliff[23] reported the best position at or close to the right angle; King and colleagues[19] concluded that fusion in a neutral position is indicated.

The position of the fused ankle was assessed clinically in eleven patients who, as is previously noted, have excellent gait (Table 16-9). All the eleven happened to be males.

Four ankles were at a right angle, six were in 5° of equinus, and one was in 10° of equinus. Fusion of the ankle in males at a right angle or in a few degrees of equinus appear to be quite satisfactory.

RETURN TO EMPLOYMENT AFTER ANKLE FUSION

Of the twenty-four patients interviewed in the follow-up group, six were retired for some years before surgery. Two were housewives who were coping with their household duties at the time of interview. Of sixteen patients employed prior to surgery, twelve kept the same type of job,

TABLE 16–8   Gait Pattern—19 Patients

Excellent	11
Mild limp	5
Marked limp	3

TABLE 16-9 Position of Ankle Fusion

11 PATIENTS WITH EXCELLENT GAIT	
Right angle	4 patients
5° of equinus	6 patients
10° of equinus	1 patient

while three had to change because of their disability. One man had a below-knee amputation as a complication of his fusion and was unemployed.

COMPLICATIONS

A high incidence of complications was reported by Wiedeman and Morrey[27] after they reviewed fifty ankle fusions. They reported a 16 per cent infection rate, 13 per cent nonunion, and 11 per cent malalignment.

Significant complications occurred less frequently in our review than in that reported by Wiedeman and Morrey. Infection occurred in three out of thirty-seven ankles (8 per cent). In two of these infections, fusion was solid at the time of the follow-up but discharge continued. The third patient had an infected pseudoarthrosis, eventually treated by below-knee amputation. Edema of the ankle was present in two patients at the time of review. Two ankles were fused in poor position (one in 20° of heel valgus and the other with medial rotation deformity of the foot on the tibia). It was noted that fusion of the ankle results in stiffness of the subtalar joint.

CONCLUSION

Successful bony fusion occurred in 84 per cent of patients. Of thirty-seven ankles fused by various methods, all failures were symptomatic. The objective and subjective results in twenty-four patients were good to excellent (75 per cent). Subtalar stiffness, although often found, was not necessarily detrimental to gait. Fusion of the ankle in neutral position or in a few degrees of equinus and a range of psuedoplantar flexion of 20° or more (occurring at the mid-

tarsal joint) were compatible with good gait and function.

Fusion is considered a good treatment for the painful post-traumatic arthritic ankle, and the resulting functional disability is minimal. Fusions for the rheumatoid ankle are beyond the scope of this review.

REFERENCES

1. Adams, J.C.: Arthrodesis of the ankle joint. *J. Bone Joint Surg.* 30B: 506, 1948.
2. Albee, F.H.: *Bone Graft Surgery.* Philadelphia: W.B. Saunders Co., 1915, p. 335.
3. Anderson, R.: Concentric arthrodesis of the ankle joint. *J. Bone Joint Surg.* 27:37, 1945.
4. Barr, J.S. and Record, E.E.: Arthrodesis of the ankle joint. Indications, operative technique and clinical experience. *New Engl. J. Med.* 248:53, 1953.
5. Bingold, A.C.: Ankle and subtalar fusion by a transarticular graft. *J. Bone Joint Surg.* 38B: 863, 1956.
6. Brittain, H.A.: *Architectural Principals in Arthrodesis.* Baltimore: The Williams and Wilkins Co., 1942, p. 58.
7. Charnley, J.: Compression arthrodesis of the ankle and shoulder. *J. Bone Joint Surg.* 33B:180, 1951.
8. Chuinard, E.G. and Peterson, R.E.: Distraction-compression bone graft arthrodesis of the ankle. A method especially applicable in children. *J. Bone Joint Surg.* 45A:481, 1963.
9. Coventry, M.B. and Tapper, E.M.: Pelvic instability. A consequence of removing iliac bone for grafting. *J. Bone Joint Surg.* 54A:83, 1972.
11. Gallie, W.E.: Arthrodesis of the ankle joint. *J. Bone Joint Surg.* 30B:619, 1948.
11. Goldthwait, J.E.: An operation for the stiffening of the ankle joint in infantile paralysis. *Am. J. Ortho. Surg.* 5:271, 1907-08.
12. Hallock, H.: Arthrodesis of the ankle joint for old painful fractures. *J. Bone Joint Surg.* 27:49, 1945.
13. Harris, W.H. and Heaney, R.P.: *Skeletal Renewal and Metabolic Bone Disease.* Boston: Little, Brown and Co., 1970.
14. Hatt, R.N.: The central bone graft in joint arthrodesis. *J. Bone Joint Surg.* 22:393, 1940.
15. Horwitz, T.: The use of the transfibular approach in arthrodesis of the ankle joint. *Am. J. Surg.* 55:550, 1942.
16. Jansen, K.: Arthrodesis of the ankle joint. *Acta Ortho. Scand.* 32:476, 1962.
17. Johnson, E.W. and Boseker, E.H.: Arthrodesis of the ankle. *Arch. Surg.* 97:766, 1968.
18. Kennedy, J.C.: Arthrodesis of the ankle with particular reference to the Gallie procedure. A review of 50 cases. *J. Bone Joint Surg.* 42A:1308, 1960.

19. King, H.A., Watkins, T.B. and Samuelson, K.M.: Analysis of foot position in ankle arthrodesis and its influence on gait. Paper read at the American Orthopaedic Foot Society Annual Meeting, San Francisco, 1979.

20. Mulfinger, G.I. and Treuta, J.: The blood supply of the talus. *J. Bone Joint Surg.* 52B:160, 1970.

21. Ottolenghi, C.E., Animoso, J. and Burgo, P.H.: Percutaneous arthrodesis of the ankle joint. *Clin. Ortho.* 68:72, 1970.

22. Pridie, K.H.: Arthrodesis of the ankle. *J. Bone Joint Surg.* 35B:152, 1953.

23. Ratliff, A.H.C.: Compression arthrodesis of the ankle. *J. Bone Joint Surg.* 41B:524, 1959.

24. Staples, S.O.: Posterior arthrodesis of the ankle and the subtalar joint. *J. Bone Joint Surg.* 38A:50, 1956.

25. Thomas, F.B.: Arthrodesis of the ankle. *J. Bone Joint Surg.* 51B:53, 1969.

26. White, A.A., III: A precision posterior ankle fusion. *Clin. Ortho. Rel. Res.* 98:239, 1974.

27. Wiedeman, G.P. and Morrey, B.F.: Complications and long term results of ankle arthrodesis. Paper read at the American Orthopaedic Foot Society Annual Meeting, San Francisco, 1979.

28. Wilson, H.: Arthrodesis of the ankle. A technique using bilateral hemimalleolar onlay grafts with screw fixation. *J. Bone Joint Surg.* 51A:775, 1969.

Chapter Seventeen

ARTHROPLASTY OF THE GREAT TOE WITH A SILICONE IMPLANT

ALFRED B. SWANSON, M.D.
ROBERT M. LUMSDEN II, M.D.
ALFRED A. BRAUNOHLER, M.D. AND
GENEVIEVE DEGROOT SWANSON, M.D.

Flexible implant resection arthroplasty of the great toe has been performed since 1968 in patients with metatarsophalangeal joint problems in rheumatoid arthritis, hallux valgus, and hallux rigidus. Until 1974 all implant resection arthroplasties involved replacement of the proximal third of the proximal phalanx with a single-stem great-toe spacer (Fig. 17-1). It is well tolerated by both the bone and the cartilage, as has been previously reported.[12, 13, 14]

The development of the high-performance silicone elastomer prompted us to use the flexible double-stem hinge implant in patients with rheumatoid arthritis and severe osteoarthritis. Others have reported favorable results using the double-stem flexible hinge (finger joint) in implant resection arthroplasty of the first metatarsophalangeal joint.[3, 9, 10] The implant is positioned upside down to correspond with the range of motion characteristics of the great toe (Fig. 17-2). The double-stem flexible hinge allows more correction of the de-formity, with bone removal possible from both articular surfaces of the first metatarsophalangeal joint. Proper capsuloligamentous repair allows improved alignement. This stability is particularly valuable in a progressive disease such as rheumatoid arthritis. The superior performance of the double-stem flexible hinge in rheumatoid

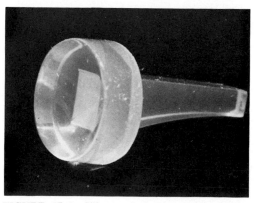

FIGURE 17-1 Silicone single-stem great toe implant.

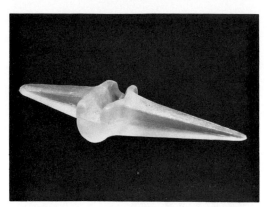

FIGURE 17-2   Silicone double-stem flexible hinged great-toe implant.

arthritis patients prompted the design of a great-toe flexible hinge (Fig. 17-3). This chapter will present the senior author's experience with these techniques and indications for each implant.

REVIEW OF LITERATURE

Until recently, only resection arthroplasty or fusion was a possible treatment for painful arthritis of the first metatarsophalangeal joint. Resection arthroplasty for first metatarsophalangeal joint destruction has been practiced since 1836, when Fricke[4] first excised the first metatarsophalangeal joint.[4] By 1886 the literature began warning of the interference in gait patterns caused by resection of the first

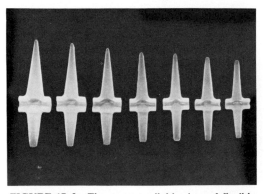

FIGURE 17-3   The seven available sizes of flexible hinged great-toe implants.

metatarsal head. In 1887 Davies-Colley recommended resection of the basal half of the proximal phalanx.[5, 9]

In 1904 Keller[8] first described his resection arthroplasty, which is the most widely used procedure for first metatarsophalangeal joint arthritis with or without hallux valgus.[8] Joplin in 1950 criticized the Keller procedure because it reduced the propulsive strength of the great toe. Others criticized the Keller procedure because of a lack of motion at the first metatarsophalangeal joint following resection of the base of the proximal phalanx. Wrighton[17] has shown that the Keller procedure will relieve the pain of hallux rigidus, but the patient will be left with a stiff toe.[17] Although many modifications have been proposed to reduce complications, little has been done to prevent shortening of the great toe. Endler in 1951 replaced the base of the proximal phalanx with an acrylic prosthesis. In 1952 Swanson designed a metatarsal head prosthetic replacement of Vitallium. There were bone absorption problems with this rigid implant and its use was abandoned. In 1965, as part of a comprehensive research program to develop flexible silicone implants for reconstructive joint surgery, a similarly shaped implant was fabricated of silicone. Because an implant on the non-weight-bearing side of the joint would have distinct mechanical advantages, an implant to be used as an adjunct to the Keller resection arthroplasty was developed. In 1967 Swanson designed a single-stem silicone implant to replace the base of the proximal phalanx. This implant has been used in many thousands of cases of arthritic disabilities in the great toe by a large variety of surgeons. Noting the recurrence of deformity in patients with rheumatoid arthritis, implant resection arthroplasty of the metatarsophalangeal joint using the double-stem flexible hinge implant was begun. There have been many encouraging preliminary reports of this procedure in the literature.[12, 13, 14] In 1974 Swanson designed a double-stem flexible hinge implant to be used in implant resection arthroplasty of the great toe in rheumatoid arthritis and severe osteoarthritis (Figs. 17-2, 17-3).

METHOD

This report involved a study of 165 single-stem implant resection arthroplasties with an average follow-up time of 48 months, and 105 double-stem flexible hinge implant resection arthroplasties with an average follow-up of 30 months. The patients in the single-stem group were divided into four diagnostic categories: rheumatoid arthritis, hallux valgus secondary to osteoarthritis, failed resection or fusion, and hallux rigidus. In the double-stem group 94 patients had rheumatoid arthritis. All others had problems similar to those mentioned.The goals of treatment were elimination of pain and improvement of deformity. Follow-up for each patient included clinical and radiologic examination from 18 months to 9 years after arthroplasty. Evaluation included the patient's freedom from pain, shoe tolerance, walking ability, gait pattern, range of motion, toe position, and subjective satisfaction. Passive range of motion was measured as approximately two pounds of force were applied in both flexion and extension. Active range of motion was also noted with the patient standing with the forefoot projecting off a stool. The active range of motion was noted to be approximately 5° less than the passive range of motion in flexion and 10° less than in passive extension. The range of motion value referred to in this paper is extension/flexion (average 60/10). In the last few years we have been adding a rubber platform to the insole of a wooden, open-toed postoperative shoe, which allows greater flexion when used in conjunction with a dynamic toe outrigger type dynamic splint (Fig. 17-4). When performing double-stem implant resection arthroplasty, a .045 inch K-wire is used to stabilize the first metatarsophalangeal joint. The following roentgenographic measurements were made: the metatarsophalangeal angle, the intermetatarsal angle, and the position of the tibial sesamoid bone. The intermetatarsal angle was related to the severity of the preoperative deformity. Evaluation of the joint per se included width of joint space, presence of erosions and cysts, and osteophyte forma-

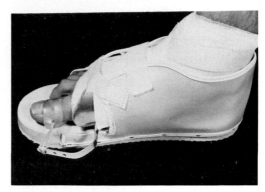

FIGURE 17-4 Wooden-soled shoe and dynamic great toe outrigger splint.

tion. The presence of bone production or bone resorption at the interface of the implant with the proximal phalanx or first metatarsal was included in the postoperative assessment of the joint. The implant itself was also evaluated on the postoperative radiograms. Hoffman procedures were performed on the lateral toes of 108 feet.[6]

OPERATIVE TECHNIQUE

The operative technique for single-stem and double-stem implant resection arthroplasty uses the same curved dorsomedial incision; a flap is developed which can be distally based in both cases, or more commonly, proximally based with the single-stem implant resection arthroplasty. In all cases the adductor tendon is released, and usually extensor hallucis longus tendon Z-lengthening is necessary, along with exostectomy of the metatarsal head. With the single-stem implant, a third of the proximal phalanx is removed and the intermedullary canal is reamed. The appropriate size implant is then inserted using testers. Then a capsulorrhaphy is performed using drill holes through the bone and 2-0 dacron sutures (Fig. 17-5).

In the double-stem implant resection arthroplasty, a partial metatarsal head resection is performed. The first metatarsal and the proximal phalanx are reamed until the appropriate size trial implant can be inserted. One-mm drill holes are placed in

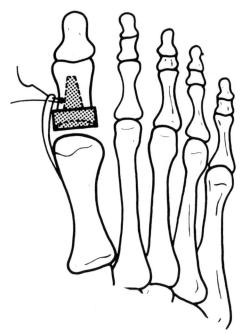

FIGURE 17–5   Single srem resection arthroplasty using a proximally based.*

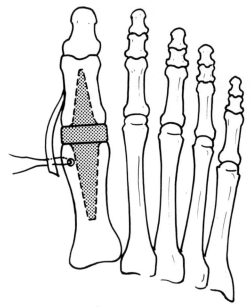

FIGURE 17–6   Double-stem flexible hinged implant resection arthroplasty using distally based medial capsular flap.*

the bone of the metatarsal neck for the medial capsulorrhaphy (Fig. 17–6).

A single-stem implant is used (1) in mild to moderate hallux valgus, (2) in hallux rigidus, and (3) after failed procedures if the metatarsal head has been preserved. The hinge is used in (1) moderate to severe rheumatoid hallux valgus with lateral toes involvement, (2) severe senile hallux valgus, and (3) revision of previous procedures if both sides of the joint are involved.

A voluminous conforming dressing is applied to the foot, which is elevated for three to five days to avoid swelling. A wooden-soled shoe and a dynamic splint are used postoperatively (Fig. 17–4).

RESULTS

IMPLANT RESECTION ARTHRO-PLASTY USING THE SINGLE-STEM GREAT-TOE SPACER. The follow-up

*From: Swanson, A.B. et al.: Silicone implant arthroplasty of the great toe. *Clin. Ortho.* 142:30–43, 1979.

was 18 months to 3 years for 59 feet, 3 to 6 years for 80 feet, and 6 to 9 years for 26 feet; the average follow-up was 48 months. The average preoperative range of motion in the rheumatoid arthritis group was 32/9°; hallux valgus group, 35/22°; hallux rigidus group, 30/10°. Postoperative range of motion for rheumatoid arthritis patients averaged 48/9°; for hallux valgus patients, 55/10°, and for hallux rigidus patients, 54/12°. The average increase in range of motion in the rheumatoid arthritis group was 16°; in the hallux valgus group, 32°; in the hallux rigidus group, 22°. The average preoperative hallux valgus angle in rheumatoid arthritis averaged 38°, 33° in hallux valgus, and 13° in hallux rigidus. The average decrease in valgus in rheumatoid arthritis was 18°, 15° in hallux valgus, and 16° in hallux rigidus.

Minimal bone production around the stem was normally present. Bone overproduction at the lateral proximal phalanx occurred in two feet; the implant was removed in one. Mild bone resorption around one stem related to poor implant collar fit concentrating forces at the stem end; the clinical result was unaffected. Moderate avascular necrosis of the head seen in one joint related to a preexisting subcortical cyst in a rheumatoid; this was not a clinical problem.

IMPLANT RESECTION ARTHROPLASTY USING THE DOUBLE-STEM FLEXIBLE HINGE IMPLANT (FINGER JOINT). The average follow-up for 105 toes operated with the flexible hinge was 30 months. The average preoperative range of motion was 33/9°, and postoperative range of motion was 42/10°. Average preoperative hallux valgus was 42°. Average postoperative hallux valgus was 12°. Average postoperative decrease in hallux valgus was 30°.

There has been no evidence of cortical bone formation, but the characteristic cancellous mineralization about the implant occurs in patients whose cancellous bone remains following implant arthroplasty.

COMPLICATIONS

In the single-stem arthroplasty, complications were noted as follows. Two postoperative infections occurred. One joint healed following conservative antibiotic therapy; the implant was removed from the other. An inflammatory reaction which subsided in four weeks and did not appear to be related to infection, was noted in one foot. This type of reaction has been reported by others and in two instances, the retrieved implants were evaluated and found to be completely inert chemically in animals. One patient known to have gout presented a similar reaction following a finger joint implant procedure; this was alleviated in 24 hours after administration of colchine. We have seen no immune-like reactions to silicone rubber when the implant was properly handled and sterilized. One implant surface had a small cut on its articular surface, which was resting on the sharp edge of the metatarsal head owing to recurrent hallux valgus. A possible tear of the implant was noted in one joint and a definitive tear was seen in another, where a trimmed radial head was inserted. The clinical results were unaffected. A tight extensor mechanism was the main contributing factor to an extension deformity noted in

seven cases and ranged from 5° to 20°. Routine sectioning of the short extensor and lengthening of the long extensor are indicated in moderate to severe deformities. Varus overcorrection from 4° to 10° was seen in six feet and was of no concern to the patients. Patients who had hallux valgus with degenerative arthritis and those with hallux rigidus presented no significant recurrence of deformity. The tendency toward recurrence seen in rheumatoid feet signifies the progressive nature of the disease; this is better controlled with the use of the hinged implant.

In the flexible hinge group, there were no implant fractures, bone absorption, or production noted postoperatively. In one patient, the implant was removed because of infection. The nine patients who were converted to a flexible hinge arthroplasty following recurrence of deformity with the single-stem implant were satisfied with both their functional and cosmetic result.

DISCUSSION

The use of implant arthroplasty for arthritic conditions of the first metatarsophalangeal joint has been useful and rewarding. The single-stem implant has proved to be a simple and safe method to improve the Keller arthroplasty in both function and cosmesis. Its proper use can make this procedure more predictable and reproducible and is the preferred method for hallux rigidus. It can also be used for patients with an arthritic hallux valgus with a mild to moderate deformity if soft tissue procedures such as tendon releases and capsulorrhaphy are properly done. If there is metatarsus primus varus of more than 15°, corrective osteotomy at the base of the first metatarsal should be considered.[16] This procedure should not be used if the hallux angle is greater than 40° or if there are erosive changes in the metatarsal head, as seen in rheumatoid arthritis.

The use of the double-stem flexible hinge implant has allowed the correction of more severe deformities with destruction on both sides of the joint. It is most useful in the rheumatoid foot and in the severe senile hallux valgus. Our experience with this method started with the adaptation of the finger joint implant of the larger size. The design and development of the toe hinge included consideration for proper anatomic sizing and application to the foot.

SUMMARY

One hundred and sixty-five feet were reconstructed with the single-stem silicone implant, including patients with hallux rigidus, hallux valgus owing to degenerative and osteoarthritic joint changes, hallux valgus secondary to rheumatoid arthritis, and patients with previous unsuccessful "bunion" procedures. Preoperative pain and intolerance to shoe wear were relieved in the great majority of patients. The amount of correction of the hallux valgus angle was directly related to the preoperative deformity. Infection occurred in two patients, and inflammatory reaction to the implant occurred in one patient. One hundred and five feet were reconstructed with a flexible hinge implant; 94 of the feet had joints destroyed by rheumatoid arthritis. Dramatic improvement in the hallux valgus angle resulted in these feet, which had relatively severe preoperative deformities. No implant fractures were recorded. The current survey of our cases and those reported by others encourages the use of these implants by surgeons who follow the suggested indications, surgical techniques, and follow-up care.

REFERENCES

1. Bonney, G. and Macnab, J.: Hallux valgus and hallux rigidus: a critical survey of operative results. *J. Bone Joint Surg.* 34:366-85, 1952.

2. Cleveland, M. and Winant, E.M.: An end-result study of the Keller operation. *J. Bone Joint Surg.* 32A:163, 1950.

3. Delagoutte, J.P.: Traitement de l'hallux valgus par prosthèse de Swanson. *Rev. Chir. Ortho.* 60: Suppl. 2, 1974.

4. Fricke, J.L.G.: Exostosis of the ball of the foot. *Dublin J. Med. Sci.* 11:497-504, 1837.

5. Giannestras, N.J.: *Foot Disorders.* Philadelphia: Lea & Febiger, 1976.

6. Hoffman, P.: An operation for severe grades of contracted or claw toes. *Am. J. Ortho. Surg.* 9:441, 1911.

7. Kelikian, H.: *Hallux Valgus, Allied Deformities of the Forefoot and Metatarsalgia.* Philadelphia: W.B. Saunders Co., 1965.

8. Keller, W.L.: The surgical treatment of bunions and hallux valgus. *N.Y. Med. J.* 80:741-42, 1904.

9. LaPorta, G. et al.: Keller implant procedure. *J. Am. Pod. Assoc.* 66 (3): 1976.

10. Michon, J.P.: L'Arthroplastie par implants en silastic dans la cure de l'hallux valgus et des arthrites aseptiques de l'articulation metatarsophalangienne premieres impressions. *Actualities de Medecine et de Chirugie de Pied,* Tome VIII. 1973.

11. Smith, W. and Meyer, T.: End result of stone bunionectomies. *Clin. Ortho. Rel. Res.* 109:144-46, 1975.

12. Swanson, A.B. et al.: A silicone rubber implant to supplement the Keller toe arthroplasty. Inter-Clinic Information Bulletin, New York University 1971, pp. 7-14.

13. Swanson, A.B.: Implant arthroplasty of the great toe. *Clin. Ortho.* 85:75-81, 1972.

14. Swanson, A.B.: *Flexible Implant Resection Arthroplasty in the Hand and Extremities.* St. Louis: C.V. Mosby Co., 1973.

15. Vidigal, E. et. al.: The foot in chronic rheumatoid arthritis, *Ann Rheu Dis* 34:292-97.

16. Wilson, J.N.: Oblique displacement osteotomy for hallux valgus. *J. Bone Joint Surg.* 45B:552-56.

17. Wrighton, J.D.: A ten-year review of Keller's operation *Clin. Ortho.* 89:207, 1972.

Chapter Eighteen

SURGICAL CORRECTION OF HALLUX VALGUS IN CEREBRAL PALSY

M. MARK HOFFER, M.D. and

JACK L. SEAQUIST, M.D.

The Cerebral Palsy Clinic at Rancho Los Amigos Hospital follows a large population of cerebral palsy patients (801 patient evaluations in 1974) who manifest a multitude of foot deformities. An analysis of 100 consecutive clinic patients revealed 47 per cent with a valgus heel of 10° or more; of those with valgus heel, almost half (43 per cent) had an associated hallux valgus of 10° or greater, and 18 per cent had a significant hallux valgus of 30° or greater. These figures indicate that the hallux valgus deformity in cerebral palsy patients is a relatively common entity.

We have noted, as have others,[3] that hallux valgus, when symptomatic, can be bothersome and occasionally disabling. The purpose of this chapter is to describe a technique both brief and simple leading to the correction of hallux valgus in cerebral palsy patients, which can be combined with other foot surgery without significantly increasing operative time or morbidity. We will also present follow-up in a series of twenty-six feet operated upon.

CLINICAL MATERIAL

Twenty-six procedures for correction of symptomatic hallux valgus deformity were carried out in nineteen patients (Table 18-1). The type of involvement was spastic diplegia in twelve, spastic hemiplegia in five, and mixed anthetoid in two. Age of the patients ranged from six to thirty-four years. All patients were ambulatory. There were ten females and nine males. Measurements were goniometric. In only one patient was this the only procedure done at operation; in the other eighteen, this procedure was combined with tendon transfers or bony stabilizations at the fore- or hindfoot.

OPERATIVE PROCEDURE

Under hemostasis, by means of a pneumatic cuff, an incision was made dorsally paralleling the lateral great toe-first metatarsal border from 1 cm distal to the metatarsol-phalangeal joint to 2 cm proximal to the joint (Fig.18-1). The conjoined tendon of the adductor hallucis muscle was then visualized and released from its insertion on the base of the proximal phalanx (Fig. 18-2), and the lateral metatarsophalangeal joint capsule was released. With the muscular and capsular release the toe could be brought to neutral and was then usually held in place with a Steinmann pin. When the medial capsule of the metatarsophalangeal joint was excessively lax it could be plicated through the same incision; this was rarely necessary. The fibular sesamoid was not removed and no bone was resected. The patient was placed in plaster for four

TABLE 18-1 Patient Profile

PATIENT	SEX	AGE	TYPE OF CP	FOOT	HEEL DEFORMITY (PREOP)	HEEL STABILIZATION	HEEL (POSTOP)	HALLUX VALGUS CORRECTION	PIN USED
1	F	7	Diplegia	Right	Valgus	Grice	Neutral	Good	Yes
				Left	Valgus	Grice	Neutral	Good	Yes
2	F	7	Diplegia	Left	Valgus	Soft tissue	5° Valgus	Good	Yes
3	M	7	Diplegia	Right	Valgus	Soft tissue	30° Valgus	Poor	Yes
				Left	Valgus	Soft tissue	5° Valgus	Good	Yes
4	F	19	Diplegia	Left	Neutral	None	Neutral	Good	Yes
5	F	7	Hemiplegia	Left	Varus	Soft tissue	5° Valgus	Good	Yes
6	F	9	Diplegia	Left	Valgus	Soft tissue	Neutral	Good	Yes
7	M	34	Total body	Right	Valgus	Soft tissue	20° Varus	Poor	No
				Left	Valgus	Soft tissue	30° Valgus	Poor	No
8	F	10	Diplegia	Right	Valgus	Soft tissue	Neutral	Good	Yes
9	M	16	Hemiplegia	Left	Varus	Soft tissue	Cavus	Poor	No
10	F	8	Total body	Right	Valgus	Soft tissue	Neutral	Good	Yes
				Left	Valgus	Soft tissue	Neutral	Good	Yes
11	F	12	Diplegia	Right	Valgus	Soft tissue	Neutral	Good	No
12	M	12	Hemiplegia	Left	Varus	Triple arthrodesis	Neutral	Good	Yes
13	M	6	Diplegia	Left	Valgus	Grice	Neutral	Good	Yes
14	M	8	Hemiplegia	Left	Varus	Soft tissue	Neutral	Good	Yes
15	F	8	Hemiplegia	Left	Valgus	Grice	Neutral	Good	Yes
16	M	12	Diplegia	Left	Valgus	Grice	5° Valgus	Good	Yes
17	M	6	Diplegia	Right	Valgus	Soft tissue	Neutral	Good	No
				Left	Valgus	Soft tissue	Neutral	Good	No
18	M	20	Diplegia	Right	Valgus	Triple arthrodesis	Neutral	Good	Yes
				Left	Valgus	Triple arthrodesis	Neutral	Good	Yes
19	F	29	Diplegia	Right	Valgus	Triple arthrodesis	20° Equinus	Poor	No
				Left	Valgus	Triple arthrodesis	20° Equinus	Poor	No

to six weeks or for as long as necessary, depending on the primary procedure's postoperative program.

RESULTS

All patients were followed personally in the Cerebral Palsy Clinic. Average follow-up was thirty-three months, with a minimum follow-up of six months. Since correction of hallux valgus was combined with other surgical procedures, analysis of gait improvement as a result of this single procedure was not possible. Desired effects were relief of pain and correction of deformity. A painless toe with less than 10° hallux valgus postoperatively was considered a good result. A painful toe or hallux valgus greater than 10° was considered a poor result. A more sophisticated breakdown into excellent, good, fair, etc. was not warranted.

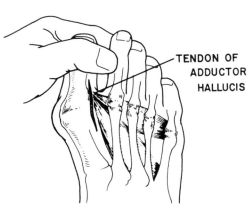

FIGURE 18-1 Skin incision over attachment of adductor hallucis tendon.

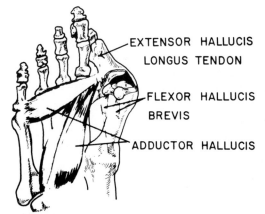

FIGURE 18-2 Plantar view of adductor hallucis attachment.

Heel Position

Preoperatively, the heel was in valgus position in twenty-one feet, in varus in four, and neutral in one. Fifteen feet had soft-tissue procedures for hindfoot correction (table 18-2), and ten feet had bony stabilizations (five triple arthrodeses and five Grice subtalar arthrodeses). In one patient no other foot surgery was done. In the twenty feet with good results postoperatively (eleven with soft-tissue procedures and eight with arthrodeses), the heel was in neutral position in sixteen, and in 5° to 10° valgus in four. When good results were obtained, the heel was never greater than 10° varus or valgus. In the six feet with poor results none of the heels were in neutral position; two were in 30° valgus, one was in 20° degrees varus, two were in 25° equinus, and one foot had cavus deformity.

Pin Stabilization Postoperatively

Of the twenty toes with good results, pins were used in seventeen. Of the six with poor results, a pin was used in only one foot.

TABLE 18-2   Soft Tissue Heel Stabilizations Used

1. Tendo achillis lengthening (Z Plasty)
2. Percutaneous tendo achillis lengthening
3. Gastrocnemius recession
4. Posterior tibial tendon release
5. Posterior tibial tendon transfer
6. Posterior tibial tendon lengthening
7. Anterior tibial tendon transfer
8. Split anterior tibial tendon transfer
9. Release of peroneus brevis tendon
10. Transfer of peroneus brevis tendon

SUMMARY

A good result was obtained in twenty of twenty-six feet (asymptomatic and less than 10° hallux valgus). (Fig. 18-3, 18-4). However, even in the six feet rated as poor, all but one toe had a lesser degree of hallux valgus postoperatively, and four of the six poor results with hallux valgus greater than 10° were asymptomatic. Two continued to be symptomatic, but both stated they were in less discomfort than preoperatively. No patient was made worse by the surgery and there were no infections.

DISCUSSION

Silver[13] and McBride[8][10] long ago

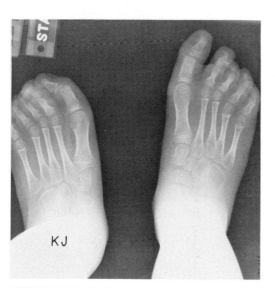
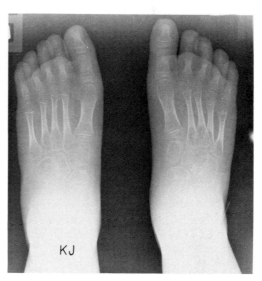

FIGURE 18-3 Patient 12, demonstrating progression of left hallux valgus deformity and result of heel stabilization and adductor hallucis release. (a) age 6; (b) age 8; (C) age 12, preop; (D) age 14, after triple arthrodesis and adductor hallucis release.

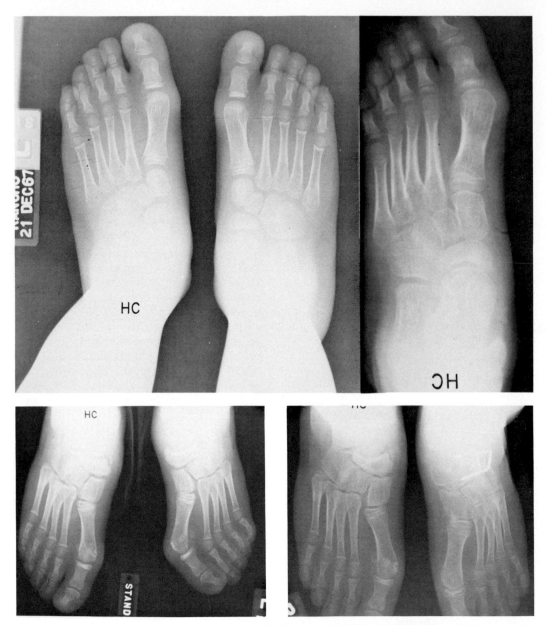

FIGURE 18-4 Patient 1, a seven-year-old spastic diplegic with bilateral deformities. (A) Preoperative radiographic appearance; (B) one year postoperative adductor release and bilateral Grice hindfoot stabilizations.

called attention to muscle imbalance of the intrinsics of the foot as a possible etiologic agent in producing the pathologic alterations of hallux valgus deformity. EMG studies revealed the predominance of the adductor hallucis muscle over the abductor hallucis in patients with "idiopathic" hallux valgus,[5] and Bassett[1] pointed out that relief of the spasticity of the adductor hallucis muscle in cerebral palsy patients can lead to correction of the hallux valgus deformity. The association of pronated feet and hallux valgus has been noted by several observers,[2,4,6,7,11,12,14] and pronated feet were present preoperatively in twenty-one feet in this study.

While hallux valgus must be considered a minor aspect in the totality of the cerebral palsy patient, it should not be ignored when symptomatic. The adductor hallucis release and lateral capsulotomy is such a benign procedure, easily combined with other surgery, that it should be employed in the relief of symptomatic hallux valgus in the cerebral palsy patient.

CONCLUSION

Nineteen cerebral palsy patients underwent correction of hallux valgus deformity in twenty-six feet, during which release of the conjoined adductor hallucis muscle insertion on the proximal phalanx, metatarsao-phalangeal lateral capsulotomy, and postoperative pin stabilization were utilized. In eighteen patients the correction of hallux valgus was secondary to another hind- or forefoot procedure. Those patients who had feet with heels stabilized at or near neutral had a good result; those whose postoperative heel position was in poor position had a poor result. Pin stabilization postoperatively increases the likelihood of a good result. With this simple, brief, reproducible procedure, overall good results were obtained in twenty of twenty-six feet.

REFERENCES

1. Bassett, F.H.: Deformities of the Feet Due to Cerebral Palsy. AAOS Instruction. Course Lectures, XX, 1971, p. 35.
2. Craigmile, D.A.: Incidence, origin, and prevention of certain foot defects. *Brit. Med. J.* 2:749, 1953.
3. DuVries, H.L.: *Surgery of the Foot.* St. Louis; C.V. Mosby Co., 1965.
4. Galland, W.I. and Jordan, H.: Hallux valgus. *Surg. Gynecol. Obstet.* 66: 95, 1938.
5. Iida, M. and Basmajian, J.V.: Electromyography of hallux valgus. *Clin. Ortho.* 101: 220, 1974.
6. Inman, V.T.: Hallux valgus: a review of etiologic factors. *Ortho. Clin. North Amer.* 5:59, 1974.
7. Mayo, C.H.: The surgical treatment of bunions. *Minn. Med.* 3:326, 1920.
8. McBride, E.D.: A conservative operation for Bunions. *J. Bone Joint Surg.* 10:735, 1928.
9. McBride, E.D.: A conservative operation for bunions. *JAMA* 105:1164, 1935.
10. McBride, E.D.: Hallux valgus, bunion deformity; its treatment in mild, moderate and severe stages. *J. Int. Coll. Surg.* 21:99, 1954.
11. Rogers, W.A. and Joplin, R.J.: Hallux valgus, weak foot and the Keller operation: an end result study. *Surg. Clin. North Amer.* 27:1295, 1947.
12. Samilson. R. I. and Hoffer, M.M.: Problems and Complications in Orthopedic Management of Cerebral Palsy. In *Orthopedic Aspects of Cerebral Palsy,* Samilson, R.L. Ed. Suffolk, England: Levenham Press, 1975.
13. Silver, D: Operative treatment of hallux valgus. *J. Bone Joint Surg.* 5:225, 1923.
14. Stein, H.C.: Hallux valgus. *Surg. Gynecol. Obstet.* 66: 889, 1938.

Chapter Nineteen

KELLER BUNIONECTOMY WITH OPENING WEDGE OSTEOTOMY OF THE FIRST METATARSAL.

DONALD R. GORE, M.D.
JAMES KNAVEL, M.D.
WENDELIN W. SCHAEFER, M.D.

The Keller buionectomy is probably the most commonly used preocedure for the alleviation of symptoms associated with degenerative arthritis of the first metatarsophalangeal joint. However, when metatarsus primus varus is also present, the Keller procedure does not correct this deformity. The purpose of this paper is to review our experience with a group of patients who had Keller bunionectomies combined with correction of metatarsus primus varus by an opening wedge osteotomy of the proximal first metatarsal.

MATERIALS AND METHODS

Patients

Sixty-eight procedures were performed on forty-four patients of whom forty-three were females. The range in age was 20 to 77 years, with a mean of 57.2 years, and the time between surgery and postoperative evaluation ranged from 2 months to 8 years with a mean of 3.3 years. Three patients with four procedures were evaluated less than one year after surgery. All patients had a painful bunion, hallux valgus, degenerative arthritis of the first metatarsophalangeal joint, and metatarsus primus varus. Five cases had previous bunion surgery: Three had removal of the bunion alone, one had a closing wedge osteotomy of the first metatarsal and an osteotomy of the proximal phalanx, and one had a Keller procedure.

Operative Technqiue

All procedures were performed in the same manner with only minor variations in technqiue. The surgical technique is outlined in Figures 19-1 and 19-2. The procedure is performed through a dorsal medial, curvilinear incision extending from the distal portion of the proximal phalanx of the great toe to the metatarsal cuneioform joint. A flap of capsule and periosteum is created on the medial side of the first metatarsophalangeal joint. The proximal one third to one half of the proximal phalanx is removed and saved for use as a

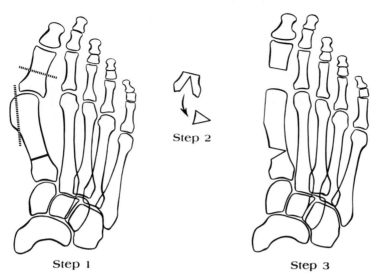

Step 1   Step 2   Step 3

FIGURE 19-1 Surgical technique. Note that wedge-shaped bone graft is cut from removed portion of proximal phalanx.

bone graft. The medial exostosis and osteophytes on the metatarsal head are removed and discarded. Using a high-speed cutting bur, an incomplete osteotomy at the base of the first metatarsal is performed approximately 1 cm distal to the metatarsal cuneiform joint. The plantar, medial, and dorsal cortices are cut, leaving only the lateral cortex intact. A wedge of bone is then fasioned from the removed bone of the proximal phalanx using a table-mounted circular saw. The medial surface of the graft is composed of cortical bone about 5 mm in length, but the exact size of the wedge depends upon the amount of correction desired. The osteotomy is opened by inserting a thin osteotome into the osteotomy and using a gentle prying action to bend but not destroy the continuity of the lateral cortex.

To further open the osteotomy, a small periosteal elevator is placed directly opposite the osteotomy on the lateral surface of the first metatarsal, and pressure is applied in a medial direction with the elevator while the distal end of the first metatarsal is simultaneously pushed laterally. When the osteotomy is opened, the assistant inserts the bone graft. The surgeon firmly taps the graft into place, countersinking the medial edge of the graft with respect to the medial surface of the metatarsal shaft. Any portions of the graft protruding superiorly or inferiorly from the cortex of the metatarsal are removed with a rongeur. It is important to insert the graft exactly on the medial side of the metatarsal to prevent deviation of the distal portion of the metatarsal in either a plantar or dorsal direction. Internal fixa-

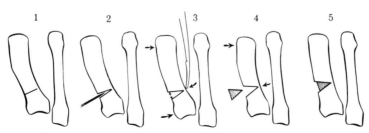

1   2   3   4   5

FIGURE 19-2 Osteotomy technique. (1) An incomplete osteotomy is performed. (2) Osteotomy is pried open with thin osteotome. (3) Osteotomy is further opened by providing counterpressure with periosteal elevator. (4) Graft is inserted. (5) Graft is countersunk.

tion of the osteotomy or graft is not used. Soft tissue is closed over the osteotomy site, and the capsule and soft tissue are closed over the distal first metatarsal while the great toe is held in a corrected position. After the skin is closed, a soft, bulky dressing is applied with the great toe held in the desired position. When the pain subsides a few days after surgery, a firm-soled cast shoe is provided and the patients are allowed to ambulate with or without external support as they choose. The dressing is left in place for two weeks, at which time the sutures are removed.

Patient Review

All charts were reviewed to determine the occurrence of postoperative complications. The results of the procedures were evaluated by patient interview and by comparison of pre- and postoperative roentgenograms. All the results relating to the patient's assessment of their procedure were obtained by personal interviews conducted by one of the three authors (usually not the operating surgeon). The interview was based on a uniform set of questions designed to determine the patient's satisfaction with the procedure in terms of pain relief, correction of deformity, and cosmetic effect, and all patients were asked to rate their feet as improved, the same, or worse after surgery, taking all aspects of the result into consideration. An attempt was made to contact all patients to return for this personal interview. Thirty-seven patients with fifty-nine procedures returned. Of the seven patients who did not return, three refused and gave no reason, one had moved out of the state, one had a serious medical problem unrelated to her foot, and two had died.

Roentgenographic evaluation was made by comparing pre- and postoperative films. All roentgenograms used for this portion of the study were non-weight bearing, dorsal plantar projections. The technique in the pre- and postoperative films was identical. The following measurements were made on the roentgenograms: (1) the angle between the first and second metatarsal; (2) the angle between the proximal phalanx of the great toe and the first metatarsal; and (3) the distal projection of the first metatarsal head with respect to the second metatarsal head. The method used for making the roentgenographic measurements is illustrated in Figure 19-3.

The lines used to measure the angle between the first and second metatarsals were drawn through the approximate long axes of these bones. The line in the first metatarsal was drawn parallel to the lateral

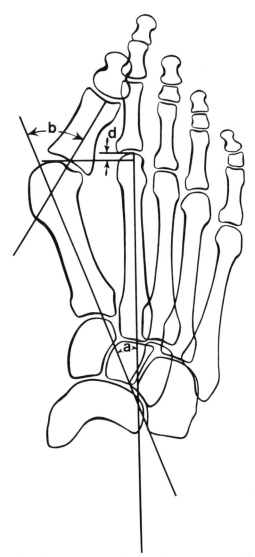

FIGURE 19-3 Technique of roentgenographic measurements.

border of the middle portion of the metatarsal, because this border was unviolated by the surgical procedure. The angle of intersection of these lines was used as a measure of the first-second metatarsal angle (angle a). The intersection of the line through the first metatarsal and the line through the long axis of the proximal phalanx was used as a measure of the degree of hallux valgus (angle b). The amount of distal projection of the first metatarsal head relative to the second was the distance (d) between two parallel lines, each perpendicular to the long axis of the second metatarsal. The first line was drawn tangent to the most distal portion of the second metatarsal, and the second line was drawn tangent to the most distal portion of the first metatarsal. This distance is not a measurement of the length of the first metatarsal but identifies the position of the first metatarsal head with respect to the second.

Analytic Methods

Mean values and standard deviations were calculated for all roentgenographic measurements. A Student's t test was used to determine the significance of differences between the pre- and postoperative measurements. A Chi Square test was used to test for significance of the frequency of patients with postoperative pain with respect to change in the distal projection of the first metatarsal. Pearson Product-Moment correlation coefficients were calculated to determine the degree of relationship between the preoperative deformity and the amount of correction obtained.

RESULTS

There was no nonunions of the meta-

tarsal osteotomies and no serious infections. Five patients had minor problems with wound healing which rapidly resolved without residuals. Pain at the first metatarsophalangeal joint or osteotomy site was uncommon. However, pain in the area of the second to the fifth metatarsal heads (lateral metatarsalgia) was reported by eleven patients with eighteen procedures (Table 19-1). Almost all patients were satisfied with the appearance of their feet and the overall result of the procedure (Table 19-2). One patient who had two procedures felt her feet were worse after surgery because of lateral metatarsalgia, and another patient who had one procedure complained of persistent swelling of her foot.

The means, standard deviations, and significance of differences between the pre- and postoperative measurements are presented in Table 19-3. The average correction of the first-second metatarsal angle was 8°, with a maximum correction of 16° in one patient the varus angle was increased 4°, and in two patients the postoperative angle was unchanged from the preoperative angle. The average correction of the metatarsophalangeal angle was 15°, with a maximum correction of 50°; in one patient the hallux valgus was increased 1°. After surgery the first metatarsal head projected a slightly further distally than before surgery.

There were statistically significant correlations indicating that the greater the preoperative deformity in the first-second metatarsal angle and the metatarsophalangeal angle, the greater the correction obtained by surgery. There was also a statistically significant correlation indicating that the greater the correction of the metatarsus primus varus, the further distal the projection of the first metatarsal head as compared with before surgery. Those patients

TABLE 19-1   Residual Pain—Fifty-nine Cases

LOCATION	PRESENT	ABSENT	% WITH PAIN
1st metatarsophalangeal joint	1	58	1.7
Osteotomy site	2	56	3.4
Lateral metatarsalgia	18	41	30.5

TABLE 19–2 Patient Satisfaction—Fifty-nine Cases

	IMPROVED	UNCHANGED	WORSE	% IMPROVED
Appearance	56	1	2	95
Overall satisfaction	56	0	3	95

who did not have more distal projection of the first metatarsal after surgery than before surgery had a significantly higher incidence of lateral metatarsalgia than the rest of the group.

DISCUSSION

For complete correction, a patient with a bunion, hallux valgus, degenerative arthritis of the first metatarsophalangeal joint, and metatarsus primus varus requires removal of the abnormal bone on the medial surface of the first metatarsal which underlies the hypertrophied soft tissue; arthroplasty of the first metatarsophalangeal joint; and reduction of the first-second intermetatarsal angle. The bunion, which is usually painful and, therefore, the patient's main complaint, is a result of chronic irritation of the soft tissue overlying an abnormally prominent medial portion of the distal first metatarsal (Fig. 19–4). This prominence results from: hallux valgus, new bone formed on the medial surface of the first metatarsal head, and metatarsus primus varus. If the hallux valgus is severe, the proximal phalanx of the great toe articulates with the lateral portion of the first metatarsal head, leaving the medial articu-

lar portion covered only by soft tissue. An exostosis is usually formed just proximal to the medial articular surface of the metatarsal as a response to chronic irritation. In addition, osteophytes may form secondary to the degenerative arthritis of the first metatarsophalangeal joint, adding to the medial prominence. Metatarsus primus varus further contributes to the prominence of the first metatarsal head because the entire first metatarsal points medially. With the standard Keller procedure an arthroplasty of the first metatarsophalangeal joint is performed, and the new bone on the distal metatarsal is removed. By adding a proximal osteotomy of the first metatarsal, the abnormal orientation of the first metatarsal is changed and the entire deformity is thereby corrected.

The amount of metatarsus primus varus required to be an important contributing factor to the deformity is not well defined. The true angle between the first and second metatarsals cannot be measured from one roentgenographic projection unless corrections are made for all factors that may result in parallactic distortion. However, comparison of two films taken in the same manner gives a reliable, although not absolute, measure of angle correction. In our study, the roentgenograms were

TABLE 19–3 Mean Values and Standard Deviations of Roentgenographic Measurements—Sixty-five Cases

	PREOPERATIVELY	POSTOPERATIVELY	DIFFERENCE PRE-HAND POSTOPERATIVELY
1st-2nd metatarsal angle	15±2.7°	7±3.9°	8.0±3.9°*
1st metatarsophalangeal angle	40±10°	25±10.5°	15.0±10.2°*
Distal projection of 1st metatarsal head with respect to 2nd	—.3±3.6 mm (more proximal)	+.4±4.0 mm (more distal)	.7±2.2 mm**

*p < .001
**p < .02

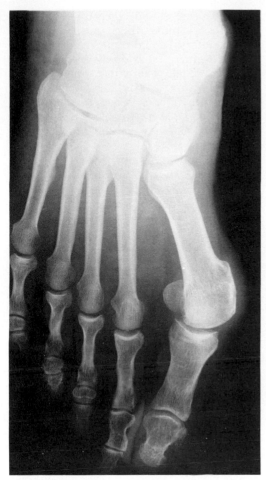

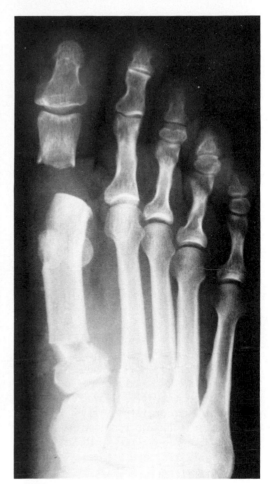

FIGURE 19-4 Preoperative roentgenogram in patient with an angle between first and second metatarsals of 15° . Note prominence of distal portion of first metatarsál caused by overgrowth of bone, hallux valgus, and metatarsus primus varus.

FIGURE 19-5 Roentgenogram of same patient as shown in Figure 19-4 two weeks after surgery. Angle betwen first and second metatarsals has been corrected to zero, graft is countersunk, and there is no displacement at osteotomy site.

taken with the patients not bearing weight, and, therefore, the deformities were minimized. We feel that a patient with an inter-metatarsal angle over 10° should be considered for an osteotomy. The opening wedge osteotomy is a simple, reliable procedure that does not require internal fixation or external immobilization, and in our experience it does not prolong the rehabilitation time, as compared with a Keller procedure alone.

The metatarsal osteotomy, as described, will provide the desired correction if done properly. A few technical points deserve emphasis. The bone wedge should be cut from the removed proximal phalanx rather than from the first metatarsal, which is usually of poor consistency and of insufficient size. The bone wedge must be fashioned with at least one cortical edge and be large enough to completely correct the deformity. Care should be taken to bend rather than completely break through the lateral cortex at the osteotomy site. Complete fracture at this point results in difficulty maintaining the position of the graft and the correction of the intermetatarsal angle. If fracture and displacement occur, internal fixation with small wires is required. Immediate postoperative roentgenograms frequently show a radiolucent line on the lateral surface of the metatarsal at the level of the osteotomy, as shown in Figure 19-4. However, the contour of the lateral cortical edge is smooth, indicating that a hinge of bone remains, preventing displacement of the metatarsal. When the graft is inserted, the medial edge should be slightly countersunk to prevent later graft displacement. In this series, unsatisfactory correction of the metatarsus primus varus was due to failure to adhere to one or more of these points.

The high incidence of metatarsalgia in patients with bunions and their associated deformities is well documented.[1,3,5,6] Although a number of causes have been assumed, as with most conditions, a combination of factors is most likely. Three of the causes of postoperative metatarsalgia suggested in the literature are pre-existing metatarsalgia, shortening of the first metatarsal, and loss of weight-bearing capacity of the great toe. Unfortunately, in this study the presence or absence of lateral metatarsalgia was not documented in every patient preoperatively. However, it was documented preoperatively in eight of the eighteen patients who reported postoperative lateral metatarsalgia. Of these eighteen patients only one rated her feet worse than before surgery.

In comparing the group with and without pain, a statistically significant higher incidence of pain was found in those patients whose first metatarsal head did not project more distally after surgery than before surgery. The opening wedge osteotomy as described here would be expected to increase the first metatarsal length as measured on the medial surface of the bone but not on the lateral surface, resulting in a more distal projection of the first metatarsal head. Failure to obtain this more distal position of the first metatarsal head could result from slippage or malposition of the graft with loss of angle correction, or from completely breaking through the lateral cortex resulting in displacement of the distal portion of the metatarsal. These are technical errors and, therefore, are preventable. A more dorsal position of the first metatarsal could result from failure to place the graft exactly on the medial side of the metatarsal. This could possibly shift weight bearing to the lateral metatarsals. However, great care was taken to avoid this error, but we were unable to effectively evaluate this factor in the postoperative review.

Another important consideration in the cause of lateral metatarsalgia is the weight-bearing ability of the great toe. Henry and Waugh[2] have pointed out that the ability to bear weight on the great toe is frequently lost in patients who have had Keller procedures in which more than one third of the proximal phalanx has been removed; this is associated with an increased incidence of metatarsalgia. Implant arthroplasty was not used in this series, but we think that reconstruction of the first metatarsophalangeal joint by this method should be considered, since it probably improves the appearance of the foot[4] and it may also reduce the incidence of metatarsalgia by restoring an articular surface and thereby retaining the weight-bearing capacity of the great toe.

REFERENCES

1. Bonney, G. and MacNab, I: Hallux valgus and hallux rigidus. *J. Bone Joint Surg.* 34B:366-85, 1952.
2. Henry, A.P.J. and Waugh, W.: The use of foot prints in assessing the results of operations for hallux valgus. A comparison of Keller's operation and arthrodesis. *J. Bone Joint Surg.* 57B:478-81, 1975.
3. Mitchell, C.L., Fleming, J.L., Allen, R., Glenney, C. and Stanford, G.G.: Osteotomy—bunionectomies for hallux valgus. *J. Bone Joint Surg.* 40A:41-60, 1958.
4. Swanson, A. B.: Implant arthroplasty for the great toe. *Clin. Ortho. Rel. Res.* 85:75-81, 1972.
5. Viladot, A.: Metatarsalgia due to biomechanical alterations of the forefoot. *Ortho. Clin. North Amer.* 4:165-78, 1973.
6. Wrighton, J.D.: A ten-year review of Keller's operation: review of Keller's operation at the Princess Elizabeth orthopaedic hospital, Exeter. *Clin. Ortho. Rel. Res.* 89:207-14, 1972.

Chapter Twenty

ORTHOPAEDIC MANAGEMENT OF RUNNERS

LOWELL D. LUTTER, M.D.

The overuse syndrome in long distance runners has only recently been noted by orthopaedists. With a large number of runners continuing past college and another group beginning to run in middle age, there are many individuals affected with foot-related overuse syndromes. It has been stated that over ten million people are running regularly.[5] Of runners going approximately thirty-five miles a week, more than 60 per cent are injured in any given year.[4] Our general experience in running injuries and specific utilization of orthoses are outlined.

One hundred and twenty-one long distance runners in a three-year period with one hundred and seventy one different injuries were seen. Injuries that were unique overuse syndromes are included. By definition, any abnormality developed by heavier than normal use can fall into an overuse syndrome category. Acute trauma, such as ankle sprains, does not fall into this group. Several runners had more than one injury, but only six had the same injury recur after healing.

Seventy-seven per cent of all injuries were of the foot or foot-related. Of the eighty-seven specific foot injuries, 50 per cent were midfoot, 30 per cent were fore-foot, and 20 percent were hindfoot injuries. Of the fifty knee injuries, 78 per cent were foot related, and of the twenty thigh-pelvis injuries, 10 per cent were foot related. No back injuries could be specifically correlated to foot problems. The greatest number of foot and foot-related injuries were strains, sprains, and inflammation, with only 6 per cent being bony injuries of the stress fracture type. In this study, we elected to look at injury patterns related to anatomic areas, rather than at specific areas as noted in other studies.[1,2,3]

The most important factor in causing running injuries occurs during the weight-bearing stage. It is this part of the running cycle which determines how and where forces are dissipated.[6]

The lower extremity injury pattern confirmed the idea that the greatest stress of running is taken up in the foot. Half of all running injuries were related to the foot. In joints successively more proximal, it was noted that there were fewer injuries. Knee injuries were 29 per cent, thigh-pelvis were 12 per cent and back injuries were 9 per cent of the cases studied.

Runners produce over five thousand foot strikes per hour and magnify even a small biomechanical deficiency. When one

155

looks at the normal lower extremity at heel strike, there is some external tibial rotation, and the midfoot is in supination. At "foot flat" position, pronation has occurred, and in conjunction with this, a small amount of internal tibial torsion occurs.[6] This pronation serves as an initial shock absorber and allows internal tibial rotation to occur. If excessive pronation occurs, force is translated rapidly to the midfoot area, producing problems here.

Forefoot problems occur when an excessively pronated foot reaches "toe off," with an abnormal stress distribution on the medial side of the foot. With excessive pronation, the tibia may internally rotate more than average prior to toe off. Excessive tibial rotation is a causal factor in many knee problems and a secondary factor in some hip and thigh problems. In the act of walking, these above- mentioned motions are present, but even if abnormal, they are not repeated as often nor are they associated with enough forces to produce injury in any but the rare individual. Decrease in the normal amount of pronation also produces abnormal stress distribution. This may occur because a tight plantar fascia, as seen in the cavus configuration, absorbs the forces which normally would be dissipated with a gentle average amount of pronation.

Cavus foot problems occur at heel strike when the foot is moving to "foot flat." The dorsiflexed toe, normal at this position, increases the windlass effect on the plantar fascia. An additional stress may be added when the foot goes to toe off, since the plantar fascia is then stretched from weight bearing through the toe.

Long-term treatment must attempt to deal with factors causing the problem, not just symptoms. Runners go back to the same mechanism and produce the same problems.

Initial treatment was symptomatic in terms of application of appropriate physical therapy, rest, and medications. Hyperpronation was a significant factor in 50 per cent of foot and 76 per cent of knee injuries. Some attempt, therefore, must be made to control this.

Long arch rigidity, as seen in the cavus foot configuration, was present in 18 per cent of the individuals. Treatment included stress reduction.

Dealing with these biomechanical difficulties, we felt that orthotic management was appropriate. We used orthotic management of pronation and cavus problems in eighty one cases. This entailed application of either ready-made, semi-flexible leather orthosis for long or metatarsal arch support, or a custom-made Orthoplast * orthosis molded to the foot in neutral position.

Sixty-one per cent of all foot problems and 56 per cent of all knee problems were treated with an orthosis. Ready-made orthoses were finished by the orthotist from pre-cut molded leather. Addition of a long arch or metatarsal arch support could be done as decided by the referring physician. These were semi-flexible with the heel cup tending to be small, and not designed to control varus or valgus at the heel.

Orthoplast orthosis production is relatively simple and can be done by the orthopaedist in the office (Fig. 20-1). A template was cut of the foot made of Orthoplast. This was dipped in water of a temperature of approximately 120°, formed into a boat shape (Fig. 20-2) and molded onto the foot, using an elastic bandage. Molding was done holding the heel in neutral position and applying whatever amount of longitudinal and metatarsal arch support was needed. The foot was dipped in cool water to allow rapid setting of the Orthoplast.* Final finishing was then done (Fig. 20-3). A rather crude product, but one that works.

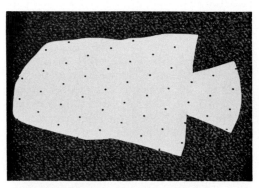

FIGURE 20-1 Template for orthosis.

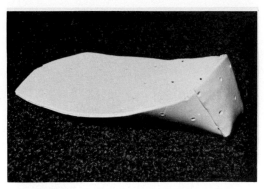

FIGURE 20-2 Molded orthosis in boot shape.

Results

The Orthoplast orthosis lasts approximately one year on 2500 running miles before breakage. The ready-made leather (Fig. 20-4) orthosis lasts approximately two years before replacement is needed. One must realize that the ready-made leather orthoses were not designed to accept the same amount of stress. Individuals treated with ready-made orthoses returned to running in, on an average, thirty-one days. Individuals treated with Orthoplast

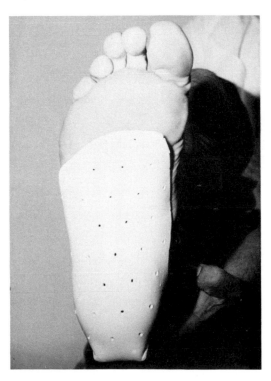

orthoses returned to running in approximately thirty-seven days. Better conformity of the foot can be obtained with the individual molded Orthoplast orthoses. The time and cost of Orthoplast orthoses are greater than for ready-made leather.

Summary

In this study, we have concentrated on specific anatomic areas of injury and their relationship to foot configuration, noting that foot and foot-related problems made up 77 per cent of the injuries we saw. Areas away from the foot are less affected.

Problems from cavus configuration are harder to treat and last longer. Initial treatment should be symptomatic but must include some plan for biomechanical foot control. A well-prescribed and well-fashioned orthosis of leather or Orthoplast works for the pronated foot. Ready-made leather orthosis were less effective for cavus configuration and we tended to use an Orthoplast support.

Orthopaedists are health care specialists uniquely trained to manage running problems. Their training, including study of biomechanics of the entire lower extremity, should allow them to better understand specific problems. Injured runners, unable to participate in their sport, are among the most anxious and agitated of patients. They never miss appointments, will wait long hours, and never return unless absolutely needed. They are highly motivated to

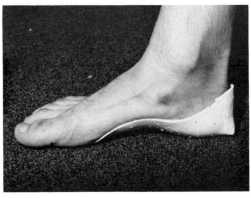

FIGURE 20-3 (A) Molded orthosis on foot, plantar view. (B) Molded orthosis, arch mold.

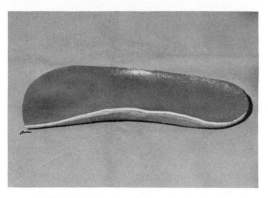

FIGURE 20-4   Leather pre-cut orthosis.

get well, following any instruction you give them.

With more and more people running, more are being injured. These are not dramatic injuries of a superstar requiring sophisticated surgery. These are nuisance injuries caused by overuse. Their seeming lack of drama does not make them less important to the injured individuals or less deserving of our attention.

REFERENCES

1. Brubaker, C. E. and James,. Injuries to runners. *J. Sports Med.* 2: 189-97, 1974.
2. Clancy, W.G.: Lower exremity injuries in the jogger and distance runner. *Phys. Sports Med.* 2:46-50, 1974.
3. Glick, J.M. and Katch, V.L.: Musculoskeletal injury in jogging. *Arch. Phys. Med.* 51:123-26, 1970.
4. Henderson, J.: First aid for the injured runner. *Runners World,* 12:32-36, 1977.
5. Jeansom, J.: *New York Times,* October 23, 1977.
6. Slocum, D. and Bowerman, W.: Biomechanics of running. *Clin. Ortho.* 23:39-45, 1962.
* Orthoplast is a trade name of the Johnson & Johnson company.

Chapter Twenty-One

FOOT INJURIES OF KARATE EXPERTS
A Study of Intentional Trauma

MICHAEL D. ROBACK, M.D.
ILAN TAMIR, M.D.
DEBRA FORRESTER, M.D.
TERRANCE BECKER, M.D.

Karate is unique as an American sport in that it developed as a reflection of the culture of Asia. For 2,500 years, the martial arts sprouted as self-defense systems of oppressed and unarmed people. It was only in the last fifteen years that the arts evolved into an international sport.

The martial arts originated in India and were introduced into China where they flourished in Buddhist and Taoist monasteries. Kung fu is the term used for the four hundred styles of the Chinese martial arts. The Chinese styles primarily use the open hands for fighting. Participants wear special soft shoes, and the foot is used mainly for pushing and tripping.

Okinawa was the link by which the fighting arts of China reached Japan. In the 1500s the nobility of Okinawa were forbidden to own weapons. Therefore, they developed an open-hand self-defense system.

In 1854 Admiral Perry sailed into Tokyo Bay and Oriental isolation ended. Asia began the road to industrialization, and the martial disciplines changed from the secret activity of a select few to a public activity that was available to all.

Open-hand fighting was not introduced to the Japanese until 1922. At first it was poorly accepted. Only during the last twenty-five years has it expanded in Japan. The word "karate" is the phonetic spelling of a Japanese word that means "empty hands." There are one hundred varieties. Karate predominantly uses a clenched fist for fighting; the bare foot is used for straight kicks.

Although a late entrant, Korea has become a world power in the martial arts since 1955. The Korean system is known as tae kwon do. Korean styles rely heavily on kicking and have many intricate kicking techniques. Shoes are not worn.

IMPACT ON AMERICAN SOCIETY AND SPORTS SCENE

Kung fu came to the United States with the Oriental migration during the gold rush. Yet it was not until 1964 that the doors were opened to nonoriental students. Karate was introduced into Hawaii in 1927; however, it did not grow in the United States until after World War II. Tae kwan do was imported after the Korean conflict and is now the most prevalent style.

The term "karate" is often used as a general term for all the different styles and will be used in that context in this chapter.

There are more than 165,000 students of karate in the United States including 42,000 children and 29,000 women. The ages of the participants ranges from 6 years to 88 years. Karate has recently expanded in special segments of American society, such as the physically handicapped. Therefore, a wide variety of injuries and orthopaedic problems are encountered by physicians who treat martial arts devotees.

FOOT TRAINING IN KARATE

Participants strengthen their feet by kicking special bags, boards, bricks and by sparring. Traditionally, body contact was avoided in sparring. In the last ten years, light contact and full contact have become accepted. Even in a noncontact situation, the kick is performed and blocked with maximum force, causing the foot to be hit repeatedly. Kicks are performed either standing or jumping. Jumping kicks are used because they increase the range and have an element of surprise.

RESEARCH PROJECT

The project consisted of an evaluation of sixteen male and four female experts. They averaged thirty three years of age, fifteen years of training, and a 3.8 degree black belt rank. The group was ethnically diverse and represented different karate styles.

Four factors were considered: (1) foot anatomy in kicking; (2) injury survey; (3) evaluation of pathology; and (4) relationship of activity to injury.

THE FOOT IN KARATE

Five areas are used in the majority of the kicks (Fig. 21-1). These are: (1) the plantar first, second, and third metatarsal heads; (2) the lateral cuboid and calcaneus; (3) the dorsal tarsals; (4) the plantar and posterior calcaneus; and (5) the medial first metatarsal base and medial tarsals.

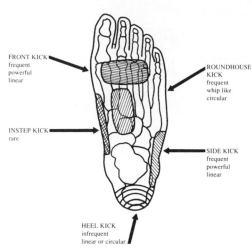

FIGURE 1: FOOT CONTACT ZONES

FIGURE 21-1   Foot contact zones.

The metatarsal heads are used in the linear front kick. The ankle is plantar flexed and the toes are pulled back. The force is directed through the extended knee and ankle to the plantar metatarsal heads. This kick delivers the greatest force (Fig. 21-2 and 21-3).

The lateral border of the foot is used in the linear lateral kick known as the knife-edge or side kick. The foot faces sideways and is pulled into maximum dorsiflex-

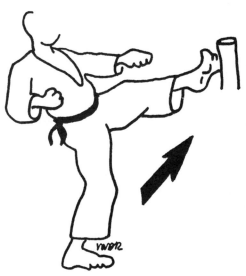

FIGURE 21-2   Front kick.

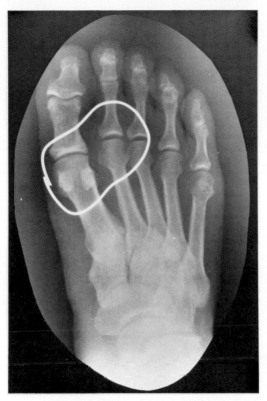

FIGURE 21–3   Front kick strike zone.

ion and varying supination (Fig. 21-4 and 21-5).

The dorsal tarsals are used with the toes flexed. They are used in straight kicks to the groin. They are also used in a foreward circular kick called a roundhouse

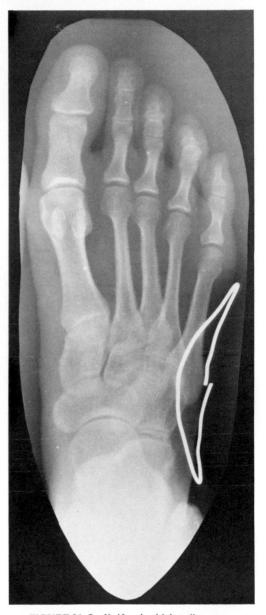

FIGURE 21–5   Knife-edge kick strike zones.

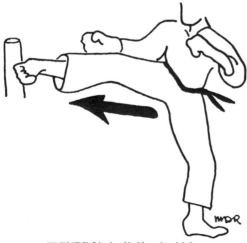

FIGURE 21–4   Knife-edge kick.

kick, which swings in a horizotal plane. The leg develops a snap similar to a whip. The foot is plantar flexed and the dorsal tissues are the striking surface. Round-house kicks are used because they attack from the periphery of the visual field and defense is difficult (Fig. 21-6 and 21-7).

The plantar and posterior surfaces of the calcaneus are used in a linear kick, or the foot can be snapped backwards in a

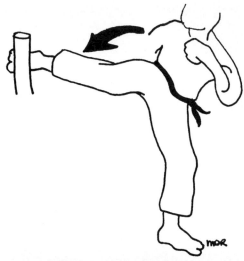

FIGURE 21–6 Roundhouse kick.

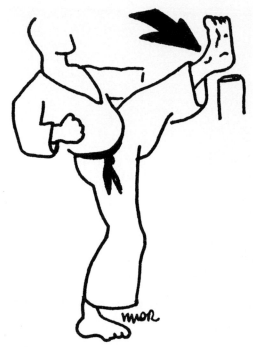

FIGURE 21–8 Spinning heel kick strike zone.

whiplike circular motion. This is called the spinning heel kick or wheel kick (Fig. 21–8 and 21–9).

The medial foot is infrequently used in karate kicks.

RETROSPECTIVE INJURY SURVEY

There were forty nine injuries in twelve participants which resulted in a one week loss, and nine that resulted in a one-month loss of training.

Forty-seven injuries involved the fore-foot. The hallux (37 per cent), second toe (28 per cent), and fifth toe (16 per cent)

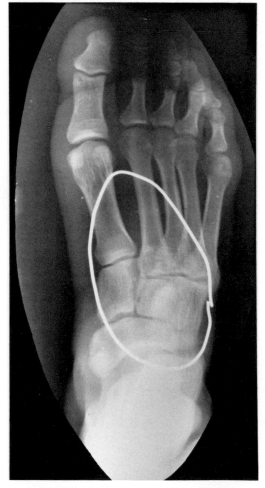

FIGURE 21–7 Roundhouse kick strike zone.

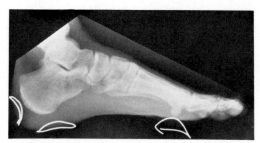

FIGURE 21–9 Heel kick strike zone.

were primarily involved. Toe injuries did not require surgery and only five required casts. Four individuals had multiple dislocations of the great or second toe. One third-degree black belt indicated that each second toe had been dislocated five times. He had bilateral Morton's toe deformities.

Two individuals sustained proximal injuries. One injured his foot while kicking a brick when he was thirty years old and a third-degree black belt with ten years' experience. The injury required surgery and he lost three months of training. He had a "chip fracture" over the lateral tarsal region. He is now forty seven years old and a tenth-degree black belt with thirty one years of experience. He noted slight foot stiffness.

A second expert "cracked all the little bones in the top" of his foot while sparring. He was treated with crutches for a month. The patient has no symptoms. He was thirty one years old and a first-degree black belt at the time of injury. He is now thirty seven years old and a second-degree black belt.

EVALUATION OF PATHOLOGIC CHANGES

Symptoms

Thirty-four experts denied foot symptoms. Four had intermittent migratory foot aches. One participant had bilateral dorsal foot aches. He was a third-degree black belt with five years of experience who frequently broke boards and bricks. X-rays showed generalized osteoarthritic changes.

One participant complained of an intermittent anterior right ankle ache. She originally sustained an injury while kicking a training bag.

There were no complaints of swelling, weakness, or instability. There were no impairments or disabilities.

Physical Examination

All participants could walk, squat, and jump without pain. There was no ankle swelling, tenderness, or ligament instability. Muscle and sensory functions were intact. Pulses were normal. Skin and hair patterns were normal. Three feet had slight varicose veins.

The heels were nontender. Four had slight posterior calcaneal prominences and seven individuals had slight ankle pronation. One foot had a scar over the sinus tarsi.

There were twelve splay feet, six decreased arches, and four pes planus. Eight feet had nontender fusiform enlargement of the proximal joint of the hallux. Five feet showed slight bunionettes.

The metatarsal heads and sesamoids were not tender. Six feet had slight Morton's toe deformity with second hammer toes. Four feet had claw toes.

X-ray Evaluation (Table 21-1)

There were six little toe phalangeal fractures. One subject lacked distal joint segmentation of the little toes.

There was hypertrophy, possibly secondary to an undisplaced fracture, of the second and/or third proximal phalanges in four subjects. There were metatarsal variations consisting of six enlargements of metatarsal heads associated with metaphyseal osteophytes; nine flattening of the second, third, or fourth metatarsal heads; one pointed first metatarsal head; and one bilateral slightly curved fifth metatarsal diaphysis. These abnormalities were not

TABLE 21-1.

CHART I: X-RAY FINDINGS

FOREFOOT	MIDFOOT
HALLUX	talonavicular spur (18)
distal phalanx spur (13)	naviculocuneiform spur (3)
lateral metatarsal spur (16)	2nd tarsometatarsal spur (2)
medial metatarsal head erosion (1)	3rd tarsometatarsal spur (2)
proximal joint subluxation (1)	4th tarsometatarsal spur (3)
2 part sesamoid (3)	5th tarsometatarsal spur (1)
minor variations of the sesamoid—	lateral cuboid calcification (1)
metatarsal area (70%)	lateral cuboid accessory
	ossification (2?)
OTHER TOES	
2nd metatarsal head spur (2)	HINDFOOT
3rd metatarsal head spur (2)	anterior tibial spur (15)
3rd and 4th metatarsal head spur (1)	dorsal tibial spur (4)
5th metatarsal head spur (4)	asymetrical bilateral os trigonum (1)
	posterior calcaneal spur (1)
	plantar calcaneal spur (1)

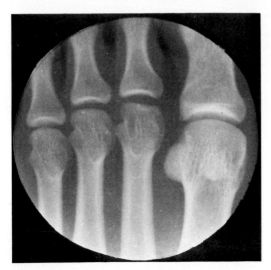

FIGURE 21-10 Asymptomatic flattening of second metatarsal head.

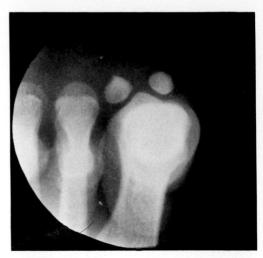

FIGURE 21-12 Asymptomatic sesamoid osteophyte.

associated with arthritic changes (Fig. 21-10).

One subject had asymptomatic bilateral os trigonum of different sizes.

There were frequent spur formations of the phalanges and distal metatarsals of the hallux which appeared to be secondary to avulsion fracture or joint disruption (Fig. 21-11). There were three halluces valgus which did not have osteoarthritic changes.

The sesamoids showed slight abnormalities in 70 per cent of patients (Fig. 21-12). There were three fragmented medial sesamoids.

Changes in the midfoot consisted of frequent dorsal osteophyte formation. These were severe in five feet (Fig. 21-13). There were three cases of radiopaque bodies at the lateral border of the cuboid. There were six cases of tarsometatarsal narrowing and osteophyte formation.

Abnormalities of the hindfoot or ankle were infrequent. There were six mild

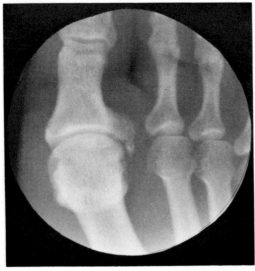

FIGURE 21-11 Asymptomatic anulsion fracture with post-traumatic changes.

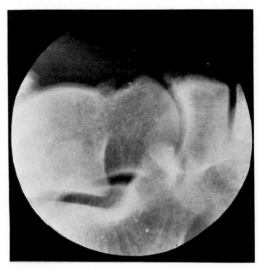

FIGURE 21-13 Symptomatic dorsal osteophytes.

TABLE 21-2.

GRAPH 1: KICK—INJURY RELATIONSHIP

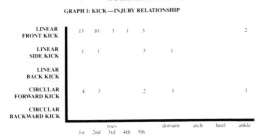

TABLE 21-3.

GRAPH 2: ACTIVITY—INJURY RELATIONSHIP

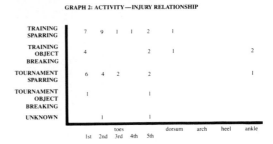

Haglund calcaneal prominences and three cases of minimal calcaneal osteophyte formation. Seventy-five per cent of ankles had anterior tibial spur formation. Four had posterior tibial spur formation, and one was associated with talar abnormalities.

Analysis of the x-ray findings indicated there were 80 per cent front kick, 40 per cent roundhouse kick, 10 per cent side kick, and 7.5 per cent heel kick strike zone abnormalities (Table 21-2).

RELATIONSHIP OF ACTIVITY TO INJURY (TABLE 21-3).

Injuries of the heel were infrequent and x-ray changes were minimal. First and second toe injuries resulted primarily from front kicks. The majority of the symptoms involved these toes. X-rays revealed frequent slight osteoarthropathy involving the sesamoids.

The little toe was vulnerable to injury in round house, front, and side kicks. It was the area of the most fractures. However, no significant symptoms were reported.

The dorsal tarsal area showed frequent osteoarthropathy. No symptoms were reported in the area. Injuries per hour of activity in tournament were eight times more prevalent than in training (Table 21-3), and injuries were not limited to the early part of the career.

CONCLUSION

Based on a small sampling of karate experts, it is concluded that one can attain karate expertise without functionally destroying the foot. Although there were frequent minor x-ray changes, there were no significant symptoms or impairments.

Chapter Twenty-Two

RUNNING, JOGGING, AND WALKING: A COMPERATIVE ELECTROMYOGRAPHIC AND BIOMECHANICAL STUDY

ROGER A. MANN, M.D.

JOHN L. HAGY, O.R.E.

This study was undertaken to obtain basic information that would enable us to compare walking, jogging, and running gaits. In order to carry out this comparison the following data were obtained: (1.) basic measurements of gait, i.e., velocity, cadence, step length, gait cycle components; (2.) range of motion of the hip, knee, and ankle joint in the sagittal plane; (3.) electromyography of eight muscles of the lower extremity and back; and (4.) force plate analysis of the ground reaction.

METHODS

The study was carried out at the Gait Analysis Laboratory at Shriners Hospital for Crippled Children in San Francisco. The motion data of the lower extremity were obtained by the photometric system of gait analysis, which is based upon bi-plane high speed photography.[1] This method enabled us to accurately determine the components of each gait, namely, velocity, cadence, step length, and time of the walking cycle. The sagittal plane range of motion of the hip, knee, and ankle joint was also obtained by using the photometric system. The electromyography was obtained by using superficial electrodes over each muscle group, recording the amplified signal, and superimposing it directly over the film of the lateral camera. With this method, accurate timing of electromyography to the position of the body is readily obtainable.

The force plate analysis of the ground reaction was determined by using a Pizo-electric force plate of which the output signal is on line to a computer. The forces measured were the vertical, fore and aft shear, and medial and lateral shear.

The study was made using five experienced joggers, three females and two males. Data on each subject were obtained three times for each speed of gait. Each set of data for each gait was then averaged. The data for each subject at each gait demonstrated minimal variation, and when compared with the other individuals, the patterns were surprisingly similar.

OBSERVATIONS

Basic measurements of the various gaits are presented in Figures 22-1 through 22-5. The walking cycle is defined as initial ground contact of the right foot until the initial ground contact of the right foot once again. *Range of motion* and *electromyography* of the hip, knee, and ankle was calculated in the sagittal plane for each speed of gait and is presented in Figures 22-6 through 22-9. Electromyography was obtained from the following muscles: gluteus maximus, hip abductors, hip adductors, quadriceps, hamstrings, gastrocsoleus, anterior tibial, and sacrospinalis. Their activity is illustrated in Figures 22-6 through 22-9 and 22-13. *Force plate* data included measurements of the vertical, fore and aft shear, and medial

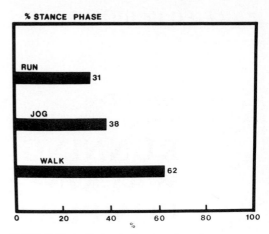

FIGURE 22-2   Percent of stance phase demonstrates that as speed of gait increases, time interval in which foot is on ground decreases.

and lateral shear. The results are presented in Figures 22-10 through 22-12.

DISCUSSION

In order to discuss so much data, we will first discuss each group of observations separately and then correlate the data. The basic measurements of gait demonstrated that as the speed of gait increases, the time of the walking cycle decreases. The stance phase which initially consumes approximately two thirds of the walking cycle is reduced to only a third for running (Figs. 22-1,21-2). As expected, the velocity,

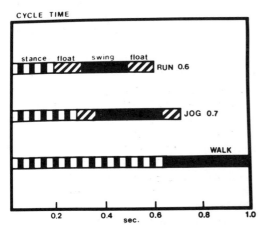

FIGURE 22-1   Comparison of cycle time for walking, jogging, and running. During walking one foot is always on the ground whereas during jogging and running there is a period in which both feet are off the ground, called float period.

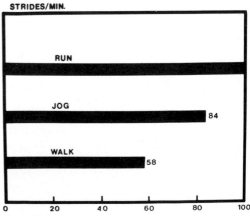

FIGURE 22-3   Strides per minute increase as speed of gait increases.

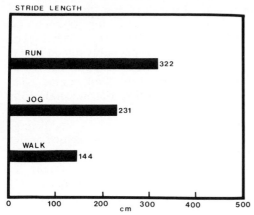

FIGURE 22-4 Stride length demonstrates progressive lengthening as speed of gait increases.

cadence, and stride length all increase considerably as the speed of gait increases (Figs. 22-3, 22-5). The float time, which is the period in which neither foot is on the ground and which does not exist during walking, consumed 20 percent of the cycle time for jogging and 40 percent for running. Therefore, as the speed of gait increases, the time the foot spends on the ground decreases.

The range of motion of the hip, knee, and ankle increased considerably as the speed of gait increased (Figs. 22-6-22-9). At the time of initial ground contact, there was a marked increase in knee flexion, which, along with dorsiflexion of the ankle, results in the lowering of the center of gravity.

During walking, full extension of the hip is reached before lift off, whereas dur-

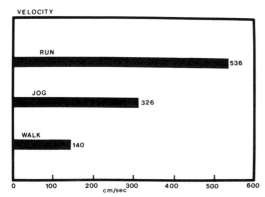

FIGURE 22-5 Velocity of gait increases with speed of gait.

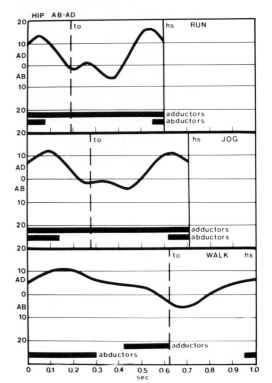

FIGURE 22-6 Comparison of hip adduction as speed of gait increases, along with superimposed electromyographic activity of adductors and abductors of hip.

ing jogging and running, full extension is not reached until after lift off has occurred (Fig. 22-7). The range of flexion during swing phase increases slightly during jogging and running. This delay in full extension of the hip in jogging and running is probably due to the fact that full extension is a passive occurrence and there isn't sufficient time during the stance phase of jogging and running for it to occur.

The range of motion of the knee joint demonstrated increased flexion at initial floor contact, from 7° for walking to 40° for jogging and running (Fig. 22-8). There was also an increased total range of motion from 60° in walking to 68° for jogging and 85° for running.

The increased flexion at initial floor contact is most likely a shock-absorption mechanism. The increased initial knee flexion is followed by still further flexion to about 60° by the midstance phase for jogging and running, compared with only 10°

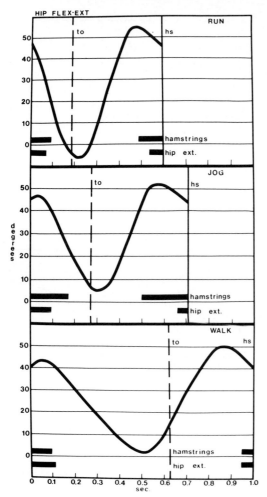

FIGURE 22-7 Comparison of hip extension and flexion as speed of gait increases, along with superimposed electromyography of hip extensors and hamstring muscles.

occurs at all speeds of gait until rapid plantar flexion begins, reaching its maximum after the foot has left the ground. This change in motion is probably due in part to the increased shock absorption needed by the body at the initial floor contact. The total range of motion of the ankle joint likewise increases as the speed of gait increases.

The force plate data demonstrated that the initial impact on the ground, which is about 85 percent of body weight for walking, increases to approximately 170 percent of body weight for jogging (Fig. 22-10). The initial impact for walking and

for walking. This markedly increased flexion is also acting as a shock-absorber mechanism; it lowers the center of gravity, as mentioned previously. The increased flexion during swing phase is caused by the rapid acceleration of the thigh after lift off, which brings about passive flexion of the knee joint.

The range of motion of the ankle joint changes most dramatically as the speed of gait increases (Fig. 22-9). During walking, plantar flexion occurs at the ankle joint on initial floor contact, but during jogging and running, dorsiflexion occurs. After the foot is firmly on the ground, dorsiflexion

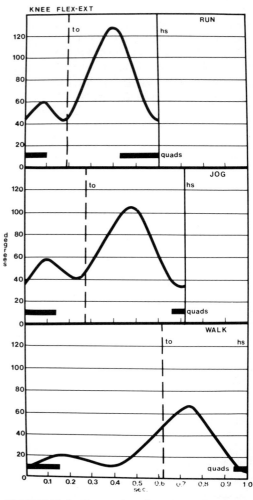

FIGURE 22-8 Range of motion of knee as speed of gait increases, with superimposed electromyography of quadricep musculature.

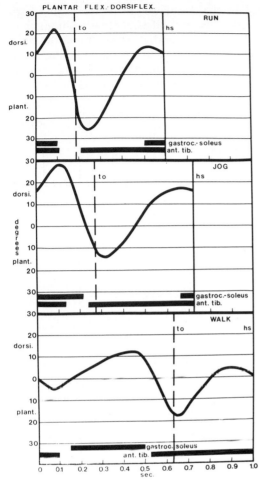

FIGURE 22-9   Comparison of range of motion of ankle during walking, jogging, and running with superimposed electromyography of anterior tibial and gastrocsoleus muscles.

body is much smoother than with jogging.

It is also possible that the center of gravity is not being elevated as high during running, and this could account for the loss of the initial spike. The first peak, which is present in all speeds of gait, represents the ground reaction to the elevation of the center of gravity after it has reached a low point at initial floor contact. The valley and second peak which are present in walking are not present in jogging or running. This change is due to the change in the weight transfer of the body. In walking,

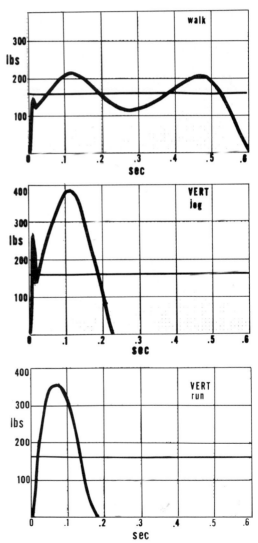

FIGURE 22-10   Vertical force curve for walking, jogging, and running.

jogging subsides slightly, following which there is a second peak in the vertical force, which is about 130 percent of body weight for walking, almost 250 percent for jogging, and slightly less for running. The loading curve for running was smooth and continuous, as compared with curves for walking and jogging. This change in the shape of the curve between jogging and running may indicate that running is a smoother type of gait and is not associated with as severe an initial impact as is jogging. It appears, based on the shape of this curve that running is a more natural event and the overall absorption of forces by the

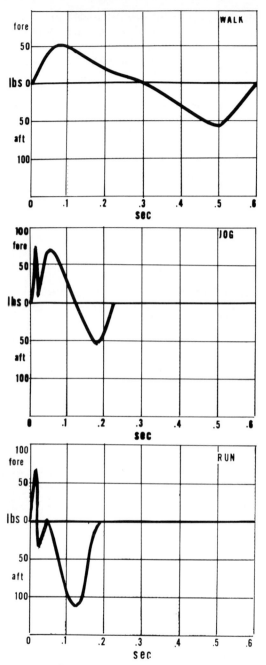

FIGURE 22-11   Fore and aft shear curve for walking, jogging, and running.

since the entire weight of the falling body strikes the ground after floating in space.

The fore and aft shear forces for walking and jogging are essentially the same, whereas in running, the aft shear is twice as great as that noted for walking and jogging

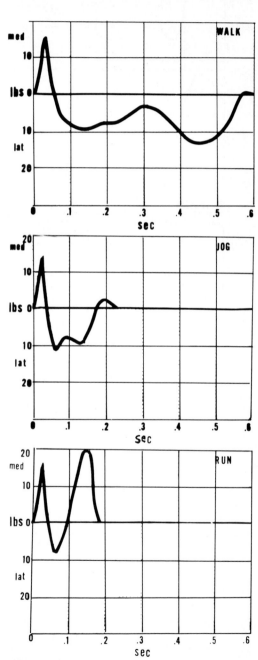

FIGURE 22-12   Medial lateral shear curve for walking, jogging, and running.

there is a smooth transition along with two periods of double weight bearing; whereas in jogging and running, these periods are lost and replaced by a float period. Therefore, the forces on the ground will increase,

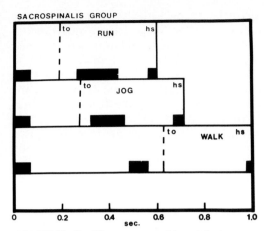

SACROSPINALIS GROUP

FIGURE 22-13 Electromyographic activity in sacro-spinalis group during walking, jogging, and running.

(Fig. 22-11). The fore and aft shear is greatly influenced by the angle the body makes with the ground. In walking, there is a slight forward body lean, but as the speed of gait increases, so does the forward lean, although we did not quantitate it in this study. These data seem to correlate fairly well with the fact that in jogging, the body is spending more time going up and down, whereas in running, the majority of the force is directed in the plane of progression.

The medial and lateral shear demonstrates that as the speed of gait increases to jogging, then running, the initial medial shear seen in walking is still present (Fig. 22-12). This correlates well with the hip abduction-adduction curve, which demonstrates that at initial floor contact, adduction of the hip occurs. The remainder of the force curve demonstrates a lateral shear for walking and jogging until lift off, but a medial shear for running. Again, this force correlates with the hip motion (abduction) for walking and jogging but not for running.

The electromyography, in general, demonstrated that in walking, the muscles are active during 20 to 30 percent of the entire cycle. During jogging and running they demonstrate, in terms of percentage, a longer period of muscular activity. Some change in the type of muscle contraction is also noted when comparing the various gaits. It should be kept in mind that a mus-

cle can undergo either a shortening contraction (concentric) or a lengthening contraction (eccentric).

Correlation of the electromyography and range of motion demonstrates some very interesting findings. The hip extensors, namely, the gluteus maximus and hamstring muscles, function at the end of swing phase and during the first 10 percent of stance during walking. During this time the hip joint, which has started to extend during the midswing phase, continues to do so under the influence of these muscles. The hip extensors are undergoing a concentric (shortening) contraction, and the hamstrings are probably undergoing an isometric type of contraction. Because it is a two-joint muscle and because the hip is extending, the knee is likewise extending. This action keeps the muscle at an almost constant length. During jogging and running, the period of activity of these muscles changes. The hip extensors are still active at the end of swing, but now they remain active through the first one third of the stance phase. During jogging the hamstrings become active before extension of the hip and probably act to decelerate the thigh and to initiate hip extension (Fig. 22-7).

During running the hamstrings become active in the last 25 percent of swing phase, just as hip joint extension begins. The activity of the hamstrings continues for the first two thirds of the stance phase for jogging and the first half for running. During this period, they are actively producing extension of the hip proximally and resisting extension of the knee distally. The longer period of activity for jogging could be due to the more constrained nature of the gait.

During normal walking the quadriceps are active during late swing and the first 15 percent of stance (Fig. 22-8). Their function is to stabilize the knee in almost full extension at initial floor contact and through the period of initial knee flexion which occurs early in stance. The quadriceps during jogging demonstrate electrical activity that is very similar to walking during swing phase, whereas during running, the quadriceps become active during the last half of swing phase, just after knee extension has begun. The quadriceps are active during running, bringing about knee extension following the swing phase. In both jogging and running they are active during the first half of stance to stabilize the knee at initial floor contact and during the period of flexion which follows. This increased period of activity is necessary because of the marked flexion in the knee joint during the stance phase of jogging and running. The knee flexion that occurs during swing phase is purely a passive event brought about by the rapid acceleration of the thigh.

The gastrocsoleus muscle group is active during walking in midstance and functions primarily to restrain the forward movement of the tibia over the fixed foot (Fig. 22-9). Previous biomechanical studies have demonstrated that there is essentially no push off to propel the body forward, and this is why "lift off" or "toe off" is the preferred terminology.[2]

However, during jogging and running the gastrocsoleus muscle becomes active at the end of swing phase, and activity continues through 80 percent of stance for jogging and 50 percent for running. This pattern of activity is a complete change from that seen in walking and is probably due to the dorsiflexion that occurs at the ankle joint after initial ground contact. The gastrocsoleus controls the progression of the tibia over the fixed foot at initial floor contact by an eccentric contraction and is acting as part of the shock absorption mechanism. During jogging the gastrocsoleus remains active during approximately 50 percent of ankle plantar flexion. It then undergoes a concentric contraction and is aiding in plantar flexion, although its activity ceases after 50 percent of the plantar flexion has occurred. During running, the gastrocsoleus function ceases just when plantar flexion of the ankle joint begins, and thus undergoes only an eccentric contraction. The difference in the period of activity for jogging and running is probably due to the increased up-and-down motion associated with jogging.

The anterior tibialis muscle is very active in walking, jogging, and running, and the electrical activity is quite similar in each gait (Fig. 22-9). In walking and jogging, it becomes active in late stance through the entire swing phase and into early stance phase for walking and the first half of stance for jogging. In running there is electrical activity just after toe off which continues through swing and through the first 60 percent of the stance phase. It is interesting to note that in walking there is plantar flexion of the ankle joint while the anterior tibialis is active, therefore, it is undergoing an eccentric contraction; whereas in jogging and running, there is dorsiflexion occurring at the ankle joint so that the muscle undergoes a concentric contraction. It appears as though the anterior tibialis is functioning to accelerate the tibia over the foot, while the gastrocsoleus is moderating the speed by undergoing an eccentric contraction. From a mechanical standpoint, it seems as though if one wanted to set up a mechanical system to provide rapid acceleration, this process of having the anterior tibialis muscle undergoing a concentric contraction is the most efficient method to increase the speed of gait.

In walking, the adductors of the hip are active during the last quarter of stance phase, whereas in jogging and running they demonstrate full phase activity (stance and swing) (Fig. 22-6). It is difficult to explain, but the adductors are probably acting to stabilize the pelvis to the thigh. This stability enables the swinging leg to impart a torque to the pelvis and hence to the stance limb. This torque ultimately is transferred down the limb and across the ankle joint to the subtalar joint to produce rotation and subsequent stability in the foot. The sacrospinalis group during walking was active from late swing through early stance and then just before and after opposite ground contact, which occurs during the stance phase (Fig. 22-13). The muscle group is functioning initially to elevate and probably help decelerate the pelvis prior to initial ground contact. The second period of activity probably helps to initiate the forward movement of the right hemipelvis, after contralateral floor contact. During jogging and running the period of activity in late swing and early stance remains the same, but a second period of activity now occurs during swing phase. It still occurs just before opposite ground contact and shortly thereafter, so that although the muscle activity takes place during swing phase, the muscle group is probably continuing to function in a similar manner.

ties, especially the knee, increases, and the period of muscle activity is prolonged. The vertical ground reaction as measured by the force plate increases significantly. The muscle function and joint motion were correlated with one another where possible.

SUMMARY

A comparative study of walking, jogging, and running has been carried out which shows that, generally, as the speed of gait increases, the stance phase decreases and the swing phase increases, the range of motion of the joints of the lower extremi-

REFERENCES

1. Sutherland, D. H. and Hagy, J. L.: Measurement of gait movements from motion picture film. *J. Bone Joint Surg.* 54A:787-97, 1967.
2. Simon, S. R., Mann, R. A., Hagy, J. L. and Larsen, L. J.: Role of the posterior calf muscles in normal gait. *J. Bone Joint Surg.* 60A:465-72, 1978.

Chapter Twenty-Three

PARTIAL EXCISION OF THE OS CALCIS IN THE TREATMENT OF LESIONS OF THE CALCANEUS

MARIO E. PORRAS M.D.
RODRIGO HIDALGO M.D.
JOSEPH QUINTANA M.S.

Osteomyelitis of the os calcis has been a relatively uncommon but persistent problem for the orthopaedic surgeon. There have been case reports in the literature describing total removal of the calcaneus for treatment of osteomyelitis as well as for other problems, including severe fracture, tuberculosis, and tumor.[13,15] Gaenslen[4] described the split heel approach for osteomyelitis of the os calcis. This allowed removal of necrotic bone and usually did not disturb the calcaneocuboid joint, but it did leave a scar on the weight-bearing portion of the heel. Wiltse[17] described resection of a major portion of the calcaneus for osteomyelitis or nonhealing ulcer of the heel in seven patients. He stressed the importance of maintaining the calcaneocuboid joint for prevention of an everted, "flipper foot" deformity which occurs at the midfoot when a total calcanectomy is performed. Other advantages of the procedure include minimal scarring, small amount of shortening, maintenance of ability to plantar flex the foot, and little danger of cutting important structures.

To verify the minimal loss of function and the importance of maintaining the calcaneocuboid joint for the transmission of weight-bearing force in any procedure involving surgery of the os calcis, an experimental model was devised. Freshly amputated lower legs and feet were used, with various stresses applied both with a normal calcaneus and after a partial resection had been performed. In addition, eight patients who had the procedure performed between 1960 and 1973 were evaluated and the clinical results were presented.

CLINICAL MATERIAL

Partial excision of the os calcis as described by Wiltse was performed on eight patients between 1960 and 1973 (Fig. 23-1). Three had refractory osteomyelitis

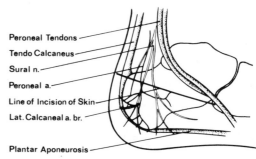

FIGURE 23-1 Line drawing illustrating approximate amount of calcaneus removed in Wiltse procedure.

Peroneal Tendons
Tendo Calcaneus
Sural n.
Peroneal a.
Line of Incision of Skin
Lat. Calcaneal a. br.
Plantar Aponeurosis

of the calcaneus (Fig. 23–2) and five had chronic nonhealing ulcers of the heel (Fig. 23–3). Ages ranged from twenty-four years to seventy-one years of age. Duration of symptoms varied from one month to five years prior to surgery. Three patients developed osteomyelitis secondary to open fractures and one to a traction pin in the calcaneus.

Five patients developed refractory decubitus ulcers of the heel during immobilization of the extremity for non-foot-related problems such as third-degree burns, severe fracture of the tibia with peroneal nerve palsy, fracture of the femur, and pain after a total hip procedure. One patient was diabetic with a chronic non-healing ulcer. Organisms were *Staphylococcus aureus*, four cases; *Pseudomonas*, two cases; and *Proteus*, two cases (Table 23–1). Length of follow-up was three months to fourteen years. One patient had postoperative drainage which cleared after five months. Five patients were completely free from pain. One patient had pain for "four or five years" which resolved to a pain-free state. Two patients had mild, nonincapacitating pain at last follow-up. All patients had a full range of motion of the ankle with plantar flexion of the foot (Fig. 23–4).

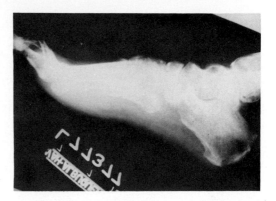

FIGURE 23–2 Lateral roentgenogram of foot with chronic osteomyelitis of calcaneus.

Only two patients required heel lifts, and one of these patients stopped wearing the lift after two months. Figure 23–5 is the x-ray of a foot after partial excision of the os calcis.

No attempt was made to classify the results in these patients as excellent, fair, or poor because of the subjectivity of the symptomatology. It was noted, however, that all had a resolution of the infection, all were ambulatory, and only two complained of pain at last follow-up.

TABLE 23–1   Patient Statistics

PATIENT	DISEASE	AGE	DURATION OF SYMPTOMS	ORGANISM	POST OPERATIVE DRAINAGE	PAIN	HEEL LIFT	LENGTH OF FOLLOWUP
E.W.	51	Osteo secondary to traction pin	8 months	*Staphylococcus aureus*	None	With activity	Wore for 2 months only	14 years
J.T.	36	Open fracture, Os calcis	1 month	*Pseudomonas*	None	Occasional, not disabling	None	7 months
J.M.	24	Shrapnel injury, Os calcis	3 + 6 years	*Staphylococcus aureus*	None	Mild	None	18 months
C.H.	51	Decubitus ulcer, heel, after multiple casting, tibia	1 year	*Staphylococcus aureus*	5 months cleared	None	None	5 months
A.M.	50	Decubitus ulcer, heel	5 years	*Proteus*	None	None	None	3 years
C.H.	71	Decubitus ulcer, heel, after immobilization for burns	4 months	*Pseudomonas*	None	None	None	3 months
W.U.	60	Osteo secondary to diabetic ulcer, heel	1 year	*Proteus*	None	None	None	5 months
H.B.	48	Decubitus ulcer, heel, secondary to pain status post total hip	1 month	*Staphylococcus aureus*	None	None	One inch	2 years

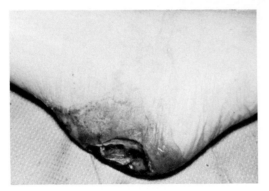

FIGURE 23-3 Chronic nonhealing ulcer of soft tissue at area of insertion of Achilles' tendon without bony involvement.

BIOMECHANICS

The weight distributing function of the foot is a dynamic relationship of bones, ligaments, tendons, and muscles. It changes with each phase from heel strike to toe off. It can, however, be analyzed both theoretically and experimentally at any given point in time by taking into account the forces acting on the foot as well as their direction of action. According to Scully,[14] the foot can be considered a bony arch or curved beam with a tension member con-

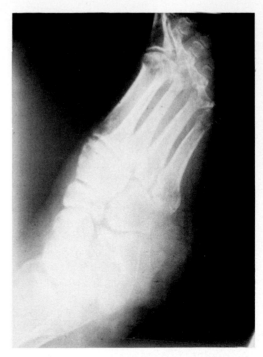

FIGURE 23-5 Lateral roentgenogram of foot showing approximately two thirds of os calcis removed.

sisting of plantar fascia and intrinsic muscles (Fig. 23-6).

This tension member serves to direct the tibial load (T) and muscle pull of the triceps surae (P) along the beam as compressive forces. These forces are then divided and transmitted through the talonavicular and calcaneocuboid joints on their

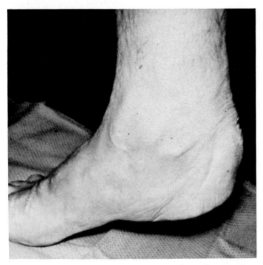

FIGURE 23-4 Patient demonstrating plantar flexion after partial excision of os calcis with reattachment of Achilles' tendon to remaining portion of bone.

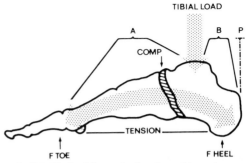

FIGURE 23-6 Schematic drawing of lateral aspect of foot showing direction of forces as compressive loads, with tension member provided by plantar fascia. Distance A is lever arm from tibial load to point of application at F toe. Distance B is lever arm from tibial load to point of application at F heel. P is point of application of Achilles' tendon muscle pull.

way to the forefoot (F toe). The percentage of force transmission through each joint can be calculated by determining the perpendicular distance from the center of each joint to the vector of the point of application of the force (T) or (P). This vector is obtained by drawing a line from (T) or (P) to the point of dispersion in the forefoot. As seen in Figures 23-7 and 23-8, the talonavicular joint bears $(\dfrac{Y}{X+Y})$ compression load arising from tibial axial loading (T), and $(\dfrac{M}{M+N})$ load arising from Achilles' tendon pull (P) (Fig. 23-7). Therefore, the force across talonavicular joint $= T(\dfrac{Y}{X+Y}) + P(\dfrac{M}{M+N})$. The same formula is used for force across the calcaneocuboid joint. This force $= T(\dfrac{X}{X+Y}) + P(\dfrac{N}{M+N})$. These forces divided by the total forces will give the theoretical percentage of force transmitted across each joint. Our calculations estimate 42 percent of the total force applied to the foot is transmitted across the calcaneocuboid joint.

The force measured at the toe and heel can, likewise, be measured by obtaining the sum of forces about a given point (Fig. 23-6). In equilibrium, the sum of forces equals zero; or $T - P - F_h - F_t = 0$. Therefore, $F \text{ heel} = T(\dfrac{A}{A+B}) - P(\dfrac{A}{A+B})$ and $F \text{ toe} = T(\dfrac{B}{A+B}) + P(\dfrac{B}{A+B})$.

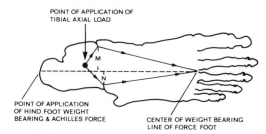

M

N

POINT OF APPLICATION
OF HIND FOOT WEIGHT
BEARING & ACHILLES FORCE

CENTER OF WEIGHT BEARING
LINE OF FORCE FOOT

FIGURE 23-8 Using skeleton and cadaver feet, it was noted that the resultant of force applied at Achilles' insertion did not pass through tibial load point of application, but rather lateral to it. This gave different values for distances M and N from Achilles' force resultant to center of the talonavicular and calcaneocuboid joints, respectively.

In our experiment, we have excised a portion of the os calcis which effectively shortens the lever arm (c) but does not otherwise change the mechanics of the system (Fig. 23-9).

METHOD

Russell Jones[8] devised a model for determining the mechanics of pressure transmission through the foot in various phases of weight bearing. A modification of his protocol was used and his values were adapted to serve as a standard for evaluation of weight-bearing changes in the longitudinal arch in stance phase before and after partial excision of the calcaneus. The static, or axial, force applied to a tibia is

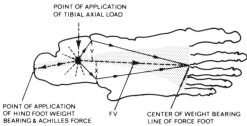

POINT OF APPLICATION
OF TIBIAL AXIAL LOAD

Y

X

POINT OF APPLICATION
OF HIND FOOT WEIGHT
BEARING & ACHILLES FORCE

FV

CENTER OF WEIGHT BEARING
LINE OF FORCE FOOT

FIGURE 23-7 Schematic drawing of anteroposterior aspect of foot showing distribution of forces from tibial axial load. Line FV is the resultant of force vectors passing through talonavicular and calcaneocuboid joints; X and Y are the distances from that resultant to those joints, respectively.

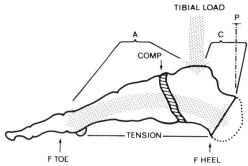

TIBIAL LOAD

P

A

C

COMP

TENSION

F TOE

F HEEL

FIGURE 23-9 Schematic drawing of foot after partial excision of os calcis. Note change in lever arm distance C from tibial load force to joint of application at F heel. Presuming maintenance of proper tension of plantar fascia, all other forces should remain the same.

equal to approximately one half of body weight when standing (T = 37 Kg). This was applied by the apparatus as demonstrated in Figure 23-10.

Extrinsic muscles of the foot also contribute a dynamic force which varies with the various phases of weight bearing. As has been shown by Jones and Morton,[8,12] a foot in stance phase bears 50 percent of the weight on the metatarsal heads or ball of the foot (Fig. 23-11).

To achieve this balance, the gastrocnemius attached to the calcaneus must exert a dynamic force equal to three fourths of the static force on the tibia.[8] In this experiment, weight equals force in kilograms. The contribution of the other extrinsic muscles was calculated according to their cross-sectional areas using the gastrocnemius as a standard. In plantar flexion, tip toes, the flexor extrinsics are active, producing forces roughly equal in proportion to their cross-sectional areas(Table 23-2).[8]

In our experiment using four freshly amputated specimens, the tendon of the flexor hallucis longus, flexor digitorum longus, posterior tibialis, peroneus longus and brevis, and the Achilles' tendon was attached to spring scales. Forces were applied as in Table 23-2. To measure the

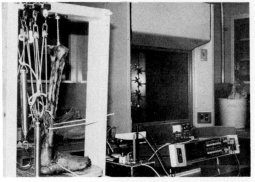

FIGURE 23-10   Force application apparatus. "Wine press" type screw assembly from top of frame applies graduated forces to tibial plateau which are read on bathroom scale below foot. Ropes and spring scales are attached to various tendons of foot used in stance phase. Compressive forces are read on digital voltmeter shown on right.

forces transmitted through the calcaneocuboid area, a strain gage module was designed and inserted after excising the calcaneocuboid joint and 9 mm of bone on either side. Measurements were then recorded in stance phase.

A partial excision of the os calcis was performed according to Wiltse. Approximately two thirds of the bone was removed in each case. The Achilles' tendon was reattached to the remaining portion of the cal-

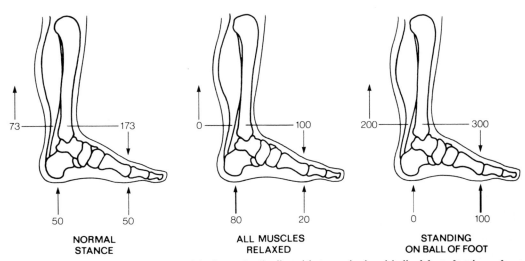

	NORMAL STANCE	ALL MUSCLES RELAXED	STANDING ON BALL OF FOOT
top	73 — 173	0 — 100	200 — 300
bottom	50 50	80 20	0 100

FIGURE 23-11   In normal stance, weight is evenly distributed between heel and ball of foot. It takes a force applied by the gastrocnemius complex of approximately 3/4 of the axial force or body weight to achieve balance. In this figure, axial force is 100 units and Achilles' force is 73. Since gastroc complex is anchored to tibia, a reactive force of 73 is added to axial force, giving a total of 173 units (lbs/kgs).

TABLE 23–2   Dynamic Force Contributions of Extrinsic Muscles of the Foot

	AVERAGE CROSS-SECTION IN SQUARE INCHES	RATIO		Kg f
			3/4 of Static Force	
Gastroc soleus	4.05	1.000	on Tibia (T) = 37 Kg	= 21.0
Posterior tibialis	0.50	0.124	21 × .124	= 2.5
Peroneus longus	0.48	0.116	21 × .116	= 2.5
Flexor hallucis longus	0.33	0.0825	21 × .082	= 1.6
Flexor digitorum communis	0.24	0.0595	21 × .059	= 1.2

caneus and plantar fascia, reproducing what occurs after healing in vivo. The above measurements were repeated with the same forces being applied. The averages of the results of all four legs was obtained.

INSTRUMENTATION

During the study, it became desirable to obtain quantitative measurements of the difference in force magnitude experienced across the calcaneocuboid joint area. Knowledge of this force under experimental conditions before and after the Wiltse procedure would reveal the degree to which the force is redistributed.

Investigation of possible methods of measuring force transmission across the joint indicated that the most efficient way would be to measure compression perpendicular to the plane of the joint.[1,2,5,6,8-10,12,15,16] This was accomplished by inserting a load sensor in the force line of the joint. This approach was implemented after theoretical verification that the major components of force under loading in stance phase under study were purely compressive (Fig. 23–6). It was observed that slight lateral and torsional motions resulted under certain load conditions; however, it was felt that the components of the transmitted forces which caused these motions were of negligible relative magnitude.

To facilitate placement of a sensor in the force line of the joint, a 9-mm section was excised from each side of the joint to provide ideal parallel surfaces perpendicular to the force line. Thus a sensor could be easily inserted in the force line to measure

the purely compressive force components. (Fig. 23–12).

The sensor devised to measure compressive forces consisted of a right circular cylinder approximately .79 cm in diameter and 1.27 cm in length, and two load surface discs approximately 1.27 cm in diameter and .32 cm thick. A load disc was bonded to each face of the cylinder to form a spool-like configuration. The bone contact surfaces of the discs were knurled to provide optimal coupling with the bone surface resulting from the saw cut.

Semiconductor strain gages were bonded on the cylinder surface to sense the compressive strain and yield the force electrical analog. The completed sensor was calibrated with a uniaxial compressive load testing machine to establish its force-to-analog ratio in kilograms. Thus, quantitative force measurements could be performed by observing the electrical analog on a digital voltmeter and converting the electrical analog level (millivolts) to kg force units.

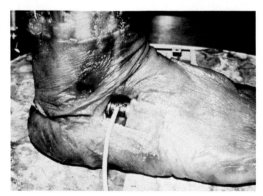

FIGURE 23–12   Calcaneocuboid joint plus 9 mm of bone on each side has been excised. Cylindrical load sensor has been placed in defect and changes in millivoltage transmitted to voltmeter.

RESULTS

Our first experiment was to load the intact foot with a progressive tibial axial load (I) but without Achilles' tendon pull (P) (Fig. 23-13). The forces transmitted were very similar (B) to the line (A) predicted theoretically if 42 percent of the total force is transmitted in the calcaneocuboid joint. Line (C) is after subtotal resection of os calcis, and a precipitous drop is noted in force transmission across the calcaneocuboid joint. This difference is due to the absence of the plantar fascia "tension member" which, although sutured to the Achilles' tendon, is not operative because of the lack of Achilles' tendon pull. Force (T) is, therefore, dissipated into the soft tissue of the mid- and hindfoot with little being transferred anteriorly.

Our second experiment was to apply both a tibial axial load (T = 37 Kg) and a progressive Achilles' tendon force (P) to an intact foot (Fig. 23-14). We then resected a portion of the os calcis and repeated our force applications (Fig. 23-15). With the intact foot, the calcaneocuboid joint was noted to transmit 49 percent of the total load. After partial resection of the os calcis, the load across the joint dropped to 35 percent.

In the experiment that followed (Fig. 23-16) we added a third force, the combined pull of the toe flexors, 4.2 Kgf;

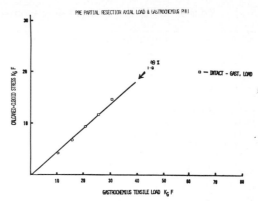

FIGURE 23-14 Application of axial load with gastrocnemius pull in an intact foot resulted in 49 percent of total force applied being transmitted through calcaneocuboid joint.

peroneals, 3.3 Kgf; and the posterior tibialis, 3.6 Kgf. These forces were estimated by making a relationship of the cross-section of each muscle to the cross-section of the gastrocsoleus complex. This ratio was then completed by using the maximal contractual force of the gastrocsoleus complex and relating it in proportion to the cross-sectional areas of the accessory muscles. This method is inexact but is reproducible and serves to provide constant force values (Table 23-2).

With the axial load, Achilles' tendon pull, and accessory muscle pull on the intact foot, it was noted that the calcane-

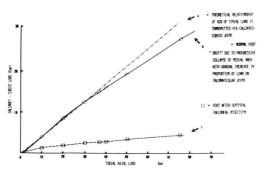

FIGURE 23-13 This graph illustrates necessity of maintaining plantar fascia as a tension member. Line B shows amount of force transmitted through calcaneocuboid joint in an intact foot. Line C is force transmitted after resection of os calcis and without Achilles' tendon pull to place tension on plantar fascia. Majority of axial load is, therefore, dissipated in hindfoot and not transmitted anteriorly.

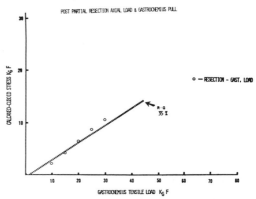

FIGURE 23-15 After partial resection of calcaneus, axial load and gastrocnemius pull are reapplied. Since plantar fascia is sutured to Achilles' tendon, a tension member is, once more, produced, and 35 percent of total force applied is transmitted through calcaneocuboid joint.

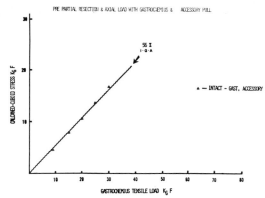

FIGURE 23-16   A third factor is added to axial load and gastrocnemius pull. This is the accessory muscles of the foot—the peroneals, tibialis posterior, and toe flexors. With these "muscles" active, this raises the force across the calcaneocuboid joint is raised to 56 percent of total force applied in intact foot.

ocuboid joint transmitted 56 percent of the total forces (Fig. 23-16). With the partial resection of the os calcis performed, the joint was noted to transmit only 20 percent of the total forces (Fig. 23-17).

DISCUSSION

It has been confirmed by several clinical studies[7,11,17] that partial resection of the os calcis for osteomyelitis of the calcaneus or for chronic nonhealing ulcer of the soft tissue over that bone is an acceptable mode of treatment. The patients are noted to

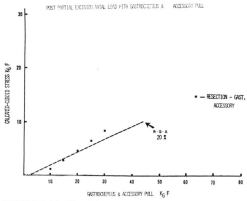

FIGURE 23-17   After partial resection of the calcaneus, the load across calcaneocuboid joint drops to 20 percent. This is the situation which most closely resembles what occurs in vivo.

have healing of the lesion, minimal scarring and pain and, most importantly, retention of an adequately functioning foot. It is postulated that the reason the foot remains so functional is the maintenance of the calcaneocuboid joint.[17] When it is removed, as in total excision of the os calcis, an everted, "flipper foot" deformity results.[18] When it is preserved, it continues to transmit compressive forces for dissipation at the forefoot as well as acting as a stabilizer of the midfoot.

In our experimental studies, we attempted to define the sources of force across the calcaneocuboid joint in stance phase in an isolated fashion and to describe how each force affected the joint in an intact foot and in one with partial excision of the os calcis. We noted that pure axial load is very poorly transmitted across the joint unless there is an intact plantar fascia tension member and, therefore, this fascia should be reattached to the remnant of the os calcis under some tension in the Wiltse procedure.

Resection of os calcis with reattachment of plantar fascia to calcaneus as well as to Achilles' tendon and subsequent application of axial and gastrocnemius forces shows a 14 percent drop in force transmission as compared with the intact foot. This drop is due to the shortened lever arm (c) of force (P) which is applied at the insertion of the Achilles' tendon to the os calcis (Fig. 23-9).

Jones[8] estimated that less than 5 percent of the force delivered to the forefoot is provided by the accessory muscles, i.e., toe flexors, peroneals, and posterior tibialis. In our last experiment, we added this force to the axial and Achilles' tendon loads on both an intact foot and on one with a partially resected os calcis. The sustentaculum tali was preserved in all cases. The force (I-G-A) transmitted across the calcaneocuboid joint was found to be 56 percent of the total force applied (Fig. 23-18).

After resection of a portion of the os calcis, however, there was a marked change in the force transmission across the calcaneocuboid joint (R-G-A). Only 20 percent of the force was measured at that joint, with the rest being transmitted via

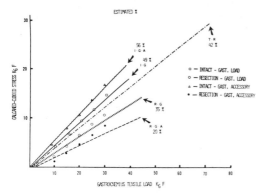

FIGURE 23-18 Composite graph showing line T-R, which is what percentage of total force should be transmitted through calcaneocuboid joint in intact foot. Note drop from 56 to 20 percent with resection of os calcis in a foot which has axial load, gastrocnemius load, and accessory muscle pull.

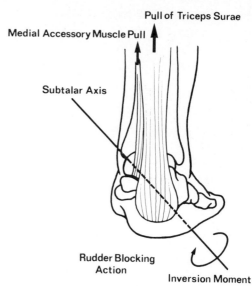

FIGURE 23-19 Body of calcaneus is in contact with flat surface, offering a "rudder type" blocking action against medial pull of accessory muscles and triceps surae. With this action removed, remaining portion of os calcis with sustentaculum tali tends to rotate around subtalar axis, increasing medial moment of force vector (F-V) of the foot. This decreases force transmitted through calcaneocuboid joint as illustrated in Figure 23-18.

the talonavicular joint. The reason for this change is probably twofold. First, as demonstrated on the previous experiment, a shortening of the (P) force level arm (b) reduced the force across the calcaneocuboid joint by 14 percent. The second reason is the shifting of the force vector to the forefoot (F-V) medially by the action of the toe flexors and posterior tibialis so that more of the force is then transmitted via the talonavicular joint (Fig. 23-7). The peroneals provide a lateral moment on the forefoot force vector, but in our experiment, 3.3 Kgf was applied through these tendons, whereas 7.8 Kgf was applied by the toe flexors and posterior tibialis. The fulcrums of the latter are in close proximity to the medial malleolus and sustentaculum tali. The rudder-type function of the posterior body of the os calcis which prevents the medial rotation of that bone around the axis of the subtalar joint is eliminated by the partial excision (Fig. 23-19). This allows the overpull of the medial tendons, thus moving the forefoot force vector medially, closer to the talonavicular joint. This last experimental model is probably that which most closely resembles what occurs in vivo. It is apparent that the major function of the calcaneocuboid joint in a foot with partial resection of the os calcis is to maintain anatomic relationship rather than actually to transmit force (Fig. 23-19).

CONCLUSION

A functional surgical procedure has been developed by Dr. Wiltse for the treatment of chronic lesions of soft tissue and bone of the heel.

Our clinical experience combined with other reports indicates that the procedure affords relief of the presenting disease without significant loss of function of the foot.

In the procedure, suture of the plantar fascia under some tension is necessary to maintain the biomechanical advantage of a curved beam.

Our experimental data show that the preservation of the calcaneocuboid joint in partial excision of the os calcis is important primarily as a spacer in maintaining anatomic relationship of the midfoot and the hindfoot. It also maintains some function as a force transmitter although much reduced in relation to its function in the normal state.

REFERENCES

1. Cochran, G.V.B.: Implantation of strain gages on bone in vivo. *J. Biomech.* 5:119-23, 1972.
2. Dorsey, J.: Semiconductor Strain Gage Handbook. Waltham, Massachusetts: BLH Electronics Inc., 1964.
3. Elftman, H.: A Cinematic study of the distribution of pressure in the human foot. *Anat. Rec.* 59:1934.
4. Gaenslen, F.J.: Split heel approach in osteomyelitis of os calcis. *J. Bone Joint Surg.* 13:759-72, 1931.
5. Hicks, J.H.: The mechanics of the foot: I. The joints. *J. Anat.* 87:345-57, 1953.
6. Hicks, J.H.: The mechanics of the foot: II. The plantar aponeurosis and the arch. *J. Anat.* (London) 88:25-31, 1954.
7. Horawitz, T.: Partial resection of the os calcis and primary closure in the treatment of resistant large ulcers of the heel with or without osteomyelitis of the os calcis. *Clin. Ortho.* 84:1972.
8. Jones, R.: The human foot—an experimental study of its mechanics and the role of its muscles and ligaments in the support of the arch. *Am. J. Anat.* 68:1-39, 1941.
9. Mann, R. and Inman, V.J.: Phasic activity of intrinsic muscles of the foot. *J. Bone Joint Surg.* 46A:469-80, 1964.
10. Manter, I.T.: Movements of the subtalar and transverse tarsal joints. *Anat. Rec.* 80:397-409, 1941.
11. Martini, M. and Martini-Benkeddache, Y., et al.: Treatment of chronic osteomyelitis of the calcaneus by resection of the calcaneus. A report of twenty cases. *J. Bone Joint Surg.* 56A:542-48, 1974.
12. Morton, D.: *Foot Biomechanics: Functional Disorders and Deformities, Medical Physics.* Chicago: Year Book Publishers, 1947, 457-66.
13. Pridie, K.: A new method of treatment for severe fractures of the os calcis. *Surg. Gynecal. Obstet.* 82:671-75, 1946.
14. Scully, T.: Personal communication.
15. Stott, J.R., Hutton, C.W. and Stokes, I.A.: Forces under the foot. *J. Bone Joint Surg.* 55B:335-44, 1973.
16. Wetzenstein, H.: A new method for assessment of the static and dynamic weightbearings of the foot. *Acta Ortho.* Scand. 30:1971.
17. Wiltse, L.L., Bateman, J.E. and Kase, S.: Resections of a major portion of the calcaneus. *Clin. Ortho.* 13:271-77, 1959.
18. Wiltse, L.L., Bateman, J.E. and Hutchinson, R.H.: Calcanectomy—partial and total. Audiovisual Program, American Academy of Orthopaedic Surgeons, Annual Meeting, San Francisco, 1967.

Chapter Twenty-Four

FORCES UNDER THE FOOT: A STUDY OF WALKING, JOGGING, AND SPRINTING FORCE DISTRIBUTION UNDER NORMAL AND ABNORMAL FEET

PIERCE E. SCRANTON, JR., M.D.
BARRY D. HOOTMAN, M.D.
JAMES H. MCMASTER, M.D.

Over the years, many attempts have been made to determine the dynamic distribution of forces under the weight-bearing foot. These efforts have resulted in a greater understanding of normal gait and of the functional pathologic factors in a variety of foot disorders. Certainly, in order to understand abnormal feet and treat them adequately, one must first comprehend the progression and transmission of forces under the normal foot. Technical difficulties in measuring these forces, however, have been the chief obstacle to gathering meaningful data. Early studies by Beely, Basler, Momberg, and others were limited by such technical difficulties and, in the final analysis, measured only the shape of the foot or the total static force during the stance phase of gait.[1,6,8,16,24] Later investigators devised electrical methods, optical devices, pressure transducers, and computerized force plates by which they were able to record momentary changes in pressure during stance phase. Their techniques, however, sometimes altered the normal gait pattern, and in no study was running gait adequately examined.[2,4,7,9,12,17,18,25,29 31,34,35] This chapter presents a study on momentary forces under the foot in which a different technique was used to record these forces.[33]

MATERIALS AND METHODS

Industrial technology has made available a new substance for monitoring temperature or pressure changes in a given environment. Commonly known as "liquid crystals," this substance has the flow properties of a liquid as well as the optical characteristics of a crystal. It can change color in response to changes in either temperature or pressure.[14,15,20,27] This study utilizes pressure-sensitive liquid crystals which change from light to dark blue as the shear force or pressure increases. Although the color change is proportional to the force applied, exact quantifications of these values was beyond the scope of this study.

The liquid crystals were enclosed in a 9x12 inch plastic sheet. A runway was laid out which passed over a viewing area set up to record the force changes on a Bolex (64 frames/sec) 16 mm camera. Figure 24-1 represents a cross-sectional illustration of the arrangement of the liquid crystals, plexiglass, supporting plywood, and Bolex camera. The crystal sheet was at ground level, and there was no limitation to runway length, so that subjects could pass over the apparatus in normal stride.

Twelve subjects were evaluated. Ten adults (five males and five females) with no history of previous injury and no clinical or roentgenographic evidence of foot abnormality were included as controls. Foot deformities were studied in two patients: One was a forty-five-year-old black female with bilateral congenital flexible pes valgus with metatarsus primus varus and hallux valgus deformities. This patient's feet were generally asymptomatic in corrective shoes with a steel arch. However, when walking in noncorrective shoes, the patient complained of metatarsalgia and aching at the midfoot. The second was a twenty-four-year-old white female with bilateral metatarsus primus varus, who had complaints of continued first-head metatarsalgia afer a Silvertype bunionectomy.

The momentary distribution of forces was studied with each of these subjects walking, jogging, and then running across the pressure plate. They were allowed to proceed at their own pace; no attempt was made to confine their stride to the beat of a metronome, which might cause an abnormal gait pattern. Multiple practice passages were made over the liquid crystal sheet so that "targeting" might be avoided. Six camera-recorded passages were made over the crystals, three walking and three running. The developed film was then studied frame by frame, using an Agfa Lupe (8x) scanner and a slow-motion analytic projector.

RESULTS

Pressure distribution under five areas of the foot was evaluated: the hindfoot, midfoot, metatarsals, great toe, and the lateral toes. The duration of forces under each area was studied as well as the progression of forces from one area to another. The first study was that of comparing the progression and duration of forces from one area to another. The next was that of comparing these forces during walking, jogging, and sprinting gait in ten normal subjects.

Although these subjects walked at their own natural pace, the average duration of walking stance phase (heel touchdown to toe pushoff) was surprisingly similar to 0.48±0.01 second. The average duration of contact when jogging was 0.17±0.04 second, and the average duration of contact for the sprinting was 0.11±0.03 second. Since the pattern of duration of forces for each type of gait was fairly similar, the data were averaged to provide a composite of each type of gait (Fig. 24-2). In addition to these measurements, photographs of the pressure changes under the walking normals were at 0.04, 0.11, 0.17, and 0.31 second after the heel strike (Fig. 24-3). The changes in progression of forces under jogging and sprinting normal feet were

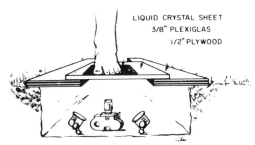

FIGURE 24-1 Diagrammatic illustration of design for recording forces under the foot. (Reprinted with permission of Pierce E. Scranton, Jr. and Pergamon Press Ltd. from *Biomechanics,* Vol. 9, 1976.)

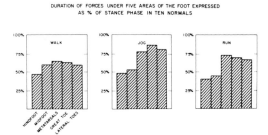

FIGURE 24- 2 Duration of walking, jogging, and sprinting forces under normal feet during stance phase.

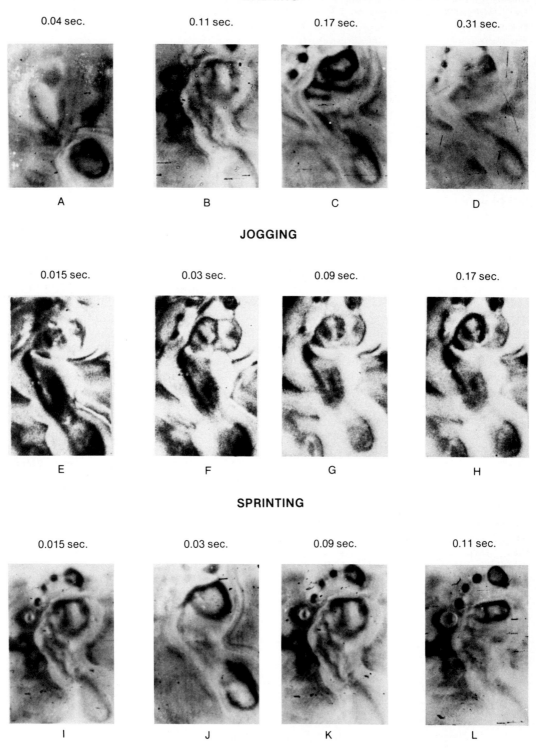

FIGURE 24-3 Comparison of progression of force under normal walking, jogging, and sprinting feet.

then compared, and these progressions were compared to those patients with foot disorders (Fig. 24-3-24-8). The time sequences for the spot photographs of the jogging and sprinting studies were not similiar to walking, however, as the duration of foot contact was considerably shorter.

DISCUSSION

Analysis of the forces under the foot during walking, jogging, and sprinting revealed different patterns of force transmission which suggested distinctly different foot functions in response to the demands of gait. During walking, there was smooth progression of forces from hindfoot, through midfoot to the metatarsals, and thence to the toes (Fig. 24-3). The distribution of these forces under the five areas of the foot was fairly even (Fig. 24-2). and suggested that during walking stance phase the main function of the foot was to provide support and balance. Forward locomotion was maintained by the gastrocnemius and soleus and the flexors and extensors of the upper thigh, as well as the forward momentum of the body mass.[21] Also to be noted was the degree of support provided by the great toe and lateral toes. Previous authors have either ignored the role of the toes during stance phase or advanced theories that the toes provided no significant weight-bearing function.[17,29] Lambrinudi, and later Barnett, were the first to stress the importance of the toes.[5,23] This study confirms their concept.

The jogging studies illustrated the pounding forces feet are subjected to when one runs without benefit of deceleration of the rate of impact. The entire foot slammed down to provide the initial platform for stance phase support (Fig. 24-3). The forefoot then functioned to initiate propulsive pushoff. Roger Mann and associates have demonstrated that jogging produces more impact forces on touchdown than any other form of gait.[23] This study supports that concept.

Considering the significant impact forces on the hindfoot of joggers it would seem that footwear for these runners would require a well-cushioned heel. Another clinical correlation concerns the observation that this form of gait is most predominant in middle-distance runners such as athletes who run the 400- and 800-meter events. It has been shown that these athletes experience "shinsplints" more commonly than any other group[10] The impact of foot strike, and the reacting forces exerted by the tibialis posterior muscle to maintain arch integrity are a reasonable explanation for the resultant posterior tibi-

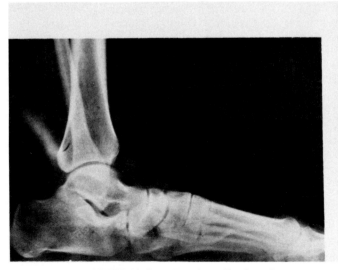
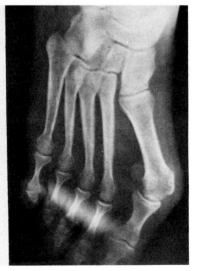

FIGURE 24-4   A-P and standing lateral roentgenograms of pes planus subject.

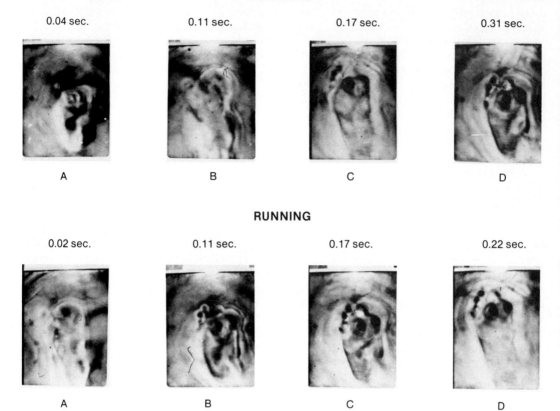

FIGURE 24-5 Comparison of walking and running forces under pes planus foot. (Reprinted with permission of Pierce E. Scranton, Jr. and Pergamon Press Ltd. from *Biomechanics* Vol. 9, 1976).

alis tendinitis, tenosynovitis, and origin periostitis.

During sprinting, an entirely different pattern of force transmission and progression was seen. Instead of the "heel-to-toe" progression seen on walking, there was rather a "forefoot-to-hindfoot-to-forefoot" progression (Fig. 24-3). The duration of hindfoot and midfoot contact also decreases as forces were shifted more to the metatarsals and toes (Fig. 24-2). In this study, forefoot strike inititated stance phase, and one can easily see the larger amount of force under the metatarsals and toes at 0.015 second after foot strike. This was because the flexors of the foot acted to decelerate the impact force before foot flat.[38] Immediately after foot flat, they again contracted to provide propulsive thrust for acceleration and pushoff.[21] Thus, during walking, the foot's function

seemed mainly to provice balance and support. During jogging the function of the forefoot increased to provide push off, but the hindfoot underwent considerable pounding without benefit of deceleration rate of impact. During running, the foot actively participated throughout stance phase by decelerating impact and later by providing propulsive push off. Again, note in both Fig. 24-2 and in the running sequence of Fig. 24-3 the large amount of force under the toes. The importance of the toes during walking and running stance phase can easily be appreciated in these normal studies and will be further emphasized in studies of those patients with disorders of the foot.

One further observation in the normal studies concerns determining the nature of the arches under the normal foot. Authors writing earlier felt that the "perfect foot"

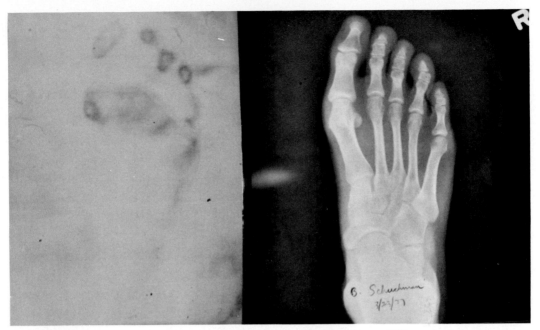

FIGURE 24-6 Standing A-P roentgenogram and midstance phase force plate study illustrating bowstrung flexor hallucis longus with abnormal force under sesamoids.

would have collapsible arches which would allow maximum foot contact at foot flat and would then spring back resiliently during swing phase.[3] Dickson and Diveley believed, rather, that there were three arches:

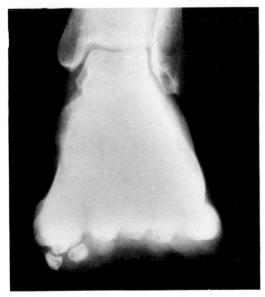

FIGURE 24-7 Skyline sesamoid view confirms diagnosis of subluxed sesamoids, the medial sesamoid riding underneath metatarsal head.

a medial and lateral longitudinal and a transverse anterior arch.[11] Morton proposed only a medial and lateral longitudinal arch with no metatarsal arch.[26] In 1889, Ellis proposed that the foot's arch during weight bearing represented a medially based "half-dome."[13] This concept was later supported by Jones and then Barnett.[5,19] The present study confirms the idea of the foot's arch functioning more as a medially based half-dome. Fig. 24-3B and C clearly show the progression of forces from the hindfoot to lateral midfoot and thence across the metatarsals. While one may observe the so-called lateral longitudinal arch in a nonweight-bearing normal foot, this is clearly not a functional entity in stance phase. In fact, the only foot in which we observed a lack of weight bearing under the lateral aspect was in a patient with pathologic congenital pes planus.

The patient with pes planus complained of first and second metatarsalgia as well as midfoot aching and fatigue when walking without corrective shoes. Roentgenographic studies revealed a medially angled talus, a subluxated navicular, an accessory navicular, flattening of the longi-

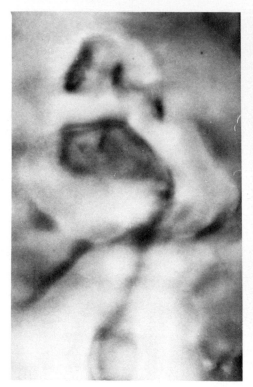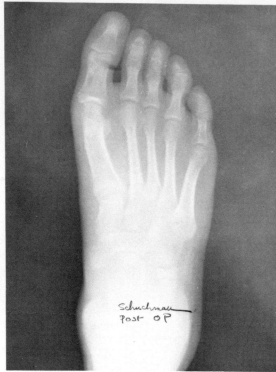

FIGURE 24-8 Postoperative standing A-P roentgenogram and midstance phase force plate study illustrating even pressure distribution under metatarsal heads.

tudinal arch, and mild metatarsus primus varus with hallux valgus (Fig. 24-4). These deformities caused an unusual distribution of forces under the foot (Fig. 24-5). For either walking or running, contact was initiated by the midfoot. Because the great toe was laterally deviated and rotated, the flexor hallucis longus was mechanically unable to provide flexion support and push off during stance phase. The forces were therefore abnormally shifted to the lateral toes as well as to the first and second metatarsal heads (Fig. 24-5C,D). This patient's main complaint was of second-head metatarsalgia, and the force study clearly illustrates the disproportionate force borne by this head. Thus, although the patient structurally did not have a "Morton's foot," in a functional sense—with the absence of support under the great toe—she did.

The patient with metatarsus primus varus complained of bilateral first-head metatarsalgia. She had been treated by a podiatrist four years earlier, receiving a simple "Silver bunionectomy." She had had no relief of symptoms and felt as though she were "walking on a pea." Figure 24-6 illustrates her deformity with the sesamoids laterally displaced in the "bowstrung" flexor hallucis longus tendon. In addition, there was abnormal force under the first metatarsal head. A sesamoid "Skyline" view (Fig. 24-7) further delineates the subluxed sesamoids. This patient underwent a proximal, opening first metatarsal osteotomy. Three months later the forces were evenly distributed, and the patient was symptom-free (Fib. 24-8).

SUMMARY

The determination of the distribution and progression of forces under the foot has been one area of investigation fraught with technical difficulties. This chapter presents a technique utilizing pressure-sensitive cholesterol crystals for analysis of the momentary distribution of forces. Walking, jogging, and sprinting gaits in ten normal subjects were studied, and these findings were then compared with a variety of abnormal feet.

This study advances the concept that the foot function alters in response to the demands of gait. While walking, the foot is passive, mainly serving to provide balance and support, with forward locomotion maintained by the gastrocnemius and soleus and the upper thigh flexors and extensors, as well as by upper body momentum. During jogging the hindfoot is subjected to considerable repetitive impact forces, but the forefoot does act to provide propulsive pushoff. Whiel sprinting, the foot actively participates throughout stance phase, initially decelerating the rate of impact, then providing propulsive push off.

The role of the great toe and lateral toes appears much larger than that ascribed to them by previous authors. In addition, dysfunction in this area is seen to contribute a great deal to functional pathologic findings seen in other foot disorders presented in this study. A detailed analysis of the abnormalities in forces under the foot in these other subjects relates functional clinical pathologic findings to observed force patterns. The technique presented is quite simple and is being utilized to study a broad variety of disorders of the foot.

Appreciation is expressed to Mr. James Crawford of Medical Photography, Mrs. Diana Montgomery and Mr. Warren Thomspon of the Orthopaedic Research Laboratory, and to Mrs. Sherry Heckathorn of the Children's Hospital Department of Orthopaedics.

REFERENCES

1. Abramson, E.: Zur Kenntnis der Mechanik des Mittelfusses. *Scand. Arch. Physiol.* Bd. 175, 1927.
2. Arcan, M. and Brull, M.A.: A fundamental characteristic of the human body and foot, the foot ground pressure pattern. *J. Biomech.* 9:453, 1976.
3. Bankart, A.S.B.: The treatment of minor maladies of the foot. *Lancet* 1:249, 1935.
4. Barnett, C.H.: A plastic pedograph. *Lancet* 2:273, 1954.
5. Barnett, C.H.: The phases of human gait. *Lancet* 2:617, 1956.
6. Basler, A.: Bestimmung des auf die einzelnen Sohlenbezirke wirkended Teilgewichtes des menschlichen Korpers. Abderhalden's Handbuch, Abt. V., Teil 5A, Heft 3, S. p. 559, 1936.
7. Bauman, J. H. and Brand, P. N.: Measurement of pressure between foot and shoe *Lancet* 1:629, p. 63.
8. Beely, F.: Zur Mechanik des Stephens. *Arch. Klin. Chir.* 27:457, 1882.
9. Carlet, G.: Essai experimental sur la locomotion humaine. 1872.
10. D'Ambrosia, R.D. et al.: Interstitial pressure measurements in the anterior and posterior compartments in athletes with shin splints. *A. J. Sports Med.* 5:84-88, 1977.
11. Dickson, F.D. and Diveley, R.L.: *Functional Disorders of the Foot* (3rd Ed.,). Philadelphia: J.B. Lippincott Co., 1953.
12. Elftman, H.: A cinematic study of the distribution of pressure in the human foot. *Anat. Rec.* 59:481, 1934.
13. Ellis, T.S.: *The Human Foot.* London: J. & A. Churchill, 1889.
14. Fergason, J.L. and Brown, G.H.: Liquid crystals and living systems. *J. Am. Oil Chem. Socl.* 45:120, 1968.
15. Ferguson, J. L.: Liquid crystals *Sci Am.* 211: 76, 1964.
16. Frostell, O.: Beitrag zur Kenntnis der vorderen Stutzpenke des fesses. *Z. Orthop. Chir.* 48:3, 1925.
17. Grundy, M., Tosh, P.A., McLeish, R.D. and Smidt, L.: An investigation of the centers of pressure under the foot while walking. *J. Bone Joint Surg.* 57B:98, 1975.
18. Hutton, W.C. and Drabble, G.E.: An apparatus to give the distribution of vertical load under the foot. *Rheumatol. Phys. Med.* 11:313, 1972.
19. Jones, F.W.: *Structure and Function as Seen in the Foot.* London; Bailliere, Tindall & Cox, 1944.
20. Klein, E.J. and Margozzi, A.P.: Apparatus for the calibration of shear-sensitive liquid crystals. *Rev. Sci. Instrum.* 41:238, 1970.
21. Klenerman, L. (Ed.): *The Foot and Its Disorders.* Oxford: Blackwell Scientific Publications, 1976.
22. Lambrinudi, C.: Action of the foot muscles. *Lancet* 2:1480, 1938.
23. Mann, R.: Personal communication.
24. Momberg: Der Gang des Menschen und die Fussgeschwalst. *Bibliothek von Coler.* 25:34, 1908.
25. Morton, D.: Structural factors in static disorders of the foot. *Am. J. Surg.* 9:315, 1930.
26. Morton, D.J.: The angle of gait. *J. Bone Joint Surg.* 14:741, 1932.
27. N.A.S.A.: Exploratory investigation on the measurement of skin friction by means of liquid crystals, TM-X-1774, 1969.
28. Romanes, G.J.: *Cunningham's Textbook of Anatomy.* London: Oxford University Press, 1964.

29. Schwartz, P. and Heath, A.: Some factors which influence the balance of the foot in walking. *J. BoneJoint Surg.* 19:431, 1937.

30. Schwartz, P. and Heath, A.: The definition of human locomotion on the basis of measurement. *J. Bone Joint Surg.* 29:203, 1947.

31. Schwartz, P. and Heath A.: The oscillographic recording and quantitative definition of functional disabilities of human locomotion. *Arch. Phys. Med.* 30:568, 1949.

32. Scranton, P.E., Jr., McMaster, J.H. and Kelly, E.: Dynamic fibular function. *Clin. Ortho.* 118:76, 1975.

33. Scranton, P.E., Jr. and McMaster, J.H.: Momentary distribution of forces under the foot. *J. Biomech.* 9:45, 1976.

34. Stokes, I.A.F., Stott, J.R.R. and Hutton, W.C.: Force distributions under the foot—a dynamic measuring system. *Biomed. Engin.* 9:140, 1974.

35. Stott, J.R.R. and Hutton, S.I.A.F.: Forces under the foot. *J. Bone Joint Surg.* 55B:335, 1973.

36. Weinert, C.R., Jr., McMaster, J.H. and Ferguson, R.J.: Dynamic function of the human fibula. *J. Anat.* 138:145, 1973.

37. Weinert, C.R., Jr., McMaster, J.H., Scranton, P.E., Jr. and Ferguson, R.J.: Human fibular dynamics. American Academy of Orthopaedic Surgeons Annual Meeting, Dallas, Texas, 1974.

38. Wells, K.: *Kinesiology.* Philadelphia: W.B. Saunders Co., 1971.

Chapter Twenty-Five

SUPPORT PHASE KINEMATICS OF THE FOOT

PIERCE E. SCRANTON, JR., M.D.
ROBERT RUTKOWSKI, M.D.
THOMAS D. BROWN, PH.D.

The functional foot response to the varied demands of gait has long been of interest to investigators. The recent technical advances in methods for measuring foot response have represented dramatic improvements since Beeley first asked subjects to run across fresh plaster of Paris in 1882.[6] Current techniques require the interpretation of the recordings of electrobasometers, electromyography, parallel cinephotography, accelerometers, electrogoniometers, computerized force plates, and so on.[5,10,11,18,-20,23-27,34,36] Equally important is the need to determine which data represent the true physiologic responses of the foot and which data are artifactual produced by the constraints of these recording devices.

Despite some limitations that the recording devices have placed on gait analysis, many aspects of our understanding of the functional biomechanics of the walking foot have consistently stood up to the analysis of a variety of investigators. We know, for example, that walking involves a complex integration of thoracic, pelvic, and femoral rotation, with shock absorption through knee flexion and propulsion and torque transmission through the ankle and subtalar joints.[15,34] We also know that during foot flat (support phase), arch integrity is maintained by bony architecture and the ligaments; the intrinsic and extrinsic muscles of the foot are electrically active only during early touchdown and the initiation of push off.[5,21,23] Many other components of walking gait have been described, helping to complete our understanding of walking biomechanics. These are well summarized in the recent literature.[14,15,18]

In the investigation of the various forms of running gait, however, a great deal remains to be done. The analysis of joggers or sprinters within the confines of a laboratory, or with electrodes in legs or underfoot, requires a critical appraisal of whether or not the resultant data represent the true response of a sprinting foot. In addition to the potential constraints of the recording devices, a wide variability of normal individual gait response exists. For example, it has been well documented that a runner's stride rate is affected by velocity, stride length, the capacity of the muscles to deliver energy, body mass, and limb structure and rotation.[25] Therefore, the validity of any interpretation of running gait within the limitations of a laboratory and/or analytic devices must undergo a certain degree of cautious criticism.

For several years, we have been interested in the analysis of walking, jogging, and sprinting gait at the University of Pittsburgh Department of Orthopaedic Surgery. In an effort to overcome the limitations imposed by standard analytic equipment, we have utilized several new techniques which allow unrestricted movement by an athlete and still permit qualitative recording of foot response to the varied demands of gait.[28,29] This chapter presents a further expansion of this work.

MATERIALS AND METHODS

Kinematic Studies

A Hycam Model 41-0004 high-speed camera with 16 mm Kodak Ektachrome 7242 film (30.5 rolls) was used to film the support phase of the foot during walking, jogging, and sprinting. The speed of the film was 500 frames per second, and this speed was assumed to be continuous. The filming was done outdoors on the University of Pittsburgh Tartan track. A telephoto F/2 lens was used three meters from the filming site. Three normal males with varsity collegiate athletic experience were used as subjects.

In walking gait, the subjects were required to start approximately 10 m from the filming site to achieve normal stride. In both jogging and sprinting gaits, the subjects started approximately 40 m from the site of filming.

The developed film was analyzed frame by frame. Two well-centered and focussed lateral and medial views of the foot during walking, jogging, and sprinting were chosen, and these twelve optimal filmed sequences were then spliced into a single film. The number of frames for each support phase in which the heel, midfoot, metatarsals and toes came into contact with the ground were counted. For each of these, a percentage of the stance was computed and an average compiled. Bar graphs show lateral and medial views in walking, jogging, and sprinting (Fig. 25–1).

RESULTS

For walking, the average duration of support phase lasted 0.69±0.02 second. For

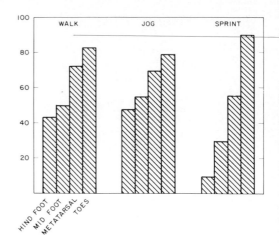

FIGURE 25–1 Bar graphs representing average duration of touchdown under each area of foot, expressed as precentage of total stance phase.

jogging, it was 0.23±0.02 second; and for sprinting, it was 0.14±0.01 second. The average duration of support under each area of the foot, expressed as a percentage of support phase, was then computed and represented in Figure 25–1.

In addition, spot photographs were made of selected frames which illustrated both well-recognized and previously unrecognized components of foot response to the variable demands of gait (Fig. 25–2 through 25–7.

DISCUSSION

Unquestionably, the accurate analysis of the functional response of the foot to the varied demands of gait has been a formidable challenge. Investigative studies have centered around three primary techniques: electrical (EMG's, electrogoniometers, etc.), optical (photographic, oscilloscopic, etc.), and pressure measurements (computerized force plates, pedography, etc.).[19] These modalities have successfully documented various aspects of the kinematics and kinetics of walking gait, despite a certain degree of natural variation during walking.

Initially, there was controversy concerning the nature and function of the

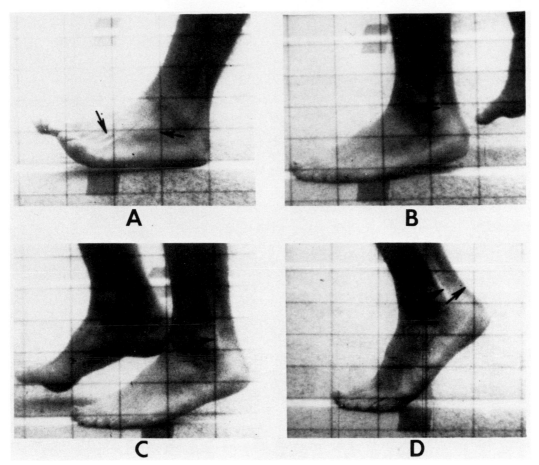

FIGURE 25-2   Sequential spot frames taken of lateral foot during walking support phase: (A) 0.04 second after heelstrike; (B) 0.29 second after heel strike; (C) 0.37 second after heel strike; and (D) 0.58 second after heel strike.

foot's arch(es). Ideas concerning the structure of the arch varied from those who believed that the "perfect foot" had no arch during weight bearing to those who believed that there were three arches: a transverse arch and medial and lateral longitudinal arches.[2,9] Recent studies utilizing pedographs, force plates, and pressure-sensitive cholesterol crystals have confirmed the initial concept of Ellis that the normal arch is best represented as a medially based "half dome."[3,13,29,33] Concerning structural support for maintenance of the arch, a second area of debate had to be resolved. Keith advanced the concept that the "sling-like" muscles, the flexors of the foot, were the first line of defense for structural stability in the arch.[17] He was opposed by Morton, who believed that static strains on the weight-bearing foot were well within the capabilities of the ligaments and bony structures.[23] This concept was later confirmed by EMG and anatomic studies which showed that the intrinsic and extrinsic muscles were electrically inactive during foot flat but exhibited early activity during touchdown and then during the initiation and completion of push off.[5,21,36] It was also noted that during running, the flexors of the foot contracted maximally throughout the stance phase.[36]

In addition to the clarification of the structure and function of the arch, as well as the phases of contraction of the intrinsic and extrinsic muscles, it was noted that during walking there was under the foot the

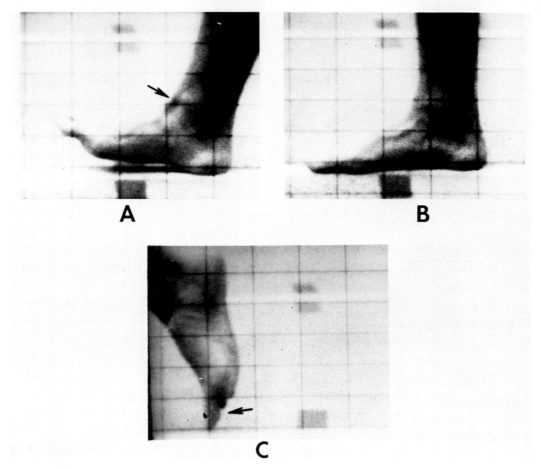

FIGURE 25-3   Sequential spot frames taken of medial foot during walking: A(0.02 second after heel- strike; (B) 0.13 second after heel-strike; and (C) 0.006 second after toe off.

smooth progression of force from hindfoot to midfoot, to metatarsals, and thence to the toes.[29,33] The walking foot seemed generally to perform its role as a "passive platform" for weight bearing in the plantigrade position, only slightly dorsiflexing to a maximum of 10° just before heel-off at midstance phase.[24,32,37,38] The initial external and the internal rotations of the tibia through support phase were converted by the subtalar joint into pronation and supination of the foot.[15] In addition, a forward shear force at the beginning of foot flat was described.[20] This would be resisted by the posterior talofibular ligament and posterior capsule. In summary, the walking foot seems mainly to provide passive balance and support, with forward locomotion maintained by upper body inertia, the momentum of the swinging of the opposite extremity, and finally by the contraction of the gastrocsoleus muscle group at pushoff.

As evidenced by our high-speed photography, however, a great deal of muscular action surrounds walking stance phase. During swing phase and heel-strike, the tendons of the tibialis anterior and long and short extensors of the toes are contracted both to clear the toes and to control evenly the descent of the forefoot (Fig. 25-2A and 25-3A). During foot flat, no tendinous activity is observed, and no muscular activity has been recorded electrically (Fig. 25-3B). As stance phase progresses, the body's center of gravity is shifted anterior to the axis of the foot. The intrinsics

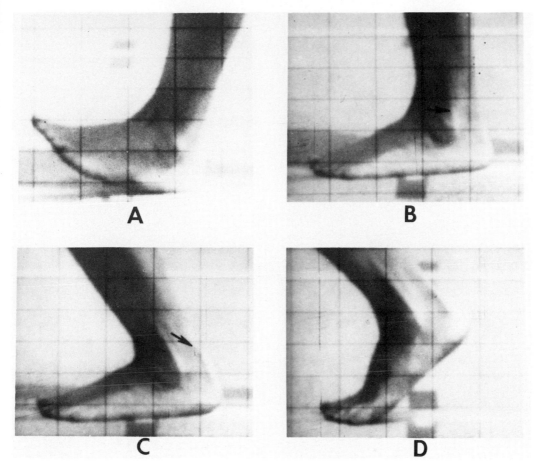

FIGURE 25–4   Sequential spot frames taken of lateral foot during jogging:(A) 0.014 second after heel- strike; (B) 0.05 second after heel-strike; (C) 0.12 second after heel-strike; and (D) 0.22 second after heel-strike.

contract, as well as the flexors of the toes, to prevent uncontrolled dorsiflexion at the metatarsophalangeal joints.[20] At the initiation of push off, the peroneus longus and Achilles' tendons are observed to become taut as they support the first metatarsal and provide a push-off force, respectively (Fig. 25-2B, C, and D). Push off occurs, but there is no follow-through by the great toe, indicating that it does not assist in providing propulsive push off (Fig. 25-3C). Rather, the foot is simply lifted off the ground by the hamstrings.

Efforts to document the kinetics and kinematics of jogging and sprinting, however, have not resulted in the same clarity as reported with walking. Perhaps the best descriptions of running mechanics are found in articles by Slocum and by James and Brubaker.[16,31] These authors recognized that there are primarily two forms of running gait: that of a sprinter running "up on the toes" and that of the runner who lands with the foot flat or on the heel. They felt that during running the foot served five primary functions: to support the body, to provide motive force, to overcome inertia, to maintain desired velocity, to accelerate the center of gravity against internal and also external resistance.

In addition to this descriptive work, there were other noteworthy observations. Roger Mann and associates reported that the foot was subjected to more impact force during jogging gait than during any other form of gait.[20] In separate studies uti-

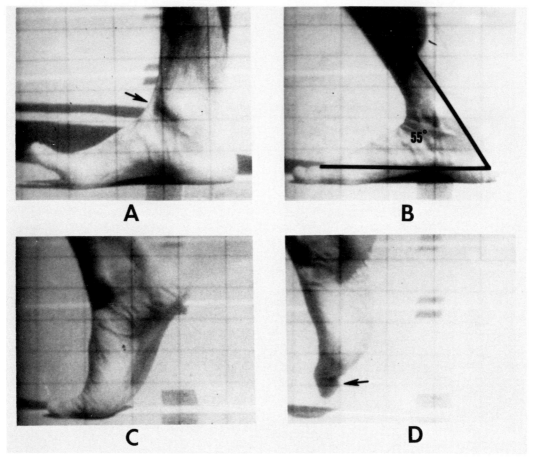

FIGURE 25–5 Sequential spot frames taken of medial foot during jogging: (A) 0.03 second after heel strike; (B) 0.13 second after heel-strike; (C) 0.20 second after heel-strike; and (D) 0.008 second after toe off.

lizing pressure-sensitive cholesterol crystals, this concept was confirmed.[28] It was also observed that the sprinting foot utilized the flexors of the foot to decelerate the rate of impact and then to provide acceleratory, propulsive push off.[29]

While these isolated observations on running mechanics were felt to be valid, there have remained clinical observations which needed further clarification. D'Ambrosia and associates investigated anterior compartmental pressures in the legs of athletes experiencing "shin splints" but found no abnormalities.[7] They did note, however, that an extremely high percentage of these subjects were so-called middle distance runners, participating in events such as the 440-meter, 880-meter, and mile run. This observation correlates with our own clinical experience, both as previous members of varsity collegiate track teams and later as team physicians involved with the track teams at the University of Pittsburgh.

Another observation concerned the high incidence in long distance runners of fibular stress fractures at the region immediately above the tibiofibular syndesmosis.[8] These fractures were originally thought to be due to a "to-and-fro" motion, described during weight bearing and non-weight bearing. Many other fibular motions, however, have been documented in recent literature.[15,30,35] Not only does the fibula move "to-and-fro," but it rotates axially as well as descends during running foot flat, pulled by the flexors of the foot

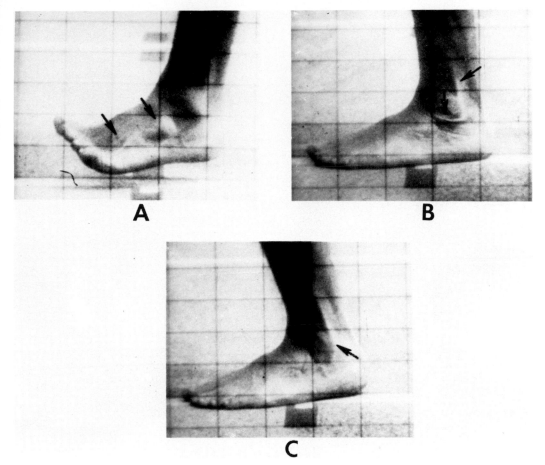

FIGURE 25-6 Sequential spot frames taken of lateral foot during sprinting: (A) 0.008 second before touchdown; (B) 0.02 second after touchdown; and (C) 0.04 second after touchdown.

as they contract to support the arch and provide propulsive push off.

With respect to the changes in angular velocity and kinematics of the jogging or sprinting foot, again very little has been written. Although it is generally accepted from an anatomic standpoint that the human ankle joint is capable of up to 30° dorsiflexion, only 10° has been described in human walking gait.[24,32,37,38] In addition, it is well known that during walking, flexion of the knee occurs at foot flat to assist in absorption of impact force.[16,20] It is also known that this knee flexion increases with running. However, middle and long distance runners experience a high incidence of shin splints and stress fractures, respectively, while sprinters complain mainly of

muscle "pulls." One would wonder, then, if the sprinter utilizes an additional means of deceleration of the rate of impact.

In our analysis of jogging and sprinting gait at 500 frames per second, we observed the following events. When jogging, both feet are unsupported during the airborne phase of gait; and the runner, in effect, is continually "falling forward" with the hindfoot breaking the fall. Since there is no ability of the hindfoot to decelerate the rate of impact, the leg is subjected to a considerable impact force, which is ultimately cushioned through flexion at the knee. Foot flat occurred, on the average, 0.05 second after heel strike; and although the anterior extensors were observed to be taut before foot flat, this 0.05-second inter-

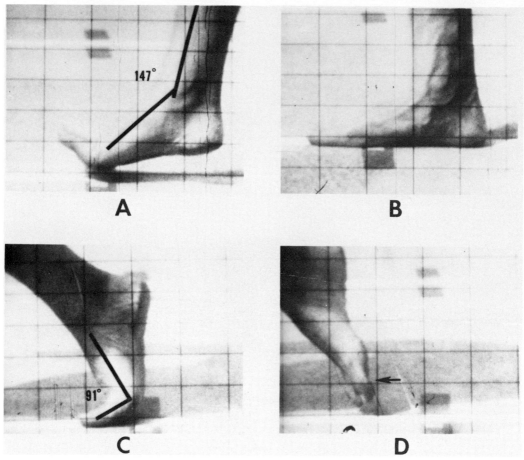

FIGURE 25-7 Sequential spot frames taken of medial foot during sprinting: (A) 0.006 second before touchdown; (B) 0.02 second after touchdown, (C) 0.14 second after touchdown; and (D) 0.008 second after toe off.

val indicates that the forefoot is not gently "let down" as in walking (Fig. 25-4A, B). A considerable shock wave passes down the leg with the impact. At 0.13 second after heel strike, there is a surprising maximum forward angulation at the ankle joint of 35° (Fig. 25-4C, B). Throughout foot flat, the peroneus longus is seen to contract, stabilizing the first metatarsal and assisting in the initiation of push off (Fig. 25-4B, C, and D). The Achilles' tendon is also observed to be taut, assisting in providing propulsive push off. There is a surprising degree of dorsiflexion of the great toe, followed by a propulsive push off in which the flexor hallucis longus actively contracts, as evidenced by the follow-

through of the great toe 0.008 second after toe off (Fig. 25-5 C, D).

For sprinting, however, an entirely different form of gait is observed. Touchdown is initiated by metatarsals, or "forefoot-strike" (Fig. 25-6A and 25-7A). The foot is plantar flexed approximately 57°. The flexors of the foot control the descent of the hindfoot, absorbing the force of impact. Foot flat occurs 0.02 second after touchdown, but the peroneus longus and Achilles' tendons are already taut, initiating push off (Fig. 25-6B). The force of contraction of the flexors of the foot at this time is evidenced by the downward migration of the fibula, producing skin folds at its inferior border (Fig. 25-6B). This downward movement deepens the ankle mortise to assist in the stabilization of the ankle. [30,35] The flexor hallucis longus is again observed to be taut, assisting in propulsive push off; and this is again confirmed by the follow-through of the great toe, 0.008 second after toe off (Fig. 25-7D). Interestingly, the great toe is dorsiflexed to a maximum of 89° during push off (Fig. 25-7C).

In summary, jogging gait was accompanied by a considerable impact force at heel strike, followed by an ankle dorsiflexion of 35°, and then propulsive push off. In sprinting gait, the rate of impact was decelerated through a controlled lengthening of the flexors of the foot, which then immediately contracted to provide propulsive push off. While there has been no reported function of the long flexors during walking gait, it was apparent during jogging and sprinting that they were assisting in propulsive push off. Though tendons of the deeper flexor digitorum longus and tibialis posterior could not be visualized in our study, it is well known through EMG studies that they also contract maximally during the stance and propulsion phases of running gait. [36]

The clinical implications of these gait patterns are quite intriguing. To begin with, the role of the foot clearly changes in response to the demands of gait. Nevertheless, if the stress is repetitive and prolonged, there are key areas of the foot prone to fatigue. The repetitive shocks of impact in jogging gait place the utmost stress upon the arch. The arch must accommodate the impact force of the acceleration of gravity on body weight, times a fulcrum gradient varying from single body weight to five times body weight across the talocrural joint. [32] The repetitive, violent impacts of gait in the competitive 440-meter, 880-meter or mile runner undoubtedly stress to the utmost the muscular "back-up" for arch stabilization, the posterior tibialis muscle. Thus in this group of runners we see the high predominance of shin splints or posterior tibial tendinitis, tenosynovitis, and origin periostitis.

In like manner, there is a high incidence of fibular stress fractures in long distance runners. In these individuals the gait is accompanied by a repetitive downward movement of the fibula, pulled distally by the flexors of the foot. It is firmly tethered, however, by the tibiofibular syndesmosis. Therefore, about 70 per cent of these fractures occur just above the syndesmosis, oriented obliquely in the anteroposterior plane. [8] Indeed, there is the so-called to-and-fro motion of the fibula, but in previous studies it occurred when the fibula moved distally, being pulled medially as well by the tether of the interosseous membrane. [30]

There are also important implications concerning the design of footwear for runners. Unquestionably, a sprinter's shoe must have a radically different design from that of a marathon runner. In the sprinter, the foot's entire response is concentrated in a rapid flexion-extension-flexion movement spread across the metatarsophalangeal, midtarsal, and talocrural joints. It is important, then, that the shoe permit free, unrestricted motion of these joints. Current advocates of special devices in the heel, such as a varus wedge or extra padding, should consider that acceleratory propulsion in the sprinting foot occurs after heel lift off, not during the brief foot flat.

Considering the case of joggers and middle distance runners, the opposite is true. Here the repetitive forces of impact dictate that the heel be fitted with a well-padded cushion. Since the hindfoot spends a considerable percentage of stance phase in surface contact (Fig. 25-1), a varus wedge may assist in maintaining optimal alignment of the midtarsal joints for efficient push off. [22] An adequate arch support is of utmost importance.

Finally, it should be emphasized that in the analysis of the kinematics and kinetics of gait there are no real absolutes. For example, one could choose to measure the percentage of duration of forces under the foot using one hundred subjects instead of three as we have done. The resultant data would certainly seem valid. If these one hundred subjects were then asked to continue walking "normally" but to increase stride length, there would be a complete alteration of the bar graphs which had earlier seemed so valid. In like manner, one may record the same vertical force deflection on a force plate when a 90-pound or 150-pound athlete jogs or sprints over it, though the impulse times would certainly differ. These inconsistencies do not invalidate either the data or the honest attempts to interpret running gait. They must be taken into consideration, however, each and every time a study points to certain conclusions concerning gait.

SUMMARY

This chapter reviews current concepts concerning the foot's functional anatomy and the kinematics and kinetics of various forms of gait. Walking, jogging, and sprinting are investigated, utilizing kinematic photography at 500 frames per second.

It is apparent that foot response alters to meet the varied demands of gait. The walking foot serves as a "passive platform" providing the balance and support for stance phase. The jogging foot is subjected to a considerable impact force, but the foot is no longer passive, as the flexors of the foot play an active role in assisting propulsive push off. During jogging, the ankle joint dorsiflexes to a maximum of 35°. The sprinting foot utilizes the flexors of the foot, through controlled lengthening, to provide a deceleration of the rate of impact. The force of contraction during this controlled deceleration and subsequent propulsive push off pulls the fibula distally, deepening the mortise, and providing greater ankle stability. During sprinting, the great toe dorsiflexes to a maximum of 89°.

Finally, this study correlates clinical disorders such as shin splints and stress fractures in competitive athletes with the functional response of the foot. Recommendations for footwear are simplified, considering these new observations.

The authors wish to acknowledge the assistance of Mr. Warren Thompson and Mrs. Diana Montgomery of the Orthopaedic Research Laboratory, and of Mr. Norman Rabinowitz of Children's Hospital Medical Illustrations.

REFERENCES

1. Andriacchi, T., Ogle, J. and Galante, J.: Walking speed as a basis for normal and abnormal gait measurements. *J. Biomech.* 10:261-68, 1977.
2. Bankart, A.: The treatment of minor maladies of the foot. *Lancet* 1:249, 1935.
3. Barnett, C.H.: The phases of human gait. *Lancet* 2:617-20, 1956.
4. Barnett, C. and Rapier, J.: The axis of rotation at the ankle joint in man. Its influence upon the form of the talus and the mobility of the fibula. *J. Anat.* 86:1-9, 1952.
5. Basmajian, J. and Stecko, G.: The role of muscles in arch support of the foot. *J. Bone Joint Surg.* 45A:1184-90, 1963.
6. Beely, F.: Zur mechanik des stehens. *Arch. Clin. Chir.* 27:457-58, 1882.
7. D'Ambrosia, R., Zelis, R., Chuinard, R. and Wilmore, J.: Interstitial pressure measurements in the anterior and posterior compartments in athletes with shin splints. *Am. J. Sports Med.* 5:172-31, 1977.
8. Devas, M.: Stress fractures of the fibula. *J. Bone Joint Surg.* 38B:818-29, 1956.
9. Dickson, F. and Diveley, R.: *Functional Disorders of the Foot* (3rd Ed.). Philadelphia: J. B. Lippincott, 1953.
10. Dubo, H., Peat, M., Winter, D., Quanbury, A., Hobson, D. and Steinke, T.: Electromyographic temporal analysis of gait: normal human locomotion. *Arch. Phys. Med. Rehabil.* 57:415-20, 1976.
11. Elftman, H.: A cinematic study of the distribution of pressures in the human foot. *Anat. Rec.* 59:481 87, 1934.
12. Elftman, H.: The transverse tarsal joint and its control. *Clin. Ortho.* 16:41-45, 1960.
13. Ellis, T.S.: *The Human Foot.* London: J. & A. Churchill, 1889.
14. Giannestras, N.: *Foot Disorders* (2nd Ed.). London: Henry Kempton, 1973.
15. Inman, V.T.: *The Joints of the Ankle:* Baltimore: Waverly Press, 1976.
16. James, S. and Brubaker, C.: Running mechanics. *J.A.M.A.* 221:1014-16, 1972.
17. Keith, A.: The history of the human foot and its bearing on orthopaedic practices. *J. Bone Joint Surg.* 11:10-32, 1929.
18. Klenerman, L. *The Foot and Its Disorders.* Oxford, England: Blackwell Scientific Publications, 1976.
19. Magora, A., Rozin, R., Robin, G., Bonen, B. and Simkin, A.: Investigation of gait, a technique of combined recording. *Electromyography* 4:385-96, 1970.
20. Mann, R.: AAOS Instructional Courses, Las Vegas, Nevada, 1977.

21. Mann, R. and Inman, V.: Phasic activity of intrinsic muscles of the foot. *J. Bone Joint Surg.* 46A:469–81, 1964.

22. Morris, J.: Biomechanics of the foot and ankle. *Clin. Ortho.* 122:10–17, 1977.

23. Morton, D. and Fuller, D.: *Human Locomotion and Body Form. A Study of Gravity and Man.* Baltimore: Williams and Wilkins Co. 1952.

24. Murray, P., Drought, B. and Kory, R.: Walking patterns of normal men. *J. Bone Joint Surg.* 46A:335–60, 1964.

25. Radford, P. and Upton, A.: Trends in speed of alternated movmenent during development and among elite sprinters. Biomechanics V-B, Baltimore: University Park Press, 1975.

26. Rasch, P. and Burke, R.: *Kinesiology and Applied Anatomy* (5th Ed.), Philadelphia: Lea & Febiger, 1974

27. Schwartz, P. and Heath, A.: The definition of human locomotion on the basis of measurement. *J. Bone Joint Surg.* 29:203–13, 1947.

28. Scranton, P.E., Hootman, B.D. and McMaster, J.H: Forces under the foot: A study of walking and running force distribution under normal and abnormal feet. Presented at the Annual Meeting of the Foot Society, Dallas, Texas, 1978.

29. Scranton, P.E. and McMaster, J.H.: Momentary distribution of forces under the foot. *J. Biomech.* 9:45–48, 1976.

30. Scranton, P.E., McMaster, J.H. and Kelly, E.: Dynamic fibular function. *Clin. Ortho.* 118:76–81, 1976.

31. Slocum, D. and James, S.: Biomechanics of running. *J.A.M.A* 205:721–28, 1968.

32. Stauffer, R., Chao, E. and Brewster, R.: Force and motion analysis of the normal, diseased, and prosthetic ankle joint. *Clin. Ortho.* 127:189–96, 1977.

33. Stott, J., Hutton, W. and Stokes, F.: Forces under the foot. *J. Bone Joint Surg.* 55B:335–44, 1973.

34. Sutherland, D. and Hagy, J.: Measurement of gait movements from motion picture film. *J. Bone Joint Surg.* 54A: 787–97, 1972.

35. Weinert, C., McMaster, J., Scranton, P. and Ferguson, R.: Human fibular dynamics. *In Foot Science.* Philadelphia: W.B. Saunders, 1976.

36. Wells, K.: *Kinesiology.* Philadelphia: W.B. Saunders Co., 1971.

37. Winter, D.A., Quanbury, A.O., Hobson, D.A.A, Sidwell, H.G., Reimer, G., Trenholm, B.G., Steinke, T. and Shlosser, H.: Kinematics of normal locomotion. A statistical study based on T.V. data. *J. Biomech.* 7:479, 1974.

38. Wright, D.G., Desai, S.M. and Henderson, W.H.: Action on the subtalar and ankle-joint complex during the stance phase of walking. *J. Bone Joint Surg.* 46A:361, 1964.

Chapter Twenty-Six

SURGICAL RECONSTRUCTION OF THE TALIPES EQUINO VARUS DEFORMITY

JOHN S. GOULD, M.D.

In 1969, Goldner[1] reported his experience with a one-stage release for congenital talipes equino varus deformity. He emphasized the anterior displacement and medial rotation of the body of the talus within the ankle mortise as noted by Hirsch[2] (1960), Settle[3] (1963), and supported by Barenfeld and Weseley[4] in 1972; and the medial and plantar deviation of the talar neck and head as demonstrated by Irani and Sherman[5] (1963) and Settle. His procedure included sectioning the tibiotalar ligaments posteriorly, medially, anteriorly, and laterally, to allow derotation of the talus. The subtalar joint is not entered as in the Turco[6] (1971) release. In addition, further releases of the medial joints, the calcaneocuboid joint, tarsometatarsal joints, excision of the plantar fascia, lengthening of the tendo Achillis, medial tendons, excision of the abductor hallucis, and cuboid wedge, and anterior tibial transfer to the middle or third cuneiform or metatarsal may all be carried out concomitantly, as each may be needed to give full correction of the deformed foot. Bleck[7] has recently reported his experience with this approach.

MATERIALS AND METHODS

Fifty-six operative procedures for the talipes equino varus deformity in forty-eight feet of thirty-one children (twenty male, eleven female) were performed at the University of Alabama Medical Center, Birmingham, Alabama from September 1975 through June 1977. The patients are all followed at the Congenital Foot Clinic of the State Crippled Children's Service and were operated upon by the author with the assistance of the orthopaedic resident staff. Patients' ages ranged from three months to seventeen years, with twenty under one year, five between age one and two years, three between two and five years, and two between five and ten years (Table 26-1). Follow-up is from six months to twenty-seven months. Four operations were performed in 1975, thirty-one in 1976, and twenty-one in 1977. The diagnosis was intrinsic club foot (a term coined by Hirsch to differentiate the malformed talus cases from those presumed secondary to malposition in utero) without associated other conditions in twenty-eight

207

TABLE 26-1   The Series

Procedures	56
Feet	48
Children	31 (20 M, 11 F)
Age < 1 Year	20
1-2	5
2-5	3
5-10	2
10-17	1

children. In three, the deformity was in myelomeningocele patients. No cases of arthrogryposis were in the series.

The basic clinical approach is to perform serial casting using the three-part (Kite)[8] clubfoot cast until it becomes apparent from x-ray and clinical examination that a plateau has been reached and further casting is without benefit. The feet are initially classified as mild, moderate, or severe for prognostic purposes, and this evaluation is modified by progress with casting and surgical findings. Many of the patients initially classified as mild and all apparent position in utero deformities are corrected with casting. Surgery is usually delayed until patients are three months of age.

The surgical approach is to correct all the apparent deformities in a one-stage procedure, utilizing Goldner's concept that the basic anomaly involves malrotation of the talus within the ankle mortise, with secondary deformities of the distal structures. All procedures are carried out using 2.5 to 4.5 times loupe magnification and hand instruments, with the feet placed on a hand (foot) table transverse to the end of the operating table. The surgeons are seated.

In this series, twenty-five tibiotalar releases including a posterior release with lengthening of the tendo Achillis, posterior tibial, flexor digitorum communis, and flexor hallucis longus, release of the talonavicular joint, navicular-first cuneiform joint, first cuneiform-first metatarsal joint, and excision of the abductor hallucis were performed. In twenty-one cases, a release of the lateral tibiotalar and calcaneocuboid joints was also necessary. The plantar fascia was excised in nine of these cases; the anterior tibial tendon transferred in twelve; and a tarsometatarsal release included in

three. In two cases the total release included the lateral portion, plantar fasciectomy, anterior tibial transfer, and tarsometatarsal release.

In the entire series, seventeen posterior releases (classic approach) were performed with or without medial tendon lengthenings. In older children, two os calcis osteotomies with metatarsal osteotomies were performed. Three cases requiring talectomies (myelomeningocele patients) concluded the series (Table 26-2). Sixteen plantar fasciectomies and nineteen anterior tibial transfers were included with the various basic procedures.

Three months of postoperative casting was standard, whereas prolonged bracing and/or special footwear has not been needed.

RESULTS

Of the seventeen classic posterior releases performed (most early in the series) for what were deemed "mild" feet, six later required a more involved release when "recurrence" or medial rotation of the talus was recognized. In four feet with "total releases," anterior tibial transfers were required at ten-month and fourteen-month postoperative intervals. Three additional feet in this category will require anterior tibial transfers, and one child with apparent peroneal dysfunction will need the transferred anterior tibials moved from the third to the fifth metatarsals. Thus, nineteen of twenty-five feet required the

TABLE 26-2   Primary Operative Procedures

Tibiotalar release with medial tendon and TA lengthening, medial release, and abductor hallucis excision	25
Including lateral release	21/25
Including plantar fascia excision	9/25
Including anterior tibial transfer	12/25
Including tarsometatarsal release	3/25
Including all of the above	2/25
Posterior release only (with or without tendon lengthening	17
Os calcis osteotomy and metatarsal osteotomies	2
Talectomies	3

transfer. One of these feet required a tarsometatarsal release and two of these required repeat distal medial releases (Table 26–3). In all of these children, the static position of stance and the weight-bearing x-rays clinically demonstrated full correction (except in the instance when tarsometatarsal release was required), while the swing phase, particularly with running, demonstrated the abnormal pull of the anterior tibial.

The patients who have undergone os calcis and and metatarsal osteotomies and talectomies have all had satisfactory results.

No infections, skin sloughs, or avascular necrosis of the talus have occurred to date. In two cases a Z-plasty of medial skin was done initially, and in one a delayed primary full-thickness graft was needed. In one case, an anterior tibial tendon pulled out of the insertion and was later replaced. Anterior displacement of the talus under the ankle mortise occurred in one case where the tibiotalar release was done (Fig. 26–1); it was explored and the talus shifted posteriorly and pinned. The x-ray appearence, however, was unchanged. In two other instances a minor anterior shift was noted postoperatively. Lateral hinging of the talus, which can be prevented by the lateral releases, accounts for this problem. Evidence of recurrence of equinus, varus, and internal rotation of the talus has not been apparent in this group. Four had somewhat pronated feet from too vigorous a release and apparent failure to reconstruct the posterior tibial tendon and calcaneonavicular ligament adequately.

Utilizing Bleck's criteria for a satisfactory result—(1) no recurrence of the equi-

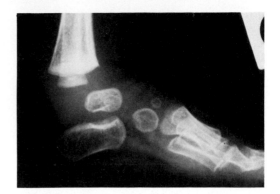

FIGURE 26–1   Anterior shift of talus.

nus or varus; (2) neutral position of the heel; (3) dorsiflexion of the ankle to at least neutral; and (4) a fairly straight forefoot so that the center line of the foot bisected either the second or third toes or passed no further laterally than the third and fourth toes—twenty-one of twenty-five total releases could be classified as fully satisfactory. (Table 26 4). Results in eleven patients who had posterior releases have remained satisfactory, and the six that required further surgery have a satisfactory result as well.

Illustrative Cases

Case 1: (A.R.) This one and one-half-year-old female was referred to the Clubfoot Clinic with a history of intermittent periods of casting since birth. Her parents had been told the right club foot was corrected at six months and she had been placed in straight-last shoes. As "recurrence" became obvious, she was placed in a reverse-last shoe and external rotation bar for "internal tibial torsion." A twister cable was utilized when she began to ambulate. At sixteen months, the patient was referred. The right foot had rigid de-

TABLE 26–3   Results

"Total" release	25
Anterior tibial transfer required later	7
Transfer performed initially	12
Transfer initially or later	19
Transfer and tarsometatarsal release required later	1
Transfer and repeat medial release required later	2
Posterior release	17
Required more extensive release later	6

TABLE 26–4   Results of "Total Release"

Anterior talar shift	3
Pronated feet	4
Satisfactory outcome (Bleck's criteria)	21/25

formities with equinus and mild varus of the hindfoot, metatarsus adductus, and equinus of the forefoot (Fig. 26-2, A–C). X-rays demonstrated the persistent deformities (Fig. 26-2 D–E).

Following tentative casting with no significant change obtained, surgery was performed. A tibiotalar release (medially, anteriorly, posteriorly, and laterally) was done, along with release of the medial talonavicular, navicular-first cuneiform, first cuneiform-first metatarsal joints, and the calcaneocuboid joint. The abductor hallucis was excised; a centimeter of the plantar fascia removed; and lengthening of the tendo Achillis, posterior tibial, flexor digitorum communis, and flexor hallucis longus tendons was performed.

A bulky dressing covered with a plaster shell was applied at surgery. Two weeks

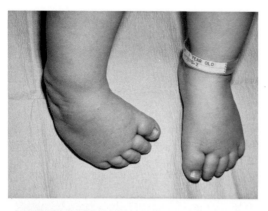

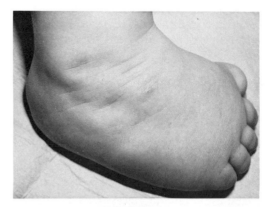

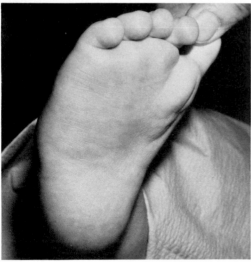

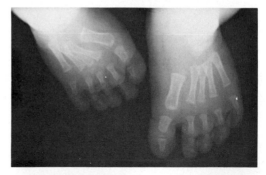

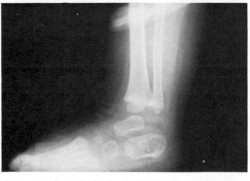

FIGURE 26–2 Intrinsic clubfoot uncorrected at age 1½ after intermittent periods of casting since birth. (B) Uncorrected clubfoot. Note lateral wrinkles and fullness of sinus tarsi. (C) Uncorrected clubfoot. Note persistent metatarsus adductus. (D) Uncorrected clubfoot. Metatarsus adductus is apparent on this film as well as foreshortening secondary to equinus position of forefoot and hindfoot. (E) Uncorrected clubfoot. Lateral view demonstrates failure of divergence of talus and calcaneus to establish a satisfactory talocalcaneal angle, indicating persistent equinus. Also note that a true lateral of talus is obtained, as indicated by its length and biconvexity, while an oblique view is seen of tibia and fibula, indicating malrotation of talus in ankle mortise.

later, under anesthesia, the foot was manipulated and a three-part clubfoot cast applied. At the six-week interval, the cast was changed and the foot appeared fully corrected. A new long leg clubfoot cast was applied for six weeks. At the three-month interval casting was discontinued and the child placed in standard footwear. Fourteen months later (Fig. 26-3A,B) the foot appeared fully corrected clinically and reasonably corrected by x-ray (Fig. 26-3C,D).

Case 2 (V.M.)   A nineteen-month-old boy was referred for evaluation of a rigid "recurrent" clubfoot. Casting had begun at two and one-half weeks of age, and at six months correction was thought to have been obtained clinically and by x-ray. He

was placed in a high-top, stiff-sole shoe and had persistent "close follow-up" for the next six months. He was lost to follow-up for seven months. At that time, he was seen with a "recurrent" deformed foot and referred to our clinic (Fig. 26-4 A–D). X-rays demonstrated the deformities (Fig. 26-4 3E,F).

A "total release" was performed including the posteromedial, medial, and lateral releases; a tarsometatarsal release; excision of the abductor hallucis, excision of 1 cm. of the plantar fascia; and transfer of the anterior tibial tendon to the third cuneiform. The tendo Achillis and medial tendons were lengthened. Our standard postoperative protocol was followed. One and one-half years later, maintenance of the

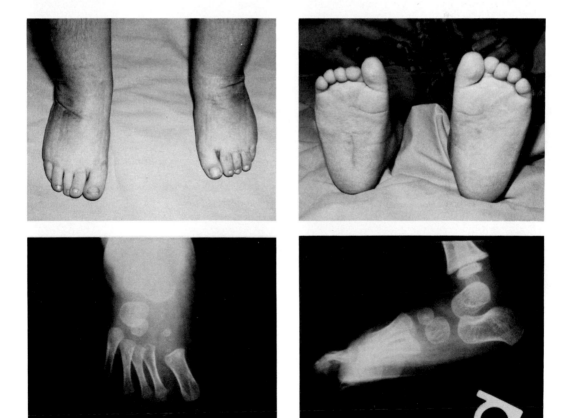

FIGURE 26–3   (A) Corrected clubfoot after a "total release." (B) Plantar view of corrected clubfoot after "total release." (C) A-P x-ray of corrected clubfoot. Note divergence of talus and calcaneus with long axis of talus pointing to first metatarsal and long axis of calcaneus pointing between fourth and fifth metatarsals. (D) Lateral x-ray of corrected clubfoot. Divergence of talus and calcaneus has been achieved. Dome of talus is convex, but bone is foreshortened with a true lateral obtained of tibia and fibula, indicating that complete derotation was not achieved, even with apparent complete clinical correction.

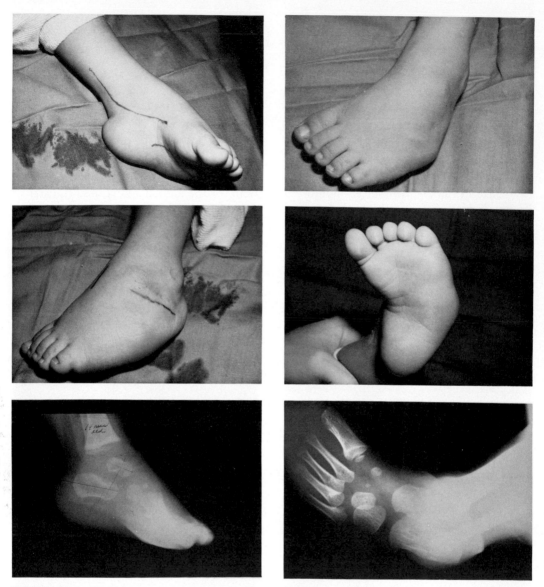

FIGURE 26-4   (A) Uncorrected clubfoot with equinus of hindfoot and forefoot at age nineteen months. Complete correction was thought to have been achieved at six months. Note markings for posteromedial and plantar incisions. (B) Uncorrected clubfoot with severe metatarsus adductus at age nineteen months. Metatarsotarsal capsulotomy was required for correction. (C) Uncorrected clubfoot. Note incision marking for lateral release and anterior tibial transfer. (D) Uncorrected clubfoot. Equinus and adductus of forefoot. (E) Lateral x-ray of uncorrected clubfoot. Note that talus and calcaneus are almost parallel, the talus forward in mortise and the forefoot in equinus and foreshortened. (F) A-P x-ray of uncorrected clubfoot. Long axis of talus and calcaneus are almost parallel; talus points to third metatarsal.

correction was demonstrated clinically and by x-ray (Fig. 26-5 A-D).

DISCUSSION AND CONCLUSION

We have been generally satisfied with the one-stage reconstruction. Complications can be avoided if details such as delicate surgical technique, use of magnification, tourniquet release, and hemostasis prior to closure are practiced. Anterior pivoting of the medial talus can be prevented

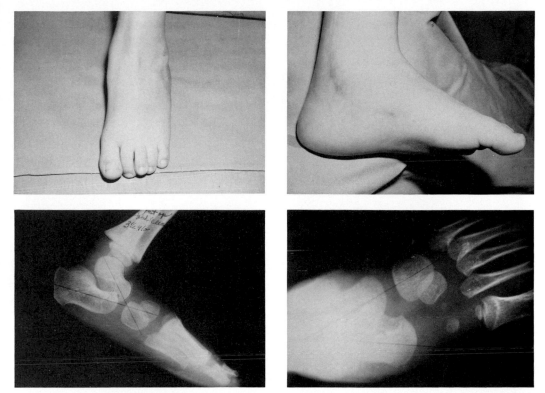

FIGURE 26–5 (A) Corrected clubfoot after "total release" (posteromedial, lateral, metatarsotarsal releases, medial tendon lengthening, excision of plantar fascia, and anterior tibial transfer). Note subcutaneous prominence of anterior tibial. (B) Lateral appearance of corrected clubfoot. Correction of hindfoot and forefoot achieved. (C) Lateral x-ray of corrected clubfoot. Talocalcaneal angle re-established Talus is biconvex, well positioned in ankle mortise. No malrotation is seen. Forefoot is well corrected. (D) Forced external rotation A-P view of corrected clubfoot. Talus and calcaneus diverge well. Note lateral notching of talus from prior alignment adjacent to calcaneus.

by the lateral release. When the extensive tibiotalar release results in instability, as with the anterior talar shift, temporary K-wire stalilization will avoid a problem. Pronation can be prevented by adequate medial reconstruction. Based on our results, anterior tibial transfer should be considered whenever the extensive release is required.

Observations of older children inherited from an earlier era in the clubfoot clinic, when posterior and medial releases and prolonged casting were the only methods of treatment, have shown extremely frequent persistence of the internally rotated talus (frequently misconstrued as internal tibial torsion) and forefoot deformities.

We conclude that the one-state recon-struction utilizing Goldner's technique is a satisfactory method to correct the talipes equino varus deformity completely and efficiently, avoiding prolonged casting, multiple surgeries, and stiff, deformed, incompletely corrected feet.

REFERENCES

1. Goldner, J.L.: Congenital equinovarus—fifteen years of surgical treatment. In *Current Practice in Orthopaedic, Surgery,* Vol. 4. St. Louis: C.V. Mosby Co., 1969, p. 61-123.
2. Hirsch, C.: Observations in early operative treatment of congenital clubfoot. *Bull. Hosp. Joint Dis.* 21:173, 1960.
3. Settle, G.W.: The anatomy of congenital talipes equinovarus: sixteen dissected specimens. *J. Bone Joint Surg.* 45A: 1341-54, 1963.

4. Weseley, M.S. and Barenfeld, P.A.: Surgical treatment of congenital clubfoot. *Clin. Ortho.* 84:79-87, 1972.

5. Irani, R.S. and Sherman, M.S.: The pathological anatomy of clubfoot. *J. Bone Joint Surg.* 45A:45-52, 1963.

6. Turco, V.: Surgical correction of the resistant clubfoot. One stage posteromedial release with internal fixation; a preliminary report. *J. Bone Joint Surg.*53A: 477-97, 1971.

7. Bleck, E.E.: Congenital clubfoot. *Clin. Ortho.* 125:119-30, 1977.

8. Kite, J.H.: *The Clubfoot.* New York, London: Grune & Stratton, 1964.

9. Kite, J.H.: Nonoperative treatment of congenital clubfoot. *Clin. Ortho.* 84:29-38, 1972.

SURGICAL CORRECTION OF THE RESISTANT CLUB FOOT

G. PAUL DeROSA, M.D.
EDWARD A. DYKSTRA, M.D.

The treatment of the resistant club foot has been the subject of considerable controversy in the orthopaedic literature during the past forty years. Although many clubfeet can be successfully managed by nonoperative means, a certain percentage will fail to respond and be classified as "resistant." This failure rate varies from 12 to 60 per cent.[2,5,7-9,11,13] The issue of "recurrence of deformity" has also been controversial. As early as 1930, Brockman stated that clubfoot deformities did not recur but were cases in which an inadequate initial correction had been accepted.[4]

The surgical treatment of resistant clubfoot during the past forty years has been quite varied. Brockman advocated an extensive soft-tissue release in an attempt to "reduce the clubfoot." His operation fell into disrepute because of a high incidence of residual stiffness and severe flattening of the foot. Thereafter, a series of limited operations were proposed. Osteotomies, tendon transfers, tendon lengthenings, talectomies, and so on, all of which have been plagued by incomplete correction and the need for additional surgery, often ending in the teenage years with a triple arthrodesis.

Recently the soft-tissue release of midfoot and hindfoot has again become popular as advocated by Bost, Schottstaedt, and Larsen,[3] Judet,[7] McCauley,[10] Reimann and Becker-Anderson,[12] and most notably in this country by Turco.[13,14] The initial problem of residual stiffness is far less serious in these recent series; this may be attributed to more meticulous surgical techniques or perhaps to the younger age of the patients at the time of surgery.

The assessment of results in clubfoot treatment has been most difficult on a clinical basis. Radiographic measures, while not without difficulties, appear more reliable as demonstrated by numerous authors.[11,13,14] To date the radiographic assessment method of Beatson and Pearson[2] appears most reliable.

This chapter presents our experience with a posteromedial release procedure for feet that are radiographically judged uncorrected. The results, though relatively short term, were graded radiographically, not clinically. In addition, an attempt was made to determine if there was any significant difference between the results in those children operated upon before twelve months age and those older than twelve months at time of procedure. No attempt was made to assess the reasons for failure of nonoperative treatment.

MATERIAL

From 1973 to 1976, sixty-four feet in forty-four patients were operated upon at the James Whitcomb Riley Hospital for

Children. The operations were performed by a single attending surgeon or by resident surgeons under his direction. Fifty feet in thirty-five patients had to have had at least an eighteen-month follow-up and adequate radiographs to be included in the study.

Group I patients (Table 27-1) were less than twelve months of age (average 7.3 months) at the time of surgery. This group comprises thirty-three feet in twenty-four patients. Group II patients were more than twelve months of age at time of surgery (average 24.6 months). This group is comprised of seventeen feet in twelve patients. It should be noted that more than 60 per cent of patients referred to our hospital or to the senior author had prior conservative therapy elsewhere which was judged unsuccessful. Only idiopathic clubfeet were included in this study. Any patient with a neurologic deficit or arthrogryposis was eliminated from the series.

METHODS

Assessment of the feet preoperatively and at time of follow-up was performed by measuring the talocalcaneal angle on both standing A-P and lateral roentgenograms. On the A-P film the lines were drawn longitudinally through the talus parallel to its medial border, and through the calcaneus parallel to its lateral border (Fig. 27-1). On the lateral film the angle was measured by a line drawn longitudinally through the center axis of the talus and parallel to the lower border of the calcaneus (Fig. 27-2). The sum of the talocalcaneal angles from the A-P and lateral films was used as the

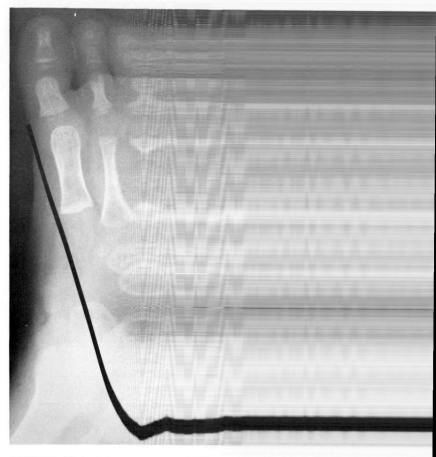

FIGURE 27-1 A-P
measurement (see text).

talocalcaneal index
and Pearson.[2] All
formed by a single
The use of st
radiographs is enc
wood has shown, i
assessment in the u

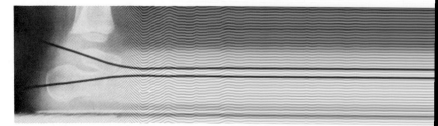

FIGURE 27-2 Later
measurement (see text).

TABLE 1   Age of patients at time of surgery and at follow-up.

	NUMBER OF PATIENTS	NUMBER OF FEET	AVERAGE AGE IN MONTHS AT TIME OF OPERATION (RANGE)	FOLLOW-UP IN MONTHS (RANGE)
Group I	24	33	7.3 (3.5-12)	31.7 (18-51)
Group II	12	17	24.6 (13-60)	26.4 (18-42)

Chapter Twenty-Seven

SURGICAL CORRECTION OF THE RESISTANT CLUB FOOT

G. Paul DeRosa, M.D.
Edward A. Dykstra, M.D.

The treatment of the resistant club foot has been the subject of considerable controversy in the orthopaedic literature during the past forty years. Although many clubfeet can be successfully managed by nonoperative means, a certain percentage will fail to respond and be classified as "resistant." This failure rate varies from 12 to 60 per cent.[2,5,7-9,11,13] The issue of "recurrence of deformity" has also been controversial. As early as 1930, Brockman stated that clubfoot deformities did not recur but were cases in which an inadequate initial correction had been accepted.[4]

The surgical treatment of resistant clubfoot during the past forty years has been quite varied. Brockman advocated an extensive soft-tissue release in an attempt to "reduce the clubfoot." His operation fell into disrepute because of a high incidence of residual stiffness and severe flattening of the foot. Thereafter, a series of limited operations were proposed. Osteotomies, tendon transfers, tendon lengthenings, talectomies, and so on, all of which have been plagued by incomplete correction and the need for additional surgery, often ending in the teenage years with a triple arthrodesis.

Recently the soft-tissue release of midfoot and hindfoot has again become popular as advocated by Bost, Schottstaedt, and Larsen,[3] Judet,[7] McCauley,[10] Reimann and Becker-Anderson,[12] and most notably in this country by Turco.[13,14] The initial problem of residual stiffness is far less serious in these recent series; this may be attributed to more meticulous surgical techniques or perhaps to the younger age of the patients at the time of surgery.

The assessment of results in clubfoot treatment has been most difficult on a clinical basis. Radiographic measures, while not without difficulties, appear more reliable as demonstrated by numerous authors.[11,13,14] To date the radiographic assessment method of Beatson and Pearson[2] appears most reliable.

This chapter presents our experience with a posteromedial release procedure for feet that are radiographically judged uncorrected. The results, though relatively short term, were graded radiographically, not clinically. In addition, an attempt was made to determine if there was any significant difference between the results in those children operated upon before twelve months age and those older than twelve months at time of procedure. No attempt was made to assess the reasons for failure of nonoperative treatment.

MATERIAL

From 1973 to 1976, sixty-four feet in forty-four patients were operated upon at the James Whitcomb Riley Hospital for

Children. The operations were performed by a single attending surgeon or by resident surgeons under his direction. Fifty feet in thirty-five patients had to have had at least an eighteen-month follow-up and adequate radiographs to be included in the study.

Group I patients (Table 27–1) were less than twelve months of age (average 7.3 months) at the time of surgery. This group comprises thirty-three feet in twenty-four patients. Group II patients were more than twelve months of age at time of surgery (average 24.6 months). This group is comprised of seventeen feet in twelve patients. It should be noted that more than 60 per cent of patients referred to our hospital or to the senior author had prior conservative therapy elsewhere which was judged unsuccessful. Only idiopathic clubfeet were included in this study. Any patient with a neurologic deficit or arthrogryposis was eliminated from the series.

METHODS

Assessment of the feet preoperatively and at time of follow-up was performed by measuring the talocalcaneal angle on both standing A-P and lateral roentgenograms. On the A-P film the lines were drawn longitudinally through the talus parallel to its medial border, and through the calcaneus parallel to its lateral border (Fig. 27–1). On the lateral film the angle was measured by a line drawn longitudinally through the center axis of the talus and parallel to the lower border of the calcaneus (Fig. 27–2). The sum of the talocalcaneal angles from the A-P and lateral films was used as the

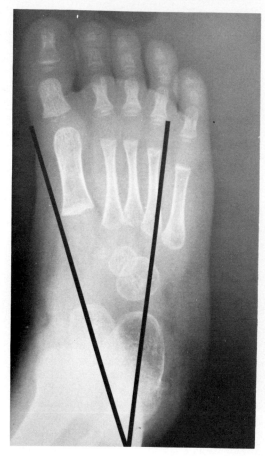

FIGURE 27–1 A-P view of talocalcaneal angle measurement (see text).

talocalcaneal index as described by Beatson and Pearson.[2] All measurements were performed by a single examiner.

The use of standing (weight-bearing) radiographs is encouraged because, as Heywood has shown, it provides a more critical assessment in the uncorrected foot.[6]

TABLE 1   Age of patients at time of surgery and at follow-up.

	NUMBER OF PATIENTS	NUMBER OF FEET	AVERAGE AGE IN MONTHS AT TIME OF OPERATION (RANGE)	FOLLOW-UP IN MONTHS (RANGE)
Group I	24	33	7.3 (3.5-12)	31.7 (18-51)
Group II	12	17	24.6 (13-60)	26.4 (18-42)

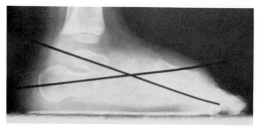

FIGURE 27–2 Lateral view of talocalconeal angle measurement (see text).

SURGICAL TECHNIQUE

The procedure is performed under tourniquet control. The skin incision begins medially and distally at the level of the tarsometatarsal joint near the insertion of the tibialis anterior tendon. The incision is continued proximally beneath the medial malleolus and then gently curved proximally toward the Achilles' tendon, ending 1 in. proximal to the superior margin of the os calcis. The Achilles' tendon is exposed and cleared of soft tissue circumferentially at its insertion into the os calcis. It is lengthened sagitally in Z-fashion, and the distal medial limb is removed from the os calcis. The neurovascular bundle is then mobilized and retracted with a rubber drain. The fibro-fatty packing tissue anterior to the Achilles' tendon and behind the tibiotalar and subtalar joints is resected. This tissue in the normal foot is fatty and pliable, whereas in the clubfoot, it is tough, fibrotic scar which is a formidable tether to the descent of the os calcis. The removal of this fibro-fatty tissue is carried laterally to expose the sheath of the peroneal tendons and identify the sural nerve and accompanying vascular structures. The subtalar joint is incised using a #64 Beaver blade. The capsule is incised from medial to lateral aspect then down the lateral aspect of the as calcis to divide the calcaneofibular ligaments. At this point a small portion of peroneal tendon sheath is excised to be certain there is no lateral tether to hinder the descent of the os calcis. Using the tendon of flexor hallucis longus as a guide, the medial aspect of the subtalar joint is opened anteriorly to the level of the sustentaculum tali. At this point the os calcis should easily descend as the foot is dorsiflexed. If it does not, any block to reduction should be determined.

Attention is then turned to the medial aspect of the foot. The neurovascular bundle is traced carefully through the hiatus in the abductor hallucis muscle. The bundle is protected as the fascial attachments of the abductor are sharply divided from the navicular and surrounding tissue. The abductor hallucis muscle belly is retracted into the sole. A plantar fasciotomy and extra periosteal Steindler strip of all muscles arising from the plantar concave surface of the os calcis are performed. The flexor hallucis longus and flexor digitorum longus tendon sheaths are opened and the master knot of Henry is excised. The tendon of tibialis posterior is Z-lengthened well above the medial malleolus. The pulley mechanism of its sheath is preserved about the medial malleolus. The flexor hallucis and flexor digitorium are Z-lengthened in the sole of the foot.

Next, the talonavicular joint is opened on its dorsal, medial, and plantar surfaces. The pseudoarticulation of the navicular with the medial malleolus is excised, taking care to preserve the insertion of tibialis posterior. A #64 Beaver blade is used with meticulous care to avoid damage to the articular cartilage. The superficial portion of the deltoid ligament is incised and the anterior part of the subtalar joint is opened. The plantar dissection of the talonavicular joint includes dividing the plantar calcaneonavicular ligament (spring ligament). This dissection is carried laterally to expose the junction of the talus and navicular superiorly, and os calcis and cuboid inferiorly. The articulation of calcaneus and cuboid is carefully and completely opened medially, plantarward, and dorsally. Any ligamentous attachments from os calcis to navicular are also incised. Once this is accomplished, the navicular and the cuboid should easily translate laterally to near normal anatomic relationship. This reduction must *not* require force. The talonavicular joint must lie in the "reduced" position without applying any external force. If it does not, then any blocks to reduction must be sought out and released.

Next the navicular cuneiform joint and cuneiform metatarsal joints are released, and a .062-inch Kirschner wire is passed anteriorly through the talus and navicular and is left subcutaneously between the first and second toes. The Z-lengthened tendons are repaired using two or three 0 chromic sutures. Very little, if any, lengthening is required of the Achilles' tendon. A threaded .062-inch Kirschner wire is passed transversely through the os calcis and allowed to protrude through the skin for incorporation into the plaster cast. Hemostasis is secured after release of the tourniquet, and routine closure accomplished. The circulation to the skin edges is checked as traction is applied to the os calcis pin, and a well-padded plaster is applied.

Two weeks postoperatively, the cast is changed under anesthesia. At this time manipulation of the os calcis may be accomplished if the skin did not permit full descent at the time of surgery. A snug plaster is then applied. Six weeks postoperatively the pins are removed and the patient is fitted with a polypropylene splint for wear at night and during naps. The splint allows for varying degrees of dorsiflexion and eversion (Fig. 27-3). This splint is retained for at least six months and preferably one year. If the child is ambulatory, straight-last shoes are worn.

RESULTS

Group I patients (less than twelve months old at time of surgical release) had an average A-P talocalcaneal angle of 13.4° (range 3° to 34°) (Table 27-2). The average preoperative lateral talocalcaneal angle was 15.2° (range 0° to 36°). The average talocalcaneal index was 27.3°. Postoperatively the average A-P angle was 24.7° (range 15° to 40°); the average lateral angle was 27.3° (range 13° to 45°); and the index was 54.4.

The index was greater than 50 in twenty-two feet and less than 40 in only two feet (Table 27-3). An index of less than 40 was considered evidence of abject failure of the procedure. An index greater than 50 was considered a good result; an index in between was considered a fair

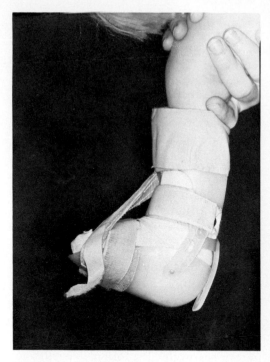

FIGURE 27-3 Night splint used for postoperative maintence of correction.

result. Group II patients (more than twelve months old at the time of the procedure) had an average preoperative A-P angle of 17.8° (range 5° to 33°), an average lateral angle of 14.8° (range 0° to 27°), and an average talocalcaneal index of 32.6. Postoperatively the average A-P angle was 20.1° (range 8° to 33°), the lateral 29° range 9°to 44°), and the index 49.6 (Table 27-2). In this group there were also two feet with an index of less than 40, i.e., the procedures were failures.

There were seven good results (index>50), eight fair (index between 40 and 50), and the two failures (index<40).

TABLE 2   Comparison of pre- and postoperative AP and talocalcaneal angles.

	AVG. PREOP AP° TALOCALCANEAL (T-C) ANGLE	AVG. PREOP LATERAL T–7C ANGLE	AVG. INDEX	AVG. POSTOP AP° T–C ANGLE	AVG. POSTOP LATERAL	AVG. INDEX
Group I	13.4° (3°-34°)	15.2° (0°-36°)	27.3° (12°-56°)	24.7° (15°-40°)	27.3° (13°-45°)	54.4° (29°-85°)
Group II	17.8° (5°-33°)	14.8° (0°-27°)	32.6° (8°-58°)	20.1° (8°-33°)	29.0° (9°-44°)	49.6° (17°-76°)

TABLE 3 Results of surgical treatment

	GOOD TALOCALCANEAL (INDEX >50) Number of Feet	FAIR (INDEX 40–50) Number of Feet	POOR (INDEX <40) Number of Feet
Group I (<12 months of age)	22	9	2
Group II (>12 months of age)	7	8	2

Careful analysis revealed the results of Group I patients to be slightly better than those in Group II patients, but the results were not statistically significant using the Student's *t*-test. To date only three feet have undergone further surgery. In each case the procedure was a repeat of the posteromedial release.

There were few complications. Skin healing was not a significant problem in any patient throughout the series; in fact, only one patient had any evidence of wound dehiscence at the time of cast removal at six weeks. This did not require any secondary procedures and did not limit the child's ability to be held in the polypropylene splint.

DISCUSSION

In the past few decades the pathologic manifestations of clubfeet have been well described by many authors including Turco,[13,14] LeNoir,[10] Fripp and Shaw,[5] Heywood,[6] and Swann, Lloyd-Roberts, and Catterall.[12] The pathologic findings can adequately be described as a subluxation of the talocalcaneonavicular triple joint complex whose ligaments and muscle become contracted, rendering the complex irreducible. Prolonged strain in the abnormally located position results in adaptive bony changes which yield permanent deformity as the child matures. If the joint capsules remain pliable, conservative efforts of stretching may relocate the joint. Limited surgical procedures, both bony and soft tissue, have been disappointing with regard to producing a complete and lasting correction of the deformity. It would appear that

a complete "open reduction" of the triple joint complex would be the ideal method of treatment, provided significant risks of damage to the foot were minimal.

A posteromedial release procedure appears to have fulfilled these requirements. Dr. Turco has given detailed description of such a procedure. The procedure described in this chapter is similar to that of Turco with the following exceptions:

1. The skin incision is longer, being carried proximally along the Achilles' tendon.

2. The tibiotalar joint is not opened posteriorly, only the subtalar joint.

3. The tibialis posterior tendon is preserved and is lengthened proximally in its sheath. The flexor hallucis and flexor digitorum are lengthened in the sole.

4. A Steindler strip and plantar fascia release is performed on all feet.

5. The calcaneocuboid joint is completely released supero-proximally to allow easy translation of the midfoot upon the hindfoot.

6. A transverse calcaneal pin is used to manipulate the os calcis and hold it in the plaster.

7. Patients are held in plaster for only six weeks and are then placed in a polypropylene splint which has a dynamic component to maintain correction.

The unreliability of clinical evaluation of completeness of correction has been shown or alluded to by numerous authors.[1,2,4,6 9,11,14,15]

Yet in most recent studies the results are expressed clinically, not radiographically. Beatson and Pearson[2] and Ashby[1] have recommended expressing results exclusively in terms of radiographic findings, as these are the most reliable indicators of completeness of correction and, as such, should also have prognostic significance.

The present study uses the measuring techniques of Beatson and Pearson, with the exception that the lateral x-rays were made in the standing or dorsiflexed position. The results of the study compare favorably with other series in which a posteromedial release procedure was used. Turco reported good or fair results in twenty-

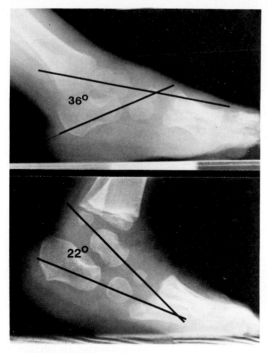

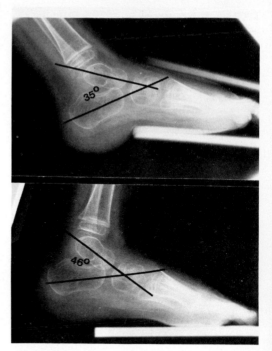

FIGURE 27-4 (Top) Uncorrected clubfoot taken in 30° plantar flexion revealing talocalcaneal angle of 36°. (Bottom) Same foot taken in dorsiflexion revealing a talocalcaneal angle of 22° (see text).

FIGURE 27-5 (Top) Normal foot taken in 30° plantar flexion revealing talocalcaneal angle of 35°. (Bottom) Same foot taken in dorsiflexion revealing a talocalcaneal angle of 46°.

seven of thirty-one feet. Reimann and Becker-Anderson reported good or fair results in one hundred, twenty-one of one hundred, forty feet. Ashby reported good or acceptable results in all twenty-six feet operated upon. Our present suudy, taking both groups as a whole, revealed good or fair results in forty-six of fifty feet, a 92 per cent success rate.

In Beatson and Pearson's study of two hundred normal feet there were no normal feet with an index less than forty. In addition, their study revealed only one *clubfoot* with an index of greater than fifty. For these reasons we chose as our level of confidence of correction a talocalcaneal index of fifty. We felt justified in using the index of forty or less as incidence of failure based upon Beatson and Pearson's work. In addition to their work, Heywood has clearly demonstrated that dorsiflexion of the foot (as our lateral x-rays were made) decreases the talocalcaneal angle in the clubfoot and increases the angle in the normal foot (Figs.

27-4 and 27-5). Thus the level of forty in our series is a far more critical assessment than in other studies.

A posteromedial release is a delicate procedure, but with care and a knowledge of both pathologic and normal anatomy it may be performed on very young children without significant risk to cartilaginous structures. Our findings suggest better results in younger children (less than twelve months old). We agree with Reimann and Becker-Anderson that it is usually possible to predict by the third month which foot will respond to conservative measures and which will not, and we agree that there is little reason for delaying surgery beyond this point. As stated earlier, many patients are referred after conservative therapy elsewhere; in addition, our surgical waiting list is nearly two months. For these and other reasons our children usually are five months old or older at the time of surgical release. If there is radiographic evidence of continuing improvement with conservative therapy there seems to be little indication for immediate surgical intervention.

An analysis of patients who do not do well usually is quite enlightening. In our series four feet were considered failures, and to date three of these four have had a repeat operation. It was obvious from the description of the procedure in the operative note that force was needed to hold the talonavicular joint reduced as it was pinned. In three of these four a release of the calcaneocuboid joint was not performed, as it was judged not necessary. Unfortunately, subsequent radiographs revealed incomplete translation of the midfoot on the hindfoot. For this reason the midfoot should be easily translated upon the hindfoot and not require force to be held. If there is any doubt an intraoperative x-ray should be made.

SUMMARY

This chapter describes our operative technique of posteromedial release which we use in resistant clubfeet to effect reduction of the talocalcaneonavicular triple joint complex. It relates our experience in fifty operative cases. The results are critically assessed by a rigorous radiographic method. The results are related to the age of the patient at the time of operation; the children less than twelve months old had slightly better results than those over twelve months of age.

REFERENCE

1. Ashby, M.E.: Roentogenographic assessment of soft tissue medial release operation in club foot deformity. Clin. Ortho. 90:146, 1973.
2. Beatson, T.R. and Pearson, J.R.: A method of assessing correction in club feet. J. Bone Joint Surg. 48B:40, 1966.
3. Bost, F.C., Schottstaedt, E.R. and Larsen, L.J.: Plantar dissection: an operation to release the soft tissues in recurrent or recalcitrant talipes equinovarus. J. Bone Joint Surg. 45A: 151, 1960.
4. Brockman, E.P.: Modern methods of treatment of club foot. Brit. Med. J. 2: 572-74, 1957.
5. Fripp, A.J. and Shaw, N.F.: Club Foot. Edinburgh: E & S Livingstone, Ltd, 1967.
6. Heywood, A.W.B.: The mechanics of the hind foot in club foot as demonstrated radiographically. J. Bone Joint Surg. 46B:102, 1964.
7. Judet, J.: New concepts in the corrective surgery of congenital talipes equinovarus and congenital and neurological flat feet. Clin. Ortho. 70:56, 1970.
8. Kite, J.H.: Principles involved in the treatment of congenital club foot. J. Bone Joint Surg. 21:595-606, 1939.
9. Kite, J.H.: Conservative treatment of the resistant recurrent club foot. Clin. Ortho. 70:93-110, 1970.
10. LeNoir, James L.: Congenital Idiopathic Talipes. Chicago: Charles C Thomas, 1960.
11. McCauley, J.C. Jr.: Clubfoot: history of the development and the concepts of pathogenesis and treatment. Clin. Ortho. 44:51, 1966.
12. Ponseti, I.V. and Smoley, E.N.: Congenital club foot: the results of treatment. J. Bone Joint Surg. 45A:261-75, 1963.
13. Reimann, I. and Becker-Anderson, H.: Early surgical treatment of congenital club foot. Clin. Ortho. 90:146-49, 1973.
14. Swann, M., Lloyd-Roberts, G.C. and Catterall, A. The anatomy of uncorrected club feet. J. Bone Joint Surg. 51B:263-69, 1969.
15. Turco, V.J.: Surgical correction of the resistant club foot. J. Bone Joint Surg. 53A:477, 1971.
16. Turco, V.J.: Resistant congenital club foot. A.A.O.S. Instructional Course Lecture (St. Louis) 24:104, 1975.

INDEX

Abductor muscles
  hallucis
    in clubfoot correction, 207, 208, 210, 211, 217
    in hallux valgus, 146
  of hip, 168, 173
Achilles tendon
  in clubfoot correction, 207, 208, 210, 211, 217
  dynamic force measurements of, 180-181
  pull of, in weight distribution in foot, 178, 179,
    182, 183
  in walking and running, 199, 202
Adams method of ankle fusion, 132
Adductor muscles
  hallucis, in hallux valgus correction, 143, 145,
    146, 147
  of hip, 168, 173, 174
Age at time of surgery
  in amputation of diabetic foot, 127
  in arthrodesis, 79-80, 120, 121, 125
  in clubfoot correction, 215, 216, 218, 219-220
  in replantation of severed foot, 70
Ambulation. See Walking
Amputation
  accidental, and replantation. See Replantation of
    foot
  after failed ankle fusion, 133, 135
  of diabetic foot, 127-130
  prosthesis after, 64, 69, 72
Anesthetics, local, in peroneal tendinitis, 103, 104-
    105, 106, 108
Ankle
  arthritis of, treatment for, 36, 39, 73, 74, 91, 131,
    132, 135
  blood supply og, 56-57
  excision of articular surfaces in foot replantation,
    65
  fractures of, 5-34
    arthrodesis in, 131
    avascular necrosis after, 52-53, 55, 56, 57, 59,
      60, 61, 62, 63
    bone implants in, 57-59, 60, 62, 63
    braces in, postoperative, 22-23
    cast immobilization in, 7, 21, 22, 24, 27, 34, 53
    classification of, 5-10, 52
    closed reduction of, 7, 8, 24-25, 34, 53, 61, 62
    degenerative changes after, 11-16
    direct violence and vertical compression in, 6, 8
    eversion injury in, 6, 7-9, 10
    forced internal rotation for reduction of, 12,

      13, 16
    Group I, 52, 53, 59
    Group II, 52, 53, 59, 62
    Group III, 52, 53, 55, 59, 62
    Hawkins sign in, 52-53, 56-57
    incomplete reduction of, mechanisms in, 11, 12,
      13
    inversion injury in, 6-7, 10
    lateral malleolus in, 8, 9, 11-16, 24-34
    leg elevation in, postoperative, 21, 22, 27
    operative procedures in, 21-22, 24-34, 52-63
    patient satisfaction with treatment of, 55
    reossification after, 57
    Type A, 6-7, 10
    Type B_1, 7-8, 10
    Type B_2, 8-9, 9-10
   fractures (continued)
    unstable, 8-9, 9-10, 11-19, 21-22
    weight-bearing after, 22, 23, 27, 28, 60-61, 62
    wire-loop fixation in, 24-34
  fusion of
    cast immobilization in, 132, 133
    surgical. See Arthrodesis
  ligament of, medial. See Deltoid ligament
  malrotation in talipes equino varus, 207, 208
  motion of, 20, 21, 23
    after arthroplasty, 36-39
    after replacement of ankle, 38, 73
    in dorsiflexion of foot, 20, 23, 170
    fibula in, 24, 34
    lateral malleolus affecting, 24, 34
    in plantar flexion, 21, 23
    tibiopedal, 36-39, 83-85, 87, 90
    in walking, running and jogging, 167, 168, 169,
      170, 174, 195, 201, 202, 203, 204
  prosthesis for
    amount of motion with, 38, 73
    arthrodesis compared to, 73, 91
  sprains of, peroneal tendinitis in, 103, 104, 105,
    109
Ankylosis, fibrous, of subtalar complex, quadruple
    arthrodesis in, 93, 94
Anthropological classification of foot, 1-2
Arch of foot
  flat. See Flatfoot
  longitudinal, 2, 3, 117, 118, 119, 179, 191, 197
  as medially-based half dome, 191, 197
  in perfect foot, 2, 190-191, 197
  structural stability of, 197

transverse, 191, 197
in weight-bearing, 179, 191, 197
Arterial repair, in foot replantation, 65-66, 70-71
Arthritis
    after tarsometatarsal joint injury, 44, 45, 46, 50
    of ankle, 36, 39, 73, 74, 91, 131, 132, 135
    arthrodesis in, 36, 73, 74, 91, 131, 132, 135
    arthroplasty in, 39, 131
        of great toe, 137, 138, 139, 140-141, 142
    gouty, 131, 132
    Keller bunionectomy in, 148, 152
    of metatarsophalangeal joint, first, 148, 152
    prosthetic joint replacement in, 73, 91
    rheumatoid, 73, 91, 135, 137, 138, 139, 140-141,
        142
    traumatic, 24, 25, 34, 73, 74, 131, 132, 135
        of subtalar joint, 52, 58, 103
    tuberculous, 131, 132
Arthrodesis, 131-135
    Adams method in, 132
    age at time of, 79-80, 120, 121, 125
    in ankle fractures, 131
    ankle replacement compared to, 73, 91
    in ankylosis, fibrous, of subtalar complex, 93, 94
    in arthritis, 36, 73, 74, 91, 131, 132, 135
    bone grafts in. See Bone grafts
    arthroplasty compared to, 36-39
    in calcaneal fractures, 93, 100, 109
    calf atrophy after, 80, 81
    Charnley procedures for, 36, 74, 75, 131, 132
    and compensatory mechanisms in gait, 82, 88, 89,
        90, 91, 99
    degenerative changes after, 75, 82
    dorsiflexion after, 36, 37, 78, 81, 82, 83-85, 90,
        134
    employment after, 79, 80, 88, 134-135
    failures in, 132-133, 135
    fibular graft in, 75, 116, 120-121, 124, 125, 132
    follow-up study of, 73-92, 131-135
    fusion time in, 133
    gait analysis after, 73-92, 133-134, 135
    Grice procedure in, 116-125, 144, 145, 146
    hallux valgus correction with, 144, 145, 146
    Hatt method of, 75, 132
    heel valgus after, 133, 145
    heel varus after, 133, 145
    indications for, 93-94, 131-132
    leg length discrepancies after, 80, 81
    midtarsal joint motion after, 133-134
    osteomyelitis after, 133
    pain after, 76, 77, 79, 88-89, 133
        relief of, 33, 93, 94, 117, 124, 144
    patient satisfaction with, 36, 37, 38, 39, 80, 133,
        135
    plantar flexion after, 36, 37, 78, 81, 82, 83-85, 90,
        102, 134
    point system in evaluation of, 76, 77-78, 79-81,
        89, 134
    position and degree of fusion in, 90-91, 134, 135
    pseudarthrosis after, 120-121, 122, 125, 133, 135
    quadruple, 93-102. See also Quadruple arthrodesis
    rotational deformity of foot after, 133
    subtalar joint motion after, 80-81, 117, 119, 124,
        133-134, 135
    tarsometatarsal, 94

tibial graft in, 116, 121, 124, 132
tibiopedal motion after, 36-39, 83-85, 87, 90
tibiotalar, 33
transfibular approach to, 75, 131, 132
triple, 94, 95, 98, 99, 105, 109, 144, 145
in valgus foot deformity, 116
weight-bearing after, 83-84, 85, 94, 101, 117
Arthrography, in tibiofibular ligament assessment,
    19
Arthoplasty
    in arthritis, 39, 131, 137, 138, 139, 140-141, 142
    arthrodesis compared to, 36-39
    bunionectomy in, 148-154, 192
    dorsiflexion after, 37
    of great toe, with silicone implant, 137-142
    Keller procedure in, 138, 142, 148-154
    literature review of, 138
    patient satisfaction with, 37, 38, 39
    plantar flexion after, 37, 139
    tibiopedal motion after, 36-39
Avulsion fracture
    of fibula, 6
    of medial malleolus, 7
    of posterior tibial lip, 8, 9-10

Back injuries, in running, 155
Ball of foot, in weight-bearing, 180
Bankhart repair, in peroneal tendon dislocation, 112
Basketball, peroneal tendon dislocations in, 110,
    113-114
Biomechanical studies, 167-204
    kinematic, 44, 47, 195-204
    limitations of, 195-196
    of normal and abnormal foot, 186-193
    in os calcis excision, 176-184
    in running, jogging and walking, 155-156, 157,
        167-175, 186-193, 195-204
Bone grafts
    in ankle fracture, 57-59, 60, 62, 63
    in arthrodesis
        absorption of, 121-122, 123, 124
        autogenous, 94
        beef bone, 94, 102
        fibular, 75, 116, 120-121, 124, 125, 132
        freeze-dried bone in, 94, 101
        in Grice procedure, 116, 120-121, 123, 124, 125
        iliac, 93-102
        tibial, 116, 121, 124, 132
        transfibular, 75, 131, 132
    in opening wedge osteotomy of first matetarsal,
        148, 153-154
Bone nails, for internal fixation, 27, 32
Bone production, after great toe arthroplasty, 139,
    140, 141
"Boplant" bone grafts, in arthrodesis, 94, 102
Braces
    after clubfoot correction, 218, 219
    after open reduction and internal fixation, 22-23
    components of, 22, 23
    custom-made, 23, 156-157
    dorsiflexion with, 22, 23
    length of time for use of, 22, 23
    plantar flexion with, 22, 23
    of ready-made semiflexible leather, 156, 157

for running problems, 156-157
Bunionectomy
  Keller, with opening wedge osteotomy of first
    metatarsal, 148-154
  Silver, 192

        Calcaneal tendon. See Achilles tendon
Calcaneocuboid joint
  in clubfoot correction, 207, 208, 210, 217, 219,
    220
  importance for minimal loss of function, 176,
    178-184
  instrumentation for study of, 181
  in partial excision of calcaneus, 176, 179-184
  in quadruple arthrodesis, 95, 97, 98, 99
  and weight distributing function of foot, 176, 178-
    184
    formula for calculation of force in, 179
Calcaneofibular ligament, 110
Calcaneotalar joint, in quadruple arthrodesis, 95
Calcaneotalocuboid-navicular fusion, in quadruple
    arthrodesis, 95, 99
Calcaneus
  angle with first metatarsal, Grice arthrodesis
    affecting, 118, 120
  as landmark in quadruple arthrodesis, 96
  fracture of
    arthrodesis in, 93, 100, 109
    peroneal tendinitis in, 103, 104, 105-106, 109
  fusion in quadruple arthrodesis, 95, 97, 98, 99,
    100, 102
  osteomyelitis of, treatment of, 176-177, 183
  partial excision of, 176-184
    in foot replantation, 65
    and weight distributing function of foot, 176,
      179-184
    Wiltse procedure in, 176, 180, 181, 183, 184
  peroneal trochlea of, 103
  surfaces used in karate kicks, 160, 161-162
  in talipes equino varus correction, 208, 209
  talocalcaneal joint. See Talocalcaneal joint
Calluses, metatarsal
  after great toe arthroplasty, 142
  after Grice arthrodesis, 122-123, 125
Cast immobilization
  in ankle fractures, 7, 21, 22, 24, 27, 34, 53
  ankle fusion in, 132, 133
  in closed reduction procedure, 24, 25, 34
  in clubfoot correction, 208, 209, 210, 211, 217-
    218, 219
  in foot replantation, 67, 68, 71
  in Grice arthrodesis, 117
  in lateral malleolus fracture, 16, 19
  in open reduction procedure, 21, 22, 25, 27, 34
  in peroneal tendon dislocation, 112, 113
  in quadruple arthrodesis, 94, 101
  in tarsometatarsal joint injury, 43, 44
Cavus deformity of foot, 156, 157. See also
    Clubfoot
Cerclage fixation, in long bone fractures, 25
Cerebral palsy, hallux valgus correction in, 143-147
Chambers procedure, in nonparalytic flatfoot
    deformities, 124-125
Charnley compression arthrodesis, 36, 74, 75, 131,

    132
Children
  clubfoot in, 207-220
  flatfoot in, asymptomatic, 4
  footwear for, 4
  replantation of severed foot, 64-72
Clawing of toes, after replantation of foot, 69, 70
Closed reduction
  in ankle fracture, 7, 8, 24-25, 34, 53, 61, 62
  disadvantages of, 24, 25, 34
  in tarsometatarsal joint injury, 43, 45
Clubfoot correction, 207-220
  age at time of, 215, 216, 218, 219-220
  cast immobilization in, 208, 209, 210, 211, 217-
    218, 219
  Goldner one-stage approach in, 207, 208, 213
  illustrative cases of, 209-212, 213
  night splint use after, 218, 219
  operative techniques for, 207, 208, 210, 211, 212-
    213, 216-218
  pin used in, 217, 218, 219
  posterior release procedure in, 208, 209, 213, 215-
    220
  radiographic assessment of, 209, 210, 211, 212,
    215, 216, 218, 219-220
  and recurrence of deformity, 215
  results of, 208-209, 212-213, 215, 218, 219-220
  shoes used in, 209
  Turco procedure in, 207, 219
  weight-bearing after, 208, 209
Crystals, pressure-sensitive, for evaluating forces
    under foot, 186-187, 193, 200
Cuboid bone, 40
  in foot replantation, 65
  in quadruple arthrodesis, 95, 97, 98, 100, 102
Cuneiform bones, 40
  in foot replantation, 65
Débridement
  of severed foot, 64-65, 70
  in tarsometatarsal joint injury, 43
Deltoid ligament
  ankle stability after division of, 11, 12, 14, 19
  detection of injury to, 19
  surgical repair of, 14, 21, 27, 30
  in Type B ankle fracture, 7
De Quervain's disease, 109
Diabetes
  foot amputation in
    Syme's procedure in, 127-130
    two-stage procedure in, 130
  juvenile, Charcot-type joint destruction in, 33
Diastasis, in ankle fracture, 8, 9
Digitorum muscles
  extensor
    in quadruple arthrodesis, 97
    in walking, 198
  flexor
    dynamic force measurements of, 180-181
    lengthening in clubfoot correction, 217, 219
    running-related injury to, 189, 200, 201, 203,
      204
    in walking, 199
Dislocation
  of metatarsal bones, 41, 42-43
  of peroneal tendons, recurrent, 110-115

of tarsometatarsal joint, 41
Distance walked, in gait analysis
    after arthrodesis, 77, 79, 88-89
    after tarsometatarsal joint injury, 44, 45, 46
Dorsalis pedis artery repair, in foot replantation, 66
Dorsiflexion of foot
    after ankle fracture, 23
    after ankle replacement, 73
    after arthrodesis, 36, 37, 78, 81, 82, 83-85, 90,
        134
    after arthroplasty, 37
    with leg brace, 22, 23
    normal, 37, 38
    position for measurement of, 20, 23, 38
    postoperative exercises for, 21-22, 23
Drop-foot deformity, ankle fusion in, 132
DuVries bone block, in peroneal tendon dislocation,
    112

E-fusion, in quadruple arthrodesis, 95, 100
Electromyography, in gait analysis, 92
    after arthrodesis, 76, 78-79, 85-87, 88
    in running, jogging and walking, 167-175
Employment
    after arthrodesis, 79, 80, 88, 134-135
    after peroneal tendinitis, 105, 106, 108
Equinus deformity of foot, 98-99, 131. See also
        Clubfoot correction
Eversion injury, in ankle fractures, 6, 7-9, 10
Exercises
    after arthrodesis, 101
    for dorsiflexion of ankle, 21-22, 23
    for limb control, 27
Extensor muscles
    digitorum
        cutting of, in quadruple arthrodesis, 97
        in walking, 198
    hallucis longus, lengthening in great toe
        arthroplasty, 139, 141
External fixation
    braces for, 22-23, 156-157, 218, 219
    casts for. See Cast immobilization
Extrinsic muscles of foot
    activity in gait, 197
    in weight-bearing, 180-181, 182, 183, 184

Fibula
    in ankle function, 24, 34
    fractures of
        Maisonneuve, 9
        in runners, 200, 203
        in Type A ankle fracture, 6
        in Type B ankle fracture, 7-9, 10
    graft with
        in arthrodesis, 76, 116, 120-121, 124, 125, 132
        and pseudarthrosis at donor site, 120-121, 125
    lateral malleolus of. See Lateral malleolus
    motion of, in running and sprinting, 200-201, 202,
        203, 204
Fibular collateral ligaments
    isolated division of, ankle stability after, 11, 12
    stretching of, with unreduced lateral malleolus,
        12, 13, 16

Fixation. See External fixation; Internal fixation
Flatfoot
    asymptomatic, in children, 4
    Chambers procedure in, 124-125
    footwear in, 116, 117, 118, 119, 124, 187, 191
    forces under, in walking and running, 190, 191-
        192
    Grice arthrodesis in, 116-125
    LeLievre operation in, 124
    quadruple arthrodesis in, 93-94, 116, 125
    roentgenogram of, 191-192
    spastic, 93-94
Flexion. See Dorsiflexion; Plantar flexion
Flexor muscles
    digitorum. See Digitorum muscles, flexor
    hallucis longus
        dynamic force measurements of, 180-181
        lengthening of, in clubfoot correction, 217, 219
        in walking and running, 192, 202, 203
Flipper foot deformity, calcaneocuboid joint in,
        176, 183
Float period, in gait cycle, 168, 169, 172
Foot
    normal, 1-4
    severed. See Replantation of foot
    support phase kinematics of, 195-204
Football, peroneal tendon dislocation in, 110, 114
Footwear
    after foot replantation, 68, 70
    after great toe arthroplasty, 139, 140, 141
    after tarsometatarsal joint injury, 46, 50
    for children, 4
    in flatfoot, 116, 117, 118, 119, 124, 187, 191
    in gait analysis, 78, 79, 81-90, 91
    inadequate fitting of, 4
    injuries due to, 28
    for runners and joggers, 189, 203, 204
    sizing measurements in, 3-4
    and stability of foot, 3
    in talipes equino varus deformity, 209
Force-plate data in gait analysis, 92
    after arthrodesis, 78-79, 87, 90
    fore and aft shear in, 168, 172-173
    medial and lateral shear in, 168, 172, 173
    in running, jogging and walking, 170-173, 175
    vertical, 168
Forefoot, 137-153
    great toe arthroplasty, 137-142
    hallux valgus correction in cerebral palsy, 143-147
    karate-related injuries to, 162-163, 165
    running-related injuries to, 155, 156
Four-hole plate, for lateral malleolus reduction, 12,
        15, 17, 18
Fractures
    of ankle. See Ankle, fractures of
    avulsion, 6, 7, 8, 9-10
    of calcaneus, 93, 100, 103, 104, 105-106, 109
    of fibula. See Fibula, fractures of
    of lateral malleolus, 16-19
    Maisonneuve, 9
    of medial malleolus, 6, 7, 15, 16, 103, 105, 106-
        108
    of metatarsals, 42, 43
    shear, 6, 7
    of tarsometatarsal joint, 40-51

of tibial posterior lip, 8, 9-10
Fusions. *See* Arthrodesis

Gait analysis
  after arthrodesis, 73-92, 133-134, 135
  after clubfoot correction, 209
  after tarsometatarsal joint injury, 44, 47-51
  ankle, hip and knee motion in, 83-87, 88, 90, 91,
    167, 168, 169-170, 173-174, 175, 195, 201-
    203, 204
  biomechanical, 155-156, 157, 167-175, 186-193,
    195-204
  calf strength in, 78, 80, 81
  compensatory mechanisms in, 82, 88, 89, 90, 91
  distance in, 44, 45, 46, 77, 79, 88-89
  electromyography in, 76, 78-79, 85-87, 88, 92,
    167-175
  float period in, 168, 169, 172
  foot switches in, 47
  footwear in, 78, 79, 81-90, 91
  force-plate data in, 78-79, 87, 90, 92, 167-175
  hills and stairs in, 77-78, 79, 89
  kinematic, 44, 47, 195-204
  limitations in, 195-196
  long-term follow-up with, 73-92
  materials and methods used in, 74-79, 92, 195-196
  midtarsal joint in, 133-134
  normal foot function in, 2
  pain in, 76, 77, 79, 88-89, 133
  in peroneal tendinitis, 103, 106, 108
  stance phase in. *See* Weight-bearing and
    distribution
  stick figure representations in, 79, 89
  stride length in, 82-83, 87-88, 89, 90, 167, 169
  subtalar joint in, 80-81, 105, 106, 108, 109, 117,
    119, 133-134
  tibiopedal motion in, 36-39, 83-85, 87, 90
  velocity in, 167-175
    after arthrodesis, 78, 79-80, 82-83, 87-88, 89, 90
    after tarsometatarsal joint injury, 47-50
  weight acceptance phase in. *See* Weight-bearing
    and distribution
Gastrocnemius muscle
  in walking, 189, 193
  in weight-bearing, 180, 182, 183, 184
Gastrocsoleus muscle group, 80, 178, 179, 184, 198
  dynamic force measurements of, 181, 182
  electromyography of, 76, 87, 168, 171, 174
  in shock absorption mechanism, 174
Gluteus muscles, in gait analysis, 76, 78, 87, 168,
    173
Goldner one-stage approach, in clubfoot correction,
    207, 208, 213
Gouty arthritis, 131, 132
Grafts, bone. *See* Bone grafts
Gravity center in running, jogging and walking, 169,
    170, 171
Great toe
  arthroplasty of
    complications from, 140, 141, 142
    double-stem flexible implant in, 137-142
    operative technique in, 139-140
    results of, 139, 140-141
    in rheumatoid arthritis, 137, 138, 139, 140-141,

      142
      with silicon implant, 137-142
      single-stem implant in, 137-142
      toe motion after, 139
  hallux rigidus, 137, 138, 139, 140, 141, 142
  hallux valgus, 137, 138, 139, 140-141, 143-147
  hallux varus, 141
  Keller bunionectomy of, 148-154
  length of, in foot classification, 1, 3
  in metatarsus primus varus, 148, 151, 152, 154,
    187, 192
  in push-off motion, 199, 202, 203, 204
  in weight-bearing and distribution, 154, 187, 189,
    192, 193
Grice arthrodesis
  adjacent joint changes after, 122, 123, 124
  age affecting results of, 120, 121, 125
  anterior tibial transfer with, 117, 119, 120, 121,
    122, 123, 125
  fibular bone graft in, 116, 120-121, 124, 125
  in flatfoot, 116-125
  graft absorption after, 121, 123, 124
  in hallux valgus correction, 144, 145, 146
  hindfoot varus deformity after, 120, 122, 124, 125
  indications for, 116, 124
  medial longitudinal arch after, 117, 118, 119
  metatarsal calluses after, 122-123, 125
  in paralytic deformities, 116, 123
  patient satisfaction with, 118-119, 122
  pseudarthroses after, 120-121, 122
  radiographic evaluation after, 117-118, 119, 120,
    121, 124
  subtalar motion after, 117, 119, 124
  symptom relief in, 117, 118-119, 124
  technique of, 116-117

Hallucis muscle
  abductor
    in clubfoot correction, 207, 208, 210, 211, 217
    in hallux valgus, 146
  adductor, in hallux valgus correction, 143, 145,
    146, 147
  extensor, in great toe arthroplasty, 139, 141
  flexor
    in clubfoot correction, 217, 219
    dynamic force measurements of, 180-181
    in walking and running, 192, 202, 203
Hallux rigidus, great toe arthroplasty in, 137, 138,
    139, 140, 141, 142
Hallux valgus, 148, 152
  abductor hallucis muscle in, 146
  adductor hallucis muscle in, 143, 145, 146, 147
  arthrodesis in, 144, 145, 146
  in cerebral palsy, correction of, 143-147
  great toe arthroplasty in, 137, 138, 139, 140, 141
  metatarsophalangeal joint capsule release in, 143,
    147
  operative technique in, 143-144
  pin stabilization in, 145, 147
  pronated feet in, 146
  soft tissue procedure in, 145
Hallux varus, after great toe arthroplasty, 141
Hamstring muscles, in gait analysis, 78, 86-87, 168,
    170, 173, 199

Hatt method of ankle fusion, 75, 132
Hawkins sign, after talus fracture, 52-53, 56-57
Heel. *See also* Calcaneus
    force measured at, 179
    in ideal normal foot, 2
    lifts in shoes, 177
    nonhealing ulcer of, 176, 177, 178, 183
    in valgus and varus positions, 133, 145
Hindfoot, 73-136. *See also* Ankle
    karate-related injuries to, 164-165
    in peroneal tendinitis, post-traumatic, 103-109
    peroneal tendon dislocation, recurrent, 110-115
    running-related injuries of, 155
    Syme's amputation of diabetic foot, 127-130
    in weight-bearing and distribution, 187, 189, 190,
        191, 193
Hips
    abductor muscles of, 168, 173
    adductor muscles of, 168, 173, 174
    motion in gait analysis
        after arthrodesis, 83, 84, 85, 86, 90
        in running, jogging and walking, 167, 168, 169,
            170, 173, 174, 195

Ice applications, in peroneal tendon
    dislocation, 112, 113
Iliac bone graft, quadruple arthrodesis with, 93-102
Infections
    after ankle fusion, 135
    after clubfoot correction, 209
    after foot amputation, 130
    after great toe arthroplasty, 141, 142
    of calcaneus, 177
Internal fixation
    arthrodesis for. *See* Arthrodesis
    bone grafts for. *See* Bone grafts
    bone nails in, 27, 32
    Kirschner wires for, 43, 52, 55, 62, 65, 213, 217
    pins for, 27, 55-56, 57, 62, 145, 217, 218, 219
    plates in, 12, 15, 17, 18, 21
    screws for, 21, 27, 28
    in tarsometatarsal joint injury, 43, 45
    wire loop, for lateral malleolus, 24-34
Intrinsic muscles
    activity in gait, 197
    as tension member of foot, 178
    in walking, 198-199
Inversion of foot
    after replantation, 68, 69
    ankle fractures due to, 6-7, 10
    in peroneal tendinitis, 103
Ischemic index, and amputation level, 129, 130

Jockeys, peroneal tendon dislocation in, 111
Jogging, 167-175, 199-204
    float period in, 168, 169, 172
    foot function in, 189, 190, 193, 204
    footwear recommended for, 189, 203
    force-plate data in, 170-173
    hip, knee and ankle motion in, 169-170, 173-174,
        175, 203, 204
    injuries related to, 189-190
    muscular activity in, 173-174, 175, 189, 202, 204

push-off in, 202, 204
weight-bearing and distribution of forces in, 186-
    193
    duration of, 196
    impact of forces in, 189, 193, 199-200, 203, 204
    kinematic study of, 196, 199, 200, 204
Jones technique, in peroneal tendon dislocation, 112-
    113

Karate
and foot areas used in kicks, 160-162, 165
foot injuries in, 159-165
    radiographic evaluation of, 163-165
foot training in, 160
Keller bunionectomy, 138, 142, 152
    in arthritis, 148, 152
    with metatarsus primus varus correction, 148, 152
    with opening wedge osteotomy of first metatarsal,
        148-154
    and weight-bearing ability of great toe, 154
Kinematic study of support phase of foot, 44, 47, 195-
    204
    interpretation of data in, 203-204
    materials and methods in, 196
Kirschner wire fixation
    in clubfoot correction, 213, 217
    in foot replantation, 65
    in talus fractures, 52, 55, 62
    in tarsometatarsal joint injury, 43
Knee
    injuries in running, 155, 156
    motion of
        after arthrodesis, 83, 84, 85, 86, 88, 90
        as shock-absorption mechanism, 169-170, 195
        in walking, running and jogging, 167, 168, 169-
            170, 173-174, 175, 195, 201

Lateral malleolus
in ankle fractures, 8, 9, 11-16, 21, 24-34
and ankle function, 11-16, 24, 34
four-hole plate in reduction of, 12, 15
incomplete reduction of, 11, 16
isolated fracture of, 16-19
manipulation in reduction of, 19
osteotomy of, ankle stability after, 11, 12, 13, 16-19
wire-loop fixation of, 24-34
Leather orthosis, for runners, 156, 157
Leg
    elevation of
        after ankle fracture repair, 21, 22, 27
        in peroneal tendon dislocation, 112, 113
        after quadruple arthrodesis, 101
    length discrepancies after arthrodesis, 80, 81
Le Lievre operation, in flatfoot correction, 124
Lidocaine, in peroneal tendinitis, 106, 108, 109
Lifestyle
    arthrodesis affecting, 74, 77, 79-80, 88-89, 91, 134-
        135
    talus fracture affecting, 53, 55, 56, 58, 61
    tarsometatarsal joint injury affecting, 44, 45-46, 50
Lift-off, in gait cycle, 174
Limp
    after arthrodesis, 74, 77, 79, 133-134

after talus fracture, 53
after tarsometatarsal joint injury, 44, 45, 46, 50
Lisfranc joint, 40. *See also* Tarsometatarsal joint
Lisfranc ligament, 41
Longitudinal arch
  after Grice arthrodesis, 117, 118, 119
  calcaneus partial excision affecting, 179
  in normal foot, 2, 3, 190-191, 197
  in pes planus foot, 187, 190, 191-192
  in weight-bearing and distribution, 179, 191, 197
Lymphatic drainage, after foot replantation, 67, 71

Maisonneuve fracture, 9
Malleolus
  lateral, of fibula. *See* Lateral malleolus
  medial, of tibia. *See* Medial malleolus
Master knot of Henry, excision of, in clubfoot
    correction, 217
Medial ankle ligament. *See* Deltoid ligament
Medial malleolus
  in ankle fractures, 6, 7
  and ankle stability, 11, 12, 14-16
  avulsion fracture of, 7
  fibrous union after fracture of, 15, 16
  manual reduction of, 11, 12
  peroneal tendinitis after fracture of, 103, 105, 106-
    108
  shear fracture of, 6
Metatarsal bones, 40
  angle between first and second, 150-151, 152-153
  arch of, 40, 41, 156
  base of, fractures of, 42, 43
  dislocation of, 41, 42-43
  karate affecting, 160, 163-164
  keystone of, 40, 42
    fracture of, 42
  length of, in foot classification, 1, 3
  ligaments joining, 40-41
  in metatarsus primus varus, 148, 151, 152, 154, 187,
    192
  osteotomy of, 192
    in clubfoot correction, 208, 209
    opening wedge, Keller bunionectomy with, 148-
      154
  in running, 156, 202
  in walking, 199
  in weight-bearing, 180, 187, 189, 190, 191, 192, 198
Metatarsal calluses
  after great toe arthroplasty, 142
  after Grice arthrodesis, 122-123, 125
Metatarsalgia
  after osteotomy, 151, 152, 154
  and karate, 163
  in metatarsus primus varus, 187, 192
  in pes planus foot, 187, 191, 192
  secondary, 142
  weight-bearing ability in, 154, 192
Metatarsophalangeal joint
  arthroplasty of, 137, 138, 142, 152
  degenerative arthritis of, 148, 152
  measurement of angle of, 151, 152
  in hallux valgus correction, 143, 147
Metatarsus primus varus foot, 187
  forces under, 192

surgical correction of, 148, 151, 152, 154
Midfoot
  karate-related injuries to, 160, 162, 163
  running-related injuries to, 155, 156
  in weight-bearing and distribution of forces, 187,
    189, 190, 191, 192, 198
Midtarsal joint motion, after ankle fusion, 133-134
Morton's foot. *See* Metatarsalgia
Myelomeningocele, and clubfoot correction, 208

Navicular bone. *See also* Talonavicular joint
  fusion in quadruple arthrodesis, 95, 97, 98, 99, 100,
    102
Naviculocalcaneal joint, in quadruple arthrodesis, 98
Naviculocuboid joint, in quadruple arthrodesis, 95,
    97, 100
Naviculo-cuneiform angle
  Grice arthrodesis affecting, 118, 120
  sag in, 124
Nerve repair, after foot replantation, 68
Normal foot, 1-4
  asymptomatic deviations in, 2-3, 4
  ideal, 2, 190-191, 197
  weight-bearing and distribution of forces in, 186-
    191, 193

Open reduction
  in ankle fractures, 21-22, 24-34, 52-63
  bone grafts in. *See* Bone grafts
  bracing after, 22-23
  casts after, 21, 22, 25, 27, 34
  in clubfoot correction, 215-220
  Kirschner wire in, 43, 52, 55, 62, 65, 213, 217
  pins in, 22, 55-56, 57, 62, 145, 217, 218, 219
  postoperative management of, 21-23, 27
  syndesmotic screws in, 21, 22
  in tarsometatarsal joint injury, 43, 45
  and wire-loop fixation of lateral malleolus, 24-34
Opening wedge osteotomy, of first metatarsal, 148-
    154
Orthoplasty orthosis, for runners, 156-157
Orthosis. *See* Braces
Os calcis. *See* Calcaneus
Osteoarthritis. *See* Arthritis
Osteoarthropathy, in karate experts, 165
Osteomyelitis
  after ankle fusion, 133
  of calcaneus, treatment of, 176-177, 183
Osteophyte formation. *See* Spur formation
Osteotomy
  of lateral malleolus, ankle stability after, 11, 12, 13,
    16-19
  of medial malleolus, ankle stability after, 11, 12, 14-
    16
  metatarsal, 192
    in clubfoot correction, 208, 209
    in metatarsus primus varus correction, 148, 151,
      152
  opening wedge
    Keller bunionectomy with, 148-154
    operative technique in, 148-150, 153-154
    patient satisfaction with, 150, 151, 152, 154
Overuse syndrome, in long-distance runners, 155-158

Pain
   after arthrodesis, 74, 75, 76, 77, 79, 88-89, 133
   after os calcis excision, 177, 183
   arthrodesis for relief of, 33, 93, 94, 117, 124, 144
   great toe arthroplasty for relief of, 139, 140, 141
   metatarsal osteotomy for relief of, 150, 151, 154
   in metatarsus. See Metatarsalgia
   in peroneal tendinitis, 103, 105, 106, 108, 109
   in peroneal tendon dislocation, 111, 113
   in talus fracture, 53, 55, 56, 58
   in tarsometatarsal joint injury, 45, 50
Palmar bone nails, for internal fixation, 27, 32
Pelvic rotation, in gait after arthrodesis, 83, 84, 90
Periostitis, in runners, 203
Peroneal muscles, 110-111
   dislocation of, 112
   dynamic force measurements of, 180-181, 183, 184
   in gait analysis, 76, 87, 199, 202
   innervation of, 110
Peroneal nerve, superficial, 97, 110
Peroneal retinaculum, 103, 110, 112-113
Peroneal tendons, 103
   dislocation of, recurrent, 110-115
      treatment of, 112-114, 115
   post-traumatic tendinitis of, 103-109
      management of, 104-105, 106, 108, 109
   shortening Z-plasty of, in foot replantation, 68, 70
Peroneal tenography, in peroneal tendinitis, 103-104,
   106, 108, 109
Peroneal trochlea, of calcaneus, 103
Pes planus foot. See Flatfoot
Pin stabilization
   in clubfoot correction, 217, 218, 219
   in hallux valgus correction, 145, 147
   Steinmann, 55-56, 57, 62
Plantar fascia
   in clubfoot correction, 207, 208, 210, 211, 217, 219
   as tension member of foot, 178, 179, 182, 183
Plantar flexion
   after ankle fracture, 23
   after ankle replacement, 73
   after arthrodesis, 36, 37, 78, 81, 82, 83-85, 90, 102,
      134
   after arthroplasty, 37, 139
   after os calcis excision, 176, 177, 178
   ankle motion in, 21, 23
   with braces, 22, 23
   normal, 37, 38
   in peroneal tendinitis, 103, 106
Plantar ligament, long, 103
Plantar nerve repair, after foot replantation, 68
Plaster casts. See Cast immobilization
Plates for internal fixation, 12, 15, 17, 18, 21
Poliomyelitis patients
   Grice arthrodesis in, 124
   quadruple arthrodesis in, 94
Pronation of foot, in running
   hyperpronation, 156, 157
   orthotic management of, 156, 157
Prosthesis
   after amputation of foot, 64, 69, 72
   ankle
      amount of motion with, 38, 73
      in arthritis, 73, 91
      arthrodesis compared to, 73, 91

Pseudarthrosis
   after arthrodesis, 120-121, 122, 125, 133, 135
   at fibular donor site, 120-121, 125
Push-off, in walking, jogging and running, 199, 202,
   203, 204
Quadriceps muscle of thigh, in gait analysis, 168, 170,
   173-174
Quadruple arthrodesis
   anatomic considerations in, 94-95
   complications of, 94, 101-102
   in flatfoot, 93-94, 116, 125
   with iliac bone graft, 93-102
   immobilization after, 94, 101, 102
   indications and contraindications for, 93-94
   operative technique in, 96-101
   postoperative management of, 94, 101
   results of, 93, 101-102

Radiography
   in arthrodesis, 75, 76, 81-82, 90
      Grice arthrodesis, 117-118, 119, 120, 121, 124
      quadruple arthrodesis, 95, 96, 97, 98, 101, 102
   in clubfoot, 209, 210, 211, 212, 215, 216, 218, 219-
      220
   foot position in, 3, 4
   in great toe arthroplasty, 139, 141
   in karate-related injuries, 163-165
   of metatarsals, 150-151, 152-154
   of normal foot, 95
   in peroneal tendon dislocation, 111-112, 113, 115
   of pes planus foot, 191-192
   in replantation of severed foot, 66, 69
   in talus fracture, 53, 55, 56, 57
   in tarsometatarsal joint injury, 44, 45, 46, 47, 50
   variations and errors in, 3, 4
Rectus muscle of thigh, in gait analysis, 76, 87
Reduction. See Closed reduction; Open reduction
Replantation of severed foot, 64-72
   arterial and venous thrombosis after, 71
   bone fixation and shortening in, 65, 70
   case report of, 64-69, 71
   factors affecting success of, 64, 70, 71
   nerve repair in, 68
   postoperative care in, 67-69, 71
   preoperative care in, 64-65, 70
   reconstruction after, 68-69
   skin closure in, 66-67, 70
   tendon repair in, 66, 68, 69, 70
   vascular repair in, 65-66, 70-71
   weight-bearing after, 67, 68, 71
Retromalleolar groove, congenitally shallow, peroneal
   tendon dislocation with, 111
Rocker-bottom foot, from arthrodesis procedure, 99,
   102
Running
   after arthrodesis, 77, 79-80, 89
   biomechanical study of, 155-156, 157, 167-175, 199-
      204
   cavus foot problems in, 156, 157
   fibular motion during, 200-201, 203
   float period in, 168, 169, 172
   foot function in, 190, 193, 199, 200
   footwear for, 189, 203, 204
   force-plate data in, 171-173

forms of gait in, 199
hip, knee and ankle motion in, 169-170, 173-174, 175, 201, 202, 203, 204
hyperpronation of foot in, 156, 157
impact forces in, 201-202
injuries related to, 155-158, 189-190, 200, 201, 203, 204
limitations in analysis of, 195
muscular activity in, 173-174, 175, 200-201, 201-202
orthopedic management of problems in, 155-158
overuse syndrome in, 155-158
push-off in, 202, 203, 204
tibial rotation in, 156
weight-bearing stage in, 155, 187, 190, 193, 200

Sacrospinalis muscle, in gait analysis, 168, 173, 174
Sclerosis
  of subchondral bone, after arthrodesis, 75
  of tarsometatarsal joint, 45, 46
Screws for internal fixation, 21, 27, 28
Shin splints, in runners, 189, 200, 201, 203, 204
Shock-absorption mechanisms
  gastrocsoleus muscle group in, 174
  knee flexion in, 169-170, 195
  in running, 190, 193, 200
  in walking, 38
Shoes. See Footwear
Silicone implant, in arthroplasty of great toe, 137-142
Silver bunionectomy, 192
Skiing, peroneal tendon dislocation from, 110, 111
Soccer, peroneal tendon dislocation from, 110, 114
Soft-tissue procedures
  in clubfoot correction, 215
  in hallux valgus correction, 144, 145
Soleus muscle. See also Gastrocsoleus muscle group
  in gait analysis, 78, 189, 193
Splints. See Braces; Cast immobilization
Sports medicine, 155-165
  karate-related injuries, 159-165
  peroneal tendon dislocation, 110, 111, 113-114
  running-related injuries, 155-158, 189-190, 200, 201, 203, 204
Sprain, ankle, 103, 104, 105, 109
Sprinting, 186-193, 199, 202-203. See also Running
  footwear for, 203
  injuries related to, 201
  muscular activity in, 202-203, 204
  push-off in, 202, 203
  weight-bearing in, 196
    and impact force, 201, 202, 203, 204
    kinematic study of, 196, 201, 202
Spur formation
  after arthrodesis, 75, 76
  in karate experts, 164, 165
  in tarsometatarsal joint injury, 45, 46
Squared foot, 1
Stance phase of gait cycle. See Weight-bearing and distribution
Steindler strip, in clubfoot correction, 217, 219
Steinmann pin fixation, in talus fracture, 55-56, 57, 62
Steroid therapy, in peroneal tendinitis, 104, 105, 109
Stress tests, in anterior tibiofibular ligament assessment, 19

Stride length in gait analysis
  after arthrodesis, 82-83, 87-88, 89, 90
  in running, jogging and walking, 167, 169
Subluxation of proximal phalanx, after great toe arthroplasty, 139, 141, 142
Subtalar joint
  arthritis of, 52, 58, 103
  in clubfoot correction, 207, 217, 219
  motion of
    after arthrodesis, 80-81, 117, 119, 124, 133-134, 135
    compensatory, 99
    in peroneal tendinitis, 103, 105, 106, 108, 109
  in quadruple arthrodesis, 93-102
Support phase of gait cycle. See Weight-bearing and distribution
Sural nerve, 97, 110
Syme amputation
  of diabetic foot, 127-130
  from severe crush injuries, 42
Sympathetic blockage, in foot replantation, 71
Syndesmotic screw fixation, 21, 22
Syndesmotic ligament, 7, 8, 21

Talectomy
  in clubfoot correction, 208, 209
  in talus fractures, 56
Talipes, 207-220. See also Clubfoot correction
  cavus, running problems in, 156, 157
  equino varus, surgical reconstruction of, 207-213
  equinus, arthrodesis in, 98-99, 131
Talocalcaneal joint
  in clubfoot assessment, 216, 218, 219-220
  Grice arthrodesis affecting, 118, 119, 120, 124
  in quadruple arthrodesis, 95, 97, 98
Talofibular ligament, posterior, 110
Talonavicular joint
  in clubfoot correction, 217, 220
  in Grice arthrodesis, 122, 124
  in quadruple arthrodesis, 95, 97, 98, 99, 102
  weight distribution through, 178-179, 184
    and formula for calculation of force, 179
Talonavicular sag, dorsoplantar, 124
Talus. See Ankle
Tarsal bones, in karate kicks, 160, 161, 165
Tarsometatarsal joint, 40-51
  arthrodesis of, 94
  in clubfoot correction, 207, 208, 209, 211
  dislocation of, 41
  stability of, 40
  trauma of, 42
    treatment of, 44-51
Tendinitis, peroneal, post-traumatic, 103-109
Tendo Achillis. See Achilles tendon
Tenography, peroneal, in peroneal tendinitis, 103-104, 106, 108, 109
Tenolysis, peroneal, in peroneal tendinitis, 105, 106, 109
Tendon repair, in replantation of foot, 66, 68, 69, 70
Tenosynovitis
  peroneal, 111
  in runners, 203
Tension member of foot, 178, 182, 183
Thrombosis, after foot replantation, 71

Tibia
    fractures of posterior lip, 8, 9-10
    graft with, in arthrodesis, 116, 121, 124, 132
    medial malleolus of. See Medial malleolus
    rotation in running, problems with, 156
    in weight-bearing and distribution of forces, 178,
        179-180, 182
Tibial muscle
    anterior, in gait analysis, 76, 86, 87, 168, 171, 174,
        198
    posterior
        dynamic force measurements of, 180-181, 183,
            184
        in jogging, 189
Tibial tendons
    in clubfoot correction, 208, 211, 213, 217, 219
    in Grice arthrodesis, 117, 119, 120, 121, 122, 123,
        125
    in replantation of foot, 68
    in runners, 203
Tibiofibular joint alignment, syndesmotic screw for,
    21
Tibiofibular ligaments
    in ankle fractures, 7, 8
    ankle stability with tears of, 16-19
    detection of injury to, 19
Tibiopedal motion, 37-38
    after arthrodesis, 36-39, 83-85, 87, 90
    after arthoplasty, 36-39
Tibiotalar joint
    arthrodesis of, 33
    in clubfoot correction, 207, 208, 209, 210, 213, 219
Toe(s)
    clawing of, after replantation of foot, 69, 70
    great. See Great toe
    karate-related injuries to, 162-163, 165
    length of, in foot classification, 1
    in weight-bearing and distribution of forces, 179,
        187, 189, 190, 192, 193, 198
Toe-off, in gait cycle, 174
Tourniquet control, in clubfoot correction, 212, 216,
    217
Transverse arch of foot, in weight-bearing, 191, 197
Transverse ligaments, joining metatarsals, 40-41
Trauma, 5-72. See also Fractures
    amputation and replantation of foot, 64-72
    arthritis from, 24, 25, 34, 52, 58, 73, 74, 103, 131,
        132, 135
    in karate experts, 159-165
    peroneal tendon dislocation from, 110, 111
    peroneal tendinitis from, 103-109
    of tarsometatarsal joint, 42
Triceps surae muscle. See Gastrocsoleus muscle group
Triple arthrodesis, 94, 95, 98, 99, 105, 109, 144, 145
Tripod of foot, after great toe arthroplasty, 141-142
Tuberculous arthritis, treatment of, 131, 132
Turco procedure, in clubfoot correction, 207, 219

U-fusion
    in quadruple arthrodesis, 95, 97, 100
    in triple arthrodesis, 98
Ultrasound, Doppler, and determination of
    amputation level, 127-130

Valgus deformity of foot
    after arthrodesis, 133, 145
    arthrodesis in, 98, 99, 116, 118
Varus deformity of foot
    after arthrodesis, 120, 122, 124, 125, 133, 145
    metatarsus primus, 148, 151, 152, 154, 187, 192
Vascular repair, in foot replantation, 65-66, 70-71
Velocity of gait, 167-175. See also Running; Walking
    after arthrodesis, 82-83, 87-88, 90

Walking
    after open reduction and internal fixation, 22, 23
    after opening wedge osteotomy of first metatarsal,
        150
    after replantation of severed foot, 68
    after tarsometatarsal joint injury, 44, 47-51
    biomechanics of, 167-175, 195, 198-199
    cycle in, 168
    distance of, 44, 45, 46, 77, 79, 88-89
    foot functions in, 38, 189, 190, 193, 198, 204
    force-plate data in, 170-173
    hip, knee and ankle motion in, 83-87, 88, 90, 91,
        167, 168, 169-170, 173-174, 175, 195, 201-203,
        204
    limp in, 44, 45, 46, 50, 53, 74, 77, 79, 133-134
    muscular activity in, 173-174, 175, 189, 193, 198-
        199
    push-off in, 199
    tibiopedal motion in, 38
    weight-bearing and distribution of forces in, 38,
        186-193, 196, 197, 198-199, 204
Wedge osteotomy, opening, of first metatarsal, 148-
    154
Weight-bearing and distribution
    Achilles tendon in, 178, 179, 182, 183
    after ankle fracture, 22, 23, 27, 28, 60-61, 62
    after arthrodesis, 83-84, 85, 94, 101, 117
    after clubfoot correction, 208, 209
    after os calcis excision, 176, 179-184
    after peroneal tendon dislocation, 113
    after replantation of foot, 67, 68, 71
    after tarsometatarsal joint injury, 43-44, 47-50
    arches of foot in, 179, 190-191, 197
    ball of foot in, 180
    biomechanics of, 167-204
    calcaneocuboid joint in, 176, 178-184
    distribution of forces in, 186
    duration of force in, 47, 48, 49, 50, 187, 196, 203
    extrinsic muscles in, 180-181, 182, 183, 184
    gastrocnemius muscle in, 180, 182, 183, 184
    gastrocsoleus muscle group in, 178, 179, 184
    hindfoot in, 187, 189, 190, 191, 193, 198
    impact of force in, 189, 193, 199-200, 201, 202, 203,
        204
    instrumentation for study of, 181, 186-187, 193,
        195-204
    lever arm in, 178, 179, 183
    metatarsal bones in, 180, 187, 189, 190, 191, 192,
        198
    in metatarsalgia, 154, 192
    in metatarsus primus varus, 192
    midfoot in, 187, 189, 190, 191, 192, 198
    in normal foot, 186-191, 193

in pes planus, 190, 191-192
plantar fascia tension member in, 178, 179, 182, 183
point of application of forces in, 178, 179
progression of force in, 187-189, 190, 191, 198
in running, jogging and walking, 38, 155, 168, 173, 174, 175, 186-193, 195-204
shock-absorption mechanisms in, 38, 169-170, 174, 190, 193, 195, 200
in stance phase, 179, 180, 181, 183
talonavicular joint in, 178-179, 184
tibial load in, 178, 179-180, 182
toes in, 154, 178, 179, 187, 189, 190, 192, 193, 198
Wiltse procedure, for os calcis partial excision, 176, 180, 181, 183, 184
Wire-loop fixation of lateral malleolus, 24-34

clinical experience with, 27-33
complications of, 33
contraindications for, 26, 27
indications for, 25-26, 34
intramedullary device in, 26, 28
operative technique in, 26-27
postoperative management in, 27, 34
results with, 28, 33
Wrestling, ankle fracture from, 31

Z-fusion, in quadruple arthrodesis, 95, 98, 99, 100
Z-plasty of peroneal tendons, in foot replantation, 68, 70